Occlusion
Second edition

Occlusion

Second edition

Hamish Thomson
FDS RCS(Eng) FDS RCS(Edin) LDS RFPS(Glas) DDS (NU)
Formerly Honorary Senior Lecturer, Department of Prosthetics, Institute of Dental Surgery;
Consultant, Eastman Dental Hospital, London

With editorial assistance from
Brian J. Parkins

Wright
London   Boston   Singapore   Sydney   Toronto   Wellington

Wright
is an imprint of Butterworth Scientific

 PART OF REED INTERNATIONAL P.L.C.

First edition published by John Wright and Sons, 1975
Second edition, 1990

© **Butterworth & Co (Publishers) Ltd, 1990**

British Library Cataloguing in Publication Data

Thomson, Hamish
  Occlusion.—2nd. ed.
  1. Man. Teeth. Occlusion
  I. Title   II. Parkins, B. J.
  617.643

ISBN 0-7236-2075-X

Library of Congress Cataloging-in-Publication Data

Thomson, Hamish.
    Occlusion/Hamish Thomson; with editorial assistance
  from Brian J. Parkins.—2nd ed.
     p. cm.
  Includes bibliographical references.
  ISBN 0-7236-2075-X:
  1. Occlusion (Dentistry)   2. Malocclusion.
  I. Parkins, B. J.   II. Title
  [DNLM: 1. Dental Occlusion.   WU 440   T483o]
RK523.T45   1990
617.6'43—dc20
DNLM/DLC
for Library of Congress   90-1633
                             CIP

Composition by Genesis Typesetting, Laser Quay, Rochester, Kent
Printed and bound in Great Britain by Courier International Ltd., Tiptree, Essex

Preface to the second edition

I greeted the invitation by Butterworths to provide a second edition of this book, originally published by John Wright & Sons, with some doubts about my ability to catch up with the expanding literature on the topic of occlusion and its association with mandibular dysfunction, facial pain, articulators and new restorative materials. It was not until I had approached and persuaded my colleague and friend, Brian Parkins, already a busy and committed teacher and practitioner, to provide the current ideas necessary for such a task that I felt able to accept without misgivings. His influence has been particularly helpful in Chapters 8 and 11 on the topics of articulators and fixed prosthodontics and these chapters have been rewritten. However, he would not accept co-authorship of the book saying: 'it is your book; mine is a small contribution'. While grateful for such modesty, I hope that his suggested improvements have been correctly interpreted. I am also grateful to Professor Yemm (University of Dundee) for his constructive criticisms of Chapter 3 and to Dr Fergal Nally (Institute of Dental Surgery) for the use of his teaching notes on neurophysiology. Finally, the original help in the preparation of Chapter 3 for the first edition from Mr Alan Newton (University of Liverpool) is not forgotten.

The study and teaching of occlusion are still hindered because of the difficulty of seeing contact between the teeth in three dimensions. Too often they are seen only as line diagrams without an appreciation of overlap and without realizing that a cusp and fossa have three dimensions and not two. It is also difficult to appreciate that occlusion is a momentary function of the teeth and that the mandible which provides these various and momentary occlusions is moving in three dimensions. The three-dimensional approach, therefore, has to exist in the minds of teacher and student, of writer and reader.

There have been minor changes in nomenclature: occlusal and rest vertical *dimensions* have become occlusal and rest vertical *relations*, *temporary* crowns are now *provisional*, and *permanent* are *definitive*. It is hoped that these changes will be improvements for purposes of communication. Anterior guidance receives more emphasis and a new chapter has been written on the mandibular dysfunction syndrome, also known as the pain dysfunction syndrome, facial arthromyalgia, *et alii*. The adjectives *maxillary* and *mandibular* are used when referring to natural teeth and tissues in those arches. *Upper* and *lower* are retained for casts of teeth and for the arms of articulators. Where the teeth themselves are indicated, the two digit system will be used (e.g. lower right first molar is 46 and the upper left second premolar is 25).

The principal message remains, namely that of preserving or recreating functional occlusion of which patients, and people in general, can be unaware. Included in the message is the advice to eat on both sides at once without the teeth touching and, particularly, to avoid the teeth touching when the mouth is empty. For these objectives to be achieved, an understanding of the tissues involved, their functions, disturbances and possible disorders is required. The intentions in this book are to provide this understanding and to suggest methods of treatment when indicated. There is a growing need for dentists to consider themselves physicians of the mouth. Happily, the disease and treatment of caries is seldom our first concern and the care of the periodontal tissues is often the reason for a first appointment. Oral manifestations of systemic diseases are a rapidly increasing responsibility for the dentist in practice and now we have the establishment and maintenance of good function as a challenge to student and teacher, scientist and practitioner. The mysteries of muscle dysfunction must be solved and the art of communication with patients learned so as to provide a widening horizon of care for the contact relations between teeth.

It takes little time for enlightened dentists to make a preliminary examination of occlusal and articular relations, to ask a few questions and give some simple advice. Thus, a new line on prevention can begin, with the accompanying rewards of improved enjoyment in eating, freedom from awareness of teeth and freedom from pain and dysfunction in the masticatory system.

Acknowledgements

In addition to the colleagues mentioned in the Preface who have provided guidance and new material for this edition, there are five other important contributors. James Morgan continued to provide additional photographic material. Edward Pullen-Warner painstakingly reviewed many of the diagrams. Margaret Clennett and her staff in the British Dental Association library were always ready to ferret and find distant journals, as was Barbara Cumbers at the Eastman Dental Hospital. Not least, Judith Hook typed as expertly as ever in addition to changing jobs at the time, as well as caring for a husband and teenage family.

I should also like to acknowledge the original stimuli for study and practice in this field from my late dentist father and, while I was a student in Chicago, from J. R. Thompson, Sicher, Boucher, Ramfjord and Ash and the gnathologists McCollum, Stuart, Granger and Thomas, and from Ballard, Beyron, Brewer, Lee, Krough-Poulson and Posselt here in Europe. Nor should I like to forget the continuing critical influence for good on our profession of Gerald Leatherman, guide, philosopher and friend, as he has proved to be.

Finally, I appreciate the tolerance of home time spent on this task by my wife.

Contents

Chapter 1

Terms, influences and concepts

The functions of the masticatory system are more varied than its name implies. In addition to eating and drinking, the system provides for speaking and singing, for smiling and snarling and all the expressions which between them lie. Then there are fighting, loving, tasting, touching, looking handsome and venting rage. There is the dry mouth of fear and the watery anticipation of food. There is the mouth breathing of strenuous exercise, with the possibilities of tooth clenching. There are the early stages of digestion and the swallow which follows, thus initiating the processes of metabolism and nutrition. In the gospel according to St Matthew (8:12) there was to be weeping and gnashing of teeth. And on one occasion when this text was preached a saddened, elderly parishioner exclaimed, 'Them as 'as 'em, gnash 'em'. And so to *occlusion* which in other spheres is shutting, closing, or retaining, in teeth is touching. Whether gnashing or nibbling, grinding food or swallowing it, to occlude is to touch the teeth with the teeth.

If the term 'occlusion' can be accepted as contact between opposing teeth without food or other agencies between them, it will be obvious that several occlusions are possible, depending on the position of the mandible. To be descriptive, the term has to be qualified. The occlusal surfaces of the teeth which make contact with each other have occlusal shapes and no two are exactly similar, except that those on the left tend to be mirror images of those on the right side of their respective arches. In spite of their dissimilarities there is always one occlusion in which there is maximal contact between opposing occlusal surfaces and this is called *intercuspal occlusion* (IO). In the dentitions called normal (Angle's class I), all the teeth make contact with opposing teeth by means of cusps, fossae and marginal ridges in the posterior teeth and by incisal edges and lingual surfaces in the anterior teeth. Such a yardstick of normal is said to be limited to 60% of dentitions and the term 'intercuspal occlusion' means maximal possible contact between opposing teeth. Thus, in cases of so-called 'anterior open bite' there may only be contact between opposing molars on the intercuspal occlusion. Similarly, in 'posterior open bite' there may be contact only between incisors. The position of the mandible when the teeth are in intercuspal occlusion is called the *intercuspal position* (IP), and the mandible is in intercuspal relation to the maxilla.

The mandible is capable of many movements and positions and a limited occlusion is possible in certain of its positions. Thus, the terms *lateral occlusion*, *protruded occlusion* and *retruded occlusion* are used to describe the contact between opposing teeth while the mandible is in lateral, protruded and retruded occlusal positions. While in these positions, the mandible is in lateral, protruded or retruded relation to the maxilla.

Lateral and protruded occlusions may occur at several lateral and protruded positions of the mandible but usually one is chosen when required. The *retruded occlusal position*, however, is constant and is usually limited to one contact on each side between the teeth which are furthest back. This contact will change, however, with the loss of those teeth or the alteration of their occlusal surfaces. This occlusion is also referred to as the *retruded contact* (RC) and is the occlusion that occurs as the mandible closes on its retruded axis. Retruded contact can be experienced by pulling the mandible back from IP until the last possible contact is felt. The *Oxford English Dictionary* (1989) classes 'retruded' as obsolete but gives it the meaning 'thrust backward'. On the other hand, 'protruded' is in current use and means 'thrust forward'. It is hoped that the dental profession may continue to revive this neglected partner of protruded. For one reason the words have a common derivation (*trudere*, to thrust) and for another they may jointly help to replace the vague and abused 'centric' and 'eccentric'.

The case against centric

Centric occlusion is a synonym for intercuspal occlusion and suggests that the teeth or the mandible are centrally placed in occlusion. This is not descriptive of the teeth or the mandible, neither of which can be said to have central positions or relations. While the term 'intercuspal occlusion' may not imply maximal contact between the teeth it does describe occlusion between cusps and does not presume to indicate a position. 'Maximal occlusion' would be a better term but intercuspal is widely enough used to prevent the need to introduce a new term. Intercuspal occlusion, therefore, indicates maximal occlusion irrespective of the position of the teeth or of the mandible. Centric occlusion suggests too many misleading possibilities.

Centric relation is a synonym for the retruded relation of the mandible to the maxilla. Here, the mandible has been thrust backward and there is even less cause for the mandible to be described as centrally placed. Confusion has been added to this term by the introduction of the qualifying adjectives 'strained' or 'unstrained' and no one seems certain which should apply. For some people the thrust backward may induce a feeling of strain and for others the thrust is not possible because of tired or stiff muscles. In order to reach it, effort is required by healthy muscles and the relationship is useful because, with healthy muscles, it is reproducible. Centric relation has also been described as the backmost, midmost and uppermost position of the mandibular condyles, which describes the retruded relation of the condyles to the glenoid fossae but adds confusion to the abused centric. *Centric* is often used as a noun when it expresses hope rather than certainty that the correct mandibular position will be achieved. The words 'intercuspal' and 'retruded' are therefore preferred.

Occlusion and articulation in mastication

Occlusion is contact between opposing teeth and refers to the moment and place of contact and not to the teeth themselves. It is visualized with the mandible stationary and this is not a natural function. All occlusal positions are moments of contact in a series of movements of the mandible. The term *articulation* is given to the contact that exists between the teeth while the mandible is moving. Occlusion and articulation are usually seen as tooth contacts in the empty mouth and are used for purposes of diagnosis and treatment of the dentition. The incidence of occlusion and articulation during mastication will be discussed several times throughout the text but the only time when contact takes place for certain is during the act of swallowing food or saliva, and even this occlusion can be avoided without harm if the food is well chewed. The study of occlusion is, therefore, faced with the paradox that occlusion is not necessary for mastication. This apparent contradiction is based on the strict definition of occlusion as contact between opposing teeth. This is not to say that teeth are unnecessary for effective mastication. On the contrary, the more complete the dentition and efficient the occlusion the less the teeth need touch. Food is most efficiently masticated between well-formed cusps which slide past each other while only the bolus makes contact with the teeth. The less the teeth touch during mastication, the more efficient will be the functions of the masticatory system and the healthier its tissues.

Occlusal function, parafunction and dysfunction

The term *occlusal function* is introduced to mean the contact that exists between the teeth and between the teeth and food during the functions of mastication and swallowing. The term *parafunction* (wrong or irregular function) is also introduced to mean the contact that exists between opposing teeth in the empty mouth during the habits of clenching, tapping, grinding or sliding the teeth together and of holding or chewing pencils, pipes and other outside agencies. Parafunction is preferred to *bruxism* which, though widely used, implies forceful occlusion and an associated disturbed emotional state. *Dysfunction* in the masticatory system is defined as functional movements of the mandible which cause a disturbance or disorder (see p. 117, Figure 7.6) in the system.

Retruded condyle axis (hinge axis)

One further group of terms and definitions concerns the retruded occlusal position (or retruded contact) and the movements to and from it. While the mandible is retruded (thrust backwards) it is capable of an arc of movement about an axis that runs through its condyles. This is called the *retruded condyle axis* (RCA). If the masticatory muscles are free from disability, the midpoint of the mandibular incisors can move on an arc for a distance of up to 20 mm (Posselt, 1952) about this condyle axis. This is the *retruded arc*, having as its centre the RCA. As the teeth occlude on the retruded arc there is usually one contact on each side. The mandible then moves forwards and upwards to the intercuspal position. During this movement the inclined surfaces of the teeth first in contact maintain articular contact. Conversely, the mandible can slide backwards and downwards from IP to RC. With healthy muscles, the relationship between the mandible and maxilla on the retruded arc is reproducible and this relationship is of great value in diagnosis and treatment of occlusal disturbances, as will be evident throughout the text. As has been pointed out, the alternative term used for all mandibular positions on the retruded arc is 'centric relation' to the maxilla. The retruded condyle axis is also known as the *terminal hinge axis* or *hinge axis* or, more simply, the *retruded axis*.

Retruded intercuspal occlusion (IP at RC)

It is seldom that intercuspal occlusion exists on the retruded arc but the opinion is expressed that this does take place in childhood and that subsequently the permanent teeth move forwards as they develop. The retruded arc and axis remain unchanged but the IP of the mandible has moved forwards. Thus it can be said that all adult intercuspal positions are habitual and are in a state of potential change as teeth wear and become lost. This tendency to forward movement of the teeth is known as the *anterior vector of force* and support for the existence of this movement is to be found in the interproximal wear that can be seen in the extracted teeth of adults. An extension of this forward tooth movement throughout life is the belief that, sooner or later, the front teeth will move forwards or will be worn by parafunctional grinding.

On this topic, Ingervall (1968) has reported from a study of 42 children (mean age 11 years 3 months) that there was a reproducibility of retruded contact and intercuspal position when measured in the sagittal plane. Thus, if IO occurs on the retruded arc in childhood it must occur before the age of 11. However, this hypothesis remains to be proven.

Aspects of study

The study of occlusion involves the student not only in the shapes and relations of the teeth but also in the positions and movements of the mandible that provide the relationships. It involves a separation between occlusal function and parafunction and the effects which they may have on the tissues of the masticatory system. The student will be required to transfer attention away from the teeth and attempt to understand the muscles and neuromuscular function of the system so that he or she can appreciate the activities of the muscles that provide jaw movement and the consequent contact between the teeth. Movement of one bone in relation to another is not possible without a joint, and a study of the mandibular joint tissues and their functions will also be made in order to assess the relations between the mandibular joints, the musculature and the teeth in function.

Occlusion and gnathology

Occlusion is considered by some dentists to mean reconstruction of the dentition by crowning all its teeth or adjustment of them by grinding. These procedures are associated with costly articulators that are a source of fascination to some dentists, objects of adverse criticism to others, and of great value to those who know how to use them. This aspect of occlusion has been abused by both practitioners and critics, but it has a part to play in the treatment of a minority of patients for whom the alternative is dental and sometimes mental breakdown. The part has to be played by an expert, however, and he or she is not easily trained. This is a reference to the subject of *gnathology* which, in its simplest meaning, is the study of the jaws, especially their alveolar processes. In dentistry, this study began with attempts to transfer the movements of the mandible to instruments which could be adjusted to copy them and the names of McCollum, Stallard, Stuart and Granger will always be associated with its origins. After sixty or so years, gnathology has prospered and, although inevitably associated with affluent patients because its applications are time consuming and costly, it has provided methods of diagnosing and treating disorders of occlusion which no other approach to these problems has solved. Gnathology and its procedures, therefore, form an integral part of the study of occlusion.

Occlusion, particular and general

It has been pointed out that occlusion is contact between opposing teeth and this definition is necessary when separating occlusal contact from occlusal function and articulation. The term 'occlusion', however, has broader implications which class it as a subject for the study of tooth contacts, both stationary and mobile, both functional and parafunctional, of the tissues that provide these functions, of the disturbances that can happen to the tissues and of the treatment procedures devised to restore them to health. Occlusion, thus enlarged, provides mastication for the masticatory system and an essential part of nutrition and health. This system also includes tissues which take part in the functions of digestion, respiration, speech, facial expression and the transmission of affection. As in all other human systems the tissues and functions of the masticatory system are subject to adaptation, abuse, wear, ageing and disease. Occlusion is, therefore, a changing condition and the responses to change vary between healthy adaptation and total disorder.

Influences affecting the dentition and occlusion

The teeth and supporting tissues develop as a result of genetic influences which do not always provide for health and adequate function. The size and number of teeth are not always accommodated in the bones provided for them. The result is overcrowding and this may promote caries, lesions of the interdental epithelium and periodontium, and disturbances of the occlusion, all of which may be interrelated. The masticatory and orofacial muscles and the nervous function which controls them behave according to endogenous patterns and respond to innumerable stimuli in order to provide the movements required in the system. These movements often have to be protective and can be harmful for various reasons. The system is subject to systemic, dietetic and emotional influences and to surgical and restorative procedures that are not always helpful in providing optimal function. Genetic and environmental factors, nature and nurture, play their part in the health of the masticatory system and, in particular, of the occlusion.

The dentition in evolution

The place which the dentition occupies in the evolution of the human species has some connection with the study of occlusion. The adoption of the upright posture was the first and major change in the animal skeleton which led to human evolution. This necessitated profound changes in the structure and function of almost all parts of the body. The heart had to pump blood against gravity to the head, neck and arms. The pelvic girdle had to transmit the weight of the head and trunk to the legs; the head and trunk had to support themselves, and the adaptive problems which this created are much in evidence today, for which there is no better example than man and his aching back. The forelimbs became arms and many functions for them were found so that the upright species could survive. Then came the enlarged brain and, among many other developments, the consequent adaptive refinements of arms and hands. The loss of bodily speed and the ability to fight were thus replaced by skills, and manufactured weapons took the place of teeth. In addition, tools for agricultural and domestic crafts were evolved and the phenomenon of cooking further reduced the need for teeth. Thus, whereas the forelimbs found other functions to perform, the teeth did not, and it can be argued today that they are vestigial tissues.

With the development of cooking came the refinement of food. Eating became a pleasure as well as a requirement, and a discerning palate became a symbol of prestige in society as well as one of enjoyment in living. The refinement of food, together with certain bacteria in the flora of the mouth, led to the disease of caries. The discomfort and loss of teeth which this disease caused gave rise to further refinement of food and the vicious cycle which we know today developed. Thus, after perhaps two million years since the upright posture was adopted, the dentition was relegated to the function of mastication and even this role can be considered unnecessary. Certainly, the species can survive without it.

This diminishing function of the dentition can be used to explain the non-adaptive part played by the teeth during the past two million years of human evolution. Apart from the inevitable increase in the range of variation of almost all human traits and tissues, including the teeth, no changes have taken place in the dentition which suggest that it has had to adapt to the environment. Its nature has remained unaffected by nurture except to bow to disease.

However, the disease of caries is coming under control and current periodontal care is providing longer life for the supporting tissues of the teeth. This brings importance to the debate on the function of cusps and the relation between their form and function. Do the observations that primitive human teeth were subject to wear early in life (Figure 1.1) suggest that this was a beneficial adaptation of form to function? And should it now be promoted to prevent caries (Berry and Poole, 1974)? Or why has there not been a developmental change to accommodate this function? One may accept the teleological view that developments and changes in mammalian form are due to the purpose that is served by them but it is difficult to avoid the thesis that cells produce other cells according to preordained patterns and produce changes in mammalian form. Selection by the evolutionary process then follows, either by successful adaptation to such changes or, in failing to adapt, by allowing the species to lose its chance of survival.

Human cusps have survived for two million years and it is suggested that their function in mastication is to identify food and to shred and chew it, while letting the saliva liquefy it, whereupon the mandibular teeth close into intercuspal occlusion and allow the act of swallowing to begin. Without cusps these functions would be less efficient and, with the increasing demand for raw or partially cooked vegetables and other tough foods, cusps are assuming a new and important role.

The danger of reducing cusp form is that removal of enamel hastens the exposure of dentine, which then wears progressively and provides hollows for food stagnation and further caries. Sensitive dentine abounds and pulp exposures in middle-aged and elderly teeth subject to this type of dentine wear are not uncommon. Besides, as caries is a bacterial disease, it will continue to thrive if the environment is favourable, as it did in some primitive teeth (Figure 1.1). In addition, today's extended lifespan means that teeth may have to perform their functions for twice as long as was required of primitive teeth. The search for occlusal positions with cuspless teeth leads to further wear and this can become an untreatable state, as practitioners with ageing, impecunious and partially edentulous patients will ruefully agree.

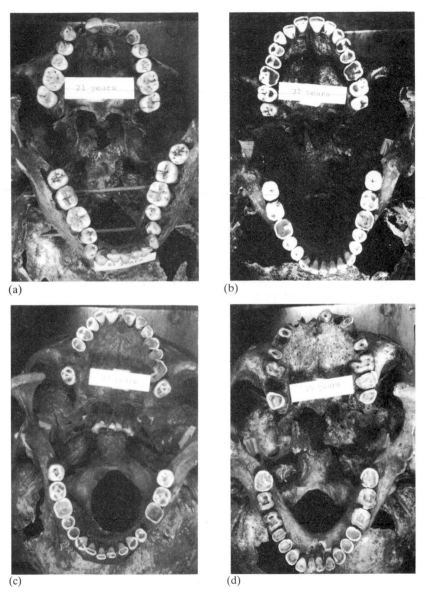

(a)   (b)

(c)   (d)

Figure 1.1 Series of dentitions photographed at the Odontological Museum of the Royal College of Surgeons of England with the permission of the Honorary Curator. They were excavated in 1950–1955 at the Anglo-Saxon cemetery at Breedon-on-the-Hill, Leicestershire. Date approximately AD 800–900. Ages as stated

The dentition today

These observations are accepted by the public and dental profession alike, partly with a shrugging acceptance by the elderly and partly with hope by the profession that the early prevention of wear as well as of caries will reduce the need to treat this problem. First, however, the cause must be investigated.

Perhaps the diminishing needs for this fully developed system have led to the development of extramasticatory functions (parafunctions) such as clenching and grinding habits in the empty mouth. These can emanate from minor upsets in the central nervous system and may be stimulated by disturbances between the teeth. Whatever the cause, this irrelevant muscle activity may be seen as a replacement for natural masticatory function or an expression of emotional tension. The alterations to tooth contacts which may be the cause or the effect of this activity make the diagnosis and treatment of occlusal disturbances an essential part of dental practice today.

Life can be sustained without teeth but contemporary humans find them a desirable if not an essential part of digestive and emotional life. There are those who become preoccupied with the function of their teeth and who are willing to spend excessive time and money on their maintenance; and there are those who look on the loss of teeth as a welcome relief from pain and disease. Between these extremes are the dentists and their patients who look upon mouth health as an integral part of general health and who place a high value on comfort and efficiency in function and a good appearance of the teeth. For them, good occlusal function is a justifiable requirement, one which is manifest by minimal awareness of teeth and the occlusion between them.

Concepts and precepts

By definition, a *concept* is an idea or general notion of a class of objects and a *precept* is a forthright maxim. Thus, there is the concept that occlusion of the teeth is contact between those of opposing arches, and the precept that occlusion should be limited to the act of swallowing. Many ideas and maxims have been expressed in the past century since Bonwill (1887) first stated his views on the articulation of human teeth. Some current views on the subject will now be expressed that will provide an outline for the text.

Occlusion is optimal when minimal. This precept provides the keynote of the text that follows and perhaps it is too much to advise that human teeth should occlude only when swallowing. However, this will help to maintain the stability and comfort of teeth in function and ranks in importance with all preventive health measures.

The *natural position for the mandible* not in function is with the teeth parted. A common misconception among patients is that the teeth should be in contact when not in use. Such a habit constitutes *irrelevant muscle activity* and will be discussed in Chapter 3.

Cusps are for function and not wear. The belief that cusps are there to be worn off is refuted. Intercuspal occlusion between the ridges that make up the cusps and the opposing ridges which make up the fossae should be on three sides and of minimal area. Thus may food be shredded and the mandible stabilized for the swallow. Worn, flattened cusps lead to inefficient chewing and an insecure intercuspal position. This in turn promotes parafunctional movements. The occlusal shapes that maintain this function will be described in the last section of Chapter 2.

Occlusal positions and articular movements are the product of muscle activity, the contours of the teeth and the function of the mandibular joints. The features of the teeth, muscles and joints that are relevant to the study of occlusion will be described in Chapter 2 and the neuromuscular function which provides efficient movement will be the subject of Chapter 3. Some of the possibilities for abnormal muscle function will also be outlined in Chapter 3.

The *positions and movements of the mandible* provide the basis for understanding occlusal function. These can be classed as a series of reproducible or habitual positions and a similar series of movements. Analyses of these movements and positions form an essential part of diagnosis and treatment of occlusal disorders. Mandibular positions and movements will be the subject of Chapter 4.

Articulation is undesirable in occlusal function of natural teeth. The teeth should be free from deflective interferences in the empty mouth. Emphasis has been placed on the classification and requirements of this phenomenon and the care given to its creation in the natural and artificial dentition should result in its minimal use. In the majority of natural dentitions there is neither need to classify articulation nor indications for correction. When the need does arise, care should be taken to ensure a clear objective. This topic will be discussed in Chapter 5.

The *forces acting on the teeth* arise from muscles through the media of food, outside agencies and opposing teeth. The response by the teeth is either by omnidirectional movement and recovery or by reposition. These phenomena will be described in the first section of Chapter 5.

Mastication is best achieved by well-shaped teeth which identify and shred food but do not themselves touch. This repetitive theme is discussed in Chapter 6 and includes the topic of tooth contacts during mastication. The phenomenon of adaptation based on an understanding of neuromuscular function is also included and will reappear many times since on it depends the healthy response of the masticatory system to the various functions it performs.

A *disturbance* of occlusal function is an alteration of its established function and a *disorder* is a pathological response to a disturbance. These terms are introduced in an attempt to classify the many interrelated conditions which affect the occlusal relations. An outline of disturbances and disorders occupies Chapter 7 and treatment has to be sought later in the book.

The *articulator* provides a means of copying mandibular positions and movements with varying accuracy. Articulators have been variously classified according to their ability to adjust to interocclusal records of jaw relations made in the mouth. The movements they provide have to be viewed in reverse since it is the upper member (the maxilla) which moves and the various interpretations of jaw movements have to be made against the obvious difficulties of copying the neuromuscular system. This will be the subject of Chapter 8.

Analysis and diagnosis are the basis of treatment and can provide an endless source of interest, questions and sometimes disillusion to the practitioner. Abuses of occlusion, either developmental, parafunctional or iatrogenic in origin, should be diagnosed, treated or prevented early in life so that disturbances do not become disorders. Of such is the content of Chapter 9.

Occlusal adjustment of the natural teeth may be indicated where cusp interferences cause a deflection of the mandible leading to an altered intercuspal position. There are indications and contraindications that should be carefully observed and the procedures used should be based on a carefully developed treatment plan. The hasty or haphazard abuses of this treatment measure can be harmful to the teeth or musculature and it should not be forgotten that dental enamel is irreplaceable. This is the subject matter of Chapter 10.

All restorations involving the occlusal surfaces of teeth require considerations of occlusion, articulation and occlusal function. Whether required to retain existing good function or to correct harmful or lost function, restorative dentistry should be directed at integrating the functions of the teeth with those of the masticatory system as a whole. From the simple alloy filling to the reconstruction of the dentition, the patient should be permitted to eat comfortably and to be unaware of teeth. These are the objectives in Chapter 11 for the natural teeth and in Chapter 12 for the artificial dentition.

The *mandibular dysfunction syndrome* is the subject of Chapter 13. This disturbance, which is often a disorder, occupies a large part of current dental literature and is still an unsolved pathological problem. A survey of this literature will be presented, together with some suggestions for treatment and preventive care.

Treatment of occlusal disorders is based on an analysis of signs, symptoms and pathological responses. Procedures can extend from complex appliances to simple advice on the correct use of muscles. They are considered for treatment in Chapter 14.

The case for intercuspal occlusion on the retruded arc as an objective in the reconstruction of the natural dentition or, in complete dentures, is one which will be advocated from time to time. It implies effort to reach the intercuspal position of the mandible but, because it is a reproducible position, it can be reached each time and therefore is reliable. The reproducibility depends on healthy muscles and the effort required implies that the position will not be maintained for longer than the time required to swallow. Thus the precept of minimal occlusion is upheld. Intercuspal occlusion on the retruded arc requires careful attention to a secure occlusion between cusps and opposing fossae. Any flatness of cusps will produce a tendency to slide out of intercuspal occlusion and to promote parafunction. In the reconstructed natural dentition this tendency is prevented by the development of articulation in the anterior segment only for all articular movements away from IP. This causes parting of the posterior teeth (disclusion) and discourages further articular movements. This is not so simple a task in complete dentures, where balanced articulation is often necessary for reasons of stability. These concepts will be discussed in Chapter 5 and in the chapters on treatment procedures.

Comment

The objective in any health measure is to prevent disease. The establishment of good function is an essential requirement in the prevention of occlusal disturbances in the masticatory system. Through the adolescent years, when the dentition is developing, the dentist has an obligation to ensure freedom from caries and periodontal diseases, to provide a pleasing appearance of the teeth, and to establish hygiene as a prevention against recurrent diseases. He also has the responsibility to provide good occlusal function and to prevent habits, both functional and parafunctional, which may disturb the various tissues of the masticatory system. Good function is good prevention.

References

Berry, D. C. and Poole, D. F. G. (1974) Masticatory function and oral rehabilitation. *Journal of Oral Rehabilitation*, **1**, 191

Bonwill, W. G. A. (1887) The geometrical and mechanical laws of the articulation of the human teeth – the anatomical articulator. *American System of Dentistry*, **3**, 486

Ingervall, B. (1968) Recording of retruded positions of mandible in children. *Odontological Review*, **19**, 65

Posselt, U. (1952) Studies in the mobility of the human mandible. *Acta Odontologica Scandinavica*, **10** (supplement 10)

Chapter 2

The muscles, joints and teeth

Occlusion of the teeth can be expressed as the product of the occlusal surfaces of the teeth (T), muscle activity (M) and the movements permitted by the mandibular joints (J). The formula O = TMJ is perhaps an oversimplification of this complex and often reflex action, especially when appreciating the nervous function which controls it and which provides for its efficiency through a lifetime of change. The muscles, the contours of the teeth and the joints are the tissues which the clinician has to know and understand when attempting to diagnose and treat disturbances of occlusal function. The muscles are subject to disturbances, the teeth to loss and change of shape and the joints to disease and dysfunction. Some relevant features of these tissues will be described and discussed in this chapter.

The muscles of mastication

There are several features of muscle function which may help the understanding of the part played by the muscles in occlusal function. First, all the muscles of mastication are in function (either contracting or relaxing) in all movements of the mandible. Secondly, there is a wide area of origin of some of the muscles compared with the area of insertion. In addition, the ability of groups of fibres within a muscle to contract make possible innumerable variations in the range of movements. Thirdly, muscles conform to patterns of movement but these are subject to alteration by adaptation, disability and disease: they can be trained, when healthy, to reproduce movements; they will fail to do this when stiff and sore. Fourthly, muscle activity is limited by ligaments but is not guided by them. Finally, muscles, and the joints about which they provide movement, are tissues and not machines and, whereas the movements can be made with precision, they are subject to alteration by stimuli, both cerebral and reflex. They are, therefore, unreliable machines and no better example of this feature, in another field of function, is the golf swing so often seemingly mechanical yet so seldom reliable as such.

The muscles of mastication and the movements which they produce can be studied in a number of ways. Electromyographic tracings of the discharge of electrical activity give precise information on degrees of contraction from localized areas of muscles but too much is perhaps made of this source of information when so little muscle activity is recorded. Dissection studies still provide new information and allow deductions to be made on mandibular movements. Histological examinations reveal muscle fibres in new directions and new places. For the clinical student interested in discerning how the mandible moves this or that way, the use of detailed descriptions with a skull to hand is well tried and worth while. This method is also helpful when attempting to visualize the mandible in function, when dealing with a tough bolus of food or, say, chewing gum, biting a piece of thread, or rotating on its retruded condyle axis.

The muscles of mastication occur bilaterally in pairs. Each muscle runs in a different direction and at different levels. Thus a wide variation of movements is possible. Some of their features relevant to the functions they perform will be described using skull photographs and related diagrams. No attempt is made to present a detailed description of these muscles nor of their nerve and blood supply.

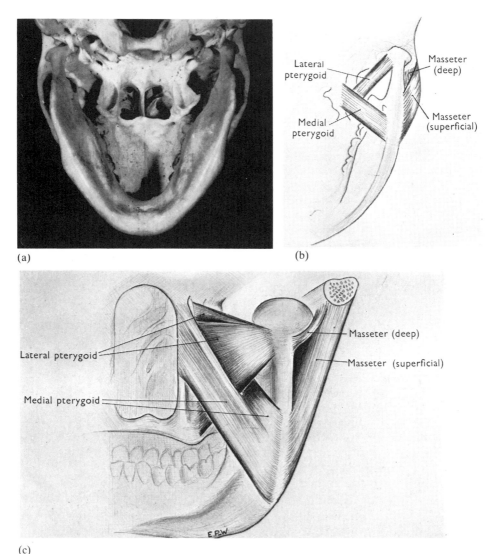

(a)

(b)

(c)

Figure 2.1 (a) Skull and mandible from below. (b) Right mandible from below. Muscles. (c) Right mandible from behind. Muscles

The masseter and medial pterygoid muscles

These are generally called the closing muscles and details of their sites of origin on the skull and insertion on the mandible can be found in any of the standard texts. When viewed from below and behind the skull (Figure 2.1a), it can be seen that the contraction of all four muscles will result in an upwards pull of the mandible. The fibres of the masseters, however, run slightly inwards as well as downwards from the zygomatic arch to the outer surface of the ramus, while the medial pterygoids run outwards as well as downwards from the medial surface of the lateral pterygoid plate to the inner surface of the ramus but at a more horizontal angle than the masseters. The direction of both muscles is also slightly backwards so that equal contraction of both pairs produces a forwards as well as an upwards movement. Stronger contraction of the left medial pterygoid and right masseter will result in an upwards and lateral movement of the mandible to the right. This involves a rotation of the right condyle and, in addition, a lateral shift outwards. This lateral shift is known as the Bennett movement and it takes place in lateral closing movements and in lateral movements from IP. In the right lateral movement the left condyle travels down and inwards; for this to happen, the lower fibres of the left lateral pterygoid have also to contract since the medial pterygoids have no fibres running upwards from their origins. This serves to emphasize the point made about all muscles being involved in all movements of the mandible.

Viewed from the side (Figure 2.2), the fibres of the masseter can be seen running downwards and backwards, thus accounting for the upwards and forwards arc of closure of the mandible with a centre of rotation in the region of the condyles.

There are two other features of the masseter muscle which have some clinical significance. First, the muscle has three parts: superficial, intermediate and deep (Last, 1966). The deep fibres, originating on the inside surface of the zygomatic arch, run slightly forwards and downwards to the region of the ramus below the coronoid process. This can produce a backwards pull on the mandible, aided by the distal fibres of the temporalis, and helps to provide the movement which pulls the mandible into its retruded relation to the maxilla, on which the retruded condyle axis rotates. Secondly, there are fibres from the inner part of the muscle which are inserted horizontally into the capsule and meniscus of the mandibular joint. Thus, a lateral pull on the meniscus is possible when the horizontal fibres are stimulated to contract. The effect on the meniscus of this contraction is to move it from its usual position on closure and to alter its path of movement on opening. This can alter the relationship between meniscus and articular eminence as the condyle moves forwards and provides a cause of joint click. The variables of condyle and eminence shapes and the number of masseter fibres inserted into the meniscus may explain why this phenomenon occurs in some people but not in others. It will be discussed again later in this chapter and in Chapter 13.

In general, the origins of the masseter muscles are more diverse than those of the medial pterygoids, which makes the masseters more varied in the movements they produce. In addition, together with the anterior fibres of the temporalis, they are the muscles that can be seen and palpated in function and this can be helpful in some aspects of occlusal function. The masseter and medial pterygoid muscles are called the power muscles of mastication and can generate considerable force when the needs or abuses of function arise. Also, being superficial, they are useful in electromyographic investigations.

14

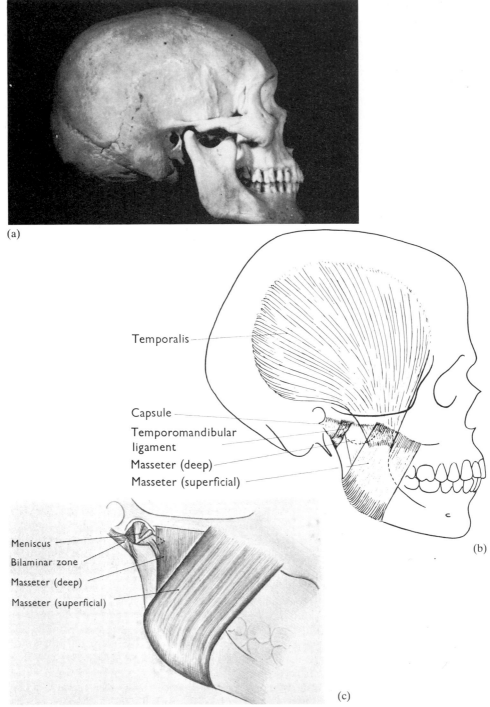

(a)

Temporalis

Capsule

Temporomandibular
ligament

Masseter (deep)

Masseter (superficial)

(b)

Meniscus

Bilaminar zone

Masseter (deep)

Masseter (superficial)

(c)

Figure 2.2 (a) Skull and mandible from side. (b) Muscles, capsule, temporomandibular ligament.
(c) Masseter muscle showing fibres from deep layer entering meniscus. Capsule removed

The temporalis and lateral pterygoid muscles

These are the muscles which provide for the horizontal movements and positioning of the condyles and mandible as the teeth come into occlusion, and for the adjustment to changes of occlusion as teeth tilt, wear and are restored. The *temporalis* muscles spread, in origin, like a fan over the side of the skull (Figure 2.2) and are inserted into the coronoid process of the mandible providing upwards and backwards movements of the mandible, with less power but with greater possibilities for fine adjustment than the closing muscles. Some temporalis fibres are inserted into the anterior part of the meniscus through the capsule and provide a source of movement for this tissue. Palpation of the anterior fibres in the region of the temples has long been a test of retruded closure of the mandible when registering jaw relations. If these fibres contract, the mandible is in its habitual IP or retruded occlusal positions. If they cannot be palpated in closure there is a protrusive component in the movement.

The wide origins of the temporalis muscles and their relatively small insertions emphasize the control they exert over the position of the mandible and, together with the lateral pterygoids, justify the term 'postural muscles' which has been applied to them. This property of control over posture is further emphasized by the ability, mentioned earlier, of groups of fibres within a muscle to contract. Thus they provide fine adjustment of position and movement in response to both voluntary and reflex stimuli.

The *lateral pterygoid* muscles, by contrast, have a more restricted area of origin but have an even smaller area of insertion compared with the temporalis (Figure 2.3). The lateral pterygoid is a more bulky and therefore more powerful muscle; it

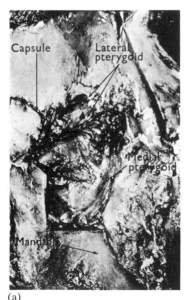

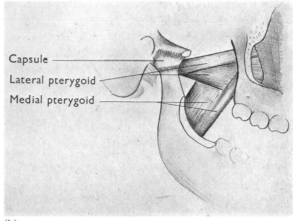

(a)   (b)

Figure 2.3 (a) Dissection. Lateral and medial pterygoid muscles. Capsule. Mandible with coronoid process removed. (Dissection performed by B. J. Parkins, by courtesy of Professor McMinn, Department of Anatomy, Royal College of Surgeons.) (b) Diagram. Lateral and medial pterygoid muscles

consists of two bellies originating on the outer surface of the lateral pterygoid plate and the infratemporal surface of the great wing of the sphenoid bone. The dissection photograph (Figure 2.3a) shows the relatively wide area of origin and emphasizes the power and control which this muscle exerts over the condyle and meniscus. The lower belly runs upwards, outwards and backwards and the upper horizontally in the same direction. Both heads merge into the area of the capsule of the joints and neck of the mandibular condyle. Fibres are inserted into the neck of the condyle, the capsule and into the meniscus itself. An investigation by Porter (1970) has shown fibres being inserted into the medial aspect of the meniscus and this feature would seem to be capable of pulling the meniscus in a medial direction.

The lateral pterygoid muscles acting together pull the condyles forwards and downwards and are two of the openers of the mandible. However, they can only pull the condyles downwards and forwards. When the left muscle contracts, while the other relaxes, the mandible moves to the right. This contraction also helps to pull the mandible bodily to the right and takes part in the production of the Bennett movement.

A significant feature of this muscle is its sole responsibility for protracting the condyles. However, there is no opposing muscle inserted into the posterior aspect of the condyles or menisci in order to retract the condyles and so impart smoothness to the closing movement. This is provided partly by contraction of the posterior fibres of the temporalis and deep fibres of the masseter muscles, both of which are inserted into the body of the ramus, and partly by the relaxation of the lateral pterygoids. This calls for a high degree of coordination, since the fine adjustment to occlusal positions and articulations (or the avoidance of them) depends on it. Equally, failure to adapt to alterations of occlusion or to an unexpected bolus can cause injury to fibres of this muscle. This has proved a common cause of mandibular joint pain (see Chapter 13).

The lateral pterygoid muscles not only play the dominant part in the fast movements of the condyles and menisci but they seldom have the opportunity fully to stretch and, as it were, rest from their labours. Stretching a muscle is an activity which allows the tension of continuous contraction to ease and is often curative of spasm. In the case of the lateral pterygoids, the habitual IP of the mandible sometimes prevents the condyles from retracting fully and it requires a conscious effort to cause the retraction necessary to stretch the muscles. This is a physiotherapeutic function often worthy of prescription (see Chapter 14).

The digastric and geniohyoid muscles

These two muscles acting together are depressors of the mandible in a downwards and backwards direction and provide the chief opening component in the retruded arc movement of the mandible. Together with the stylohyoid and mylohyoid muscles, they form the suprahyoid group of muscles.

The *digastric* muscle has two bellies, the posterior belly originating from the mastoid notch and the anterior belly from the digastric fossa of the mandible, which is close to the lower border. The two bellies are joined by a tendon which is held close to the horn of the hyoid bone by a loop of strengthened fibres of the deep cervical fascia. The length of this loop varies, as will the obtuse angle between the two bellies. This may have some effect on the angle of pull on the mandible. The anterior bellies may be joined together making one thick muscle. In order that the mandible be pulled down and back by this muscle, the hyoid bone has to be fixed;

this is achieved by the opposing contractions of the stylohyoid and infrahyoid muscles.

The *geniohyoid* muscles run down and backwards from the anterior end of the mylohyoid ridges and are inserted into the upper border of the hyoid bone. The insertion is wider than the origin and the two muscles lying together have a fan shape. Their action is to depress the mandible and it is difficult to imagine their acting without the digastric muscles. When the mandible is fixed in IP their contraction will raise the hyoid bone, which occurs during deglutition. These two pairs of muscles can be palpated in contraction when the mandible is pulled down and back; occasionally a knot of spastic muscle can be felt following a disturbance of muscle activity in this region.

Movements of the mandible

After visualizing the muscles on the mandible and skull, it may be difficult to imagine how it is that such precise and sometimes powerful movements can be carried out when the condyles seem to fit so imprecisely into the glenoid fossae. As Sicher (1964) pointed out, however, the movements of the mandible are directed by the play of the muscles and not by the shape of the bones or by the ligaments, as in many other joints.

There are essentially two movements of the condyles which account for the varied and three-dimensional mandibular movements of the mandible. These are the *rotations* and *translations* of the condyle axis. The opening and closing rotational movements are brought about by the depressor and elevator muscles and the translatory movements by the protractor and retractor muscles. It is repeated, however, that all mandibular movements involve all its muscles, either contracting or relaxing.

Opening and closing

On opening, the mandible rotates around a transverse axis which passes approximately through the centres of the two condyles; this is achieved by the action of the anterior digastric and geniohyoid muscles. At the same time, the condyles are protracted by the lateral pterygoids and the two movements continue jointly until the required amount of opening is reached. The extent of the rotatory opening is considerable and in the healthy mouth three fingers can be inserted between the incisor teeth at full opening. As the impulse to close is received, the depressors and retractors relax and the elevators begin their contraction. The condyles move back rapidly as the temporalis muscles contract. As closure approaches, the movement is slowed by the reciprocation of lateral pterygoids and temporalis when the rotation of the condyles is completed. The two elevators play the main part in this movement but the adjustment to precise closure or to the avoidance of occlusion in the chewing cycle is left to the two horizontally acting postural muscles. The movements of the meniscus in opening and closing will be described in the next section.

The opening and closing movements of the mandible, whether for mastication, speech, or other activities, all take place within a space limited by the ligaments running between mandible and maxilla and by the shape of the bones themselves.

This aspect of jaw movements will be further discussed in Chapter 4 and will be described as the parcel of mandibular movement. Meanwhile, emphasis is given to the feature of muscle activity that permits a wide range of movement through two joints.

Retruded opening and closing

With effort and patience, the mandible can be pulled back and made to rotate about an axis through the condyles which is rotational and involves no translation. This may require assistance from the dentist but can usually be practised voluntarily, provided that the muscles are healthy. The backward pull is achieved by the posterior temporalis fibres and deep belly of the masseter, with assistance from the digastrics and geniohyoids. The last two muscles will then effect opening on the retruded arc and pull the point of the chin down and backwards for a distance of up to 20 mm. Closing on this arc is achieved by the elevator muscles but with posterior fibres of temporalis and deep fibres of masseter exerting a backwards pull. As will be evident throughout the text, this movement on the retruded arc is useful in the diagnosis and treatment of occlusal disturbances because, with healthy muscles, it is reproducible.

Lateral shift (Bennett movement)

When the mandible moves to one side or the other, either in opening or closing, the condyle on the side to which the mandible is moving rotates minimally and moves slightly forwards, downwards and laterally. If, for example, the mandible moves to the right, the left condyle moves downwards, forwards and inwards while in contact with the meniscus and eminence. The right condyle is allowed only a small rotatory movement because its lateral pole is limited by the temporomandibular ligament and cannot move backwards for more than 1 mm (Sicher, 1964). It therefore moves laterally and slightly forwards and downwards due to the combined action of the left lateral and medial pterygoids and to the contact that exists between the condyles, menisci and opposing fossae. Sicher describes this as an evasive movement and the condyle as resting. Certainly, the force causing the movement comes from the left side and the right condyle moves as it can within the limits of its ligaments. If this movement is inhibited or altered by unexpected tooth contacts the pattern of muscle activity may be altered unfavourably. It should be remembered that this is only one component of an opening or closing movement. As will be described in Chapters 4 and 8, all mandibular movements can be analysed as deriving from three centres (axes) of rotation in each condyle region.

Bennett (1908) made his observations on this component of mandibular movement using bent wire and candle-light and they remained in the gloom of insignificance for twenty years. Pantographic tracings of the mandible then revealed that they still existed and have some significance in the analysis of tooth articulations and restorative dentistry. This asymmetrical lateral shift has now been separated into *immediate* and *progressive* components, as observed on pantographic tracings (see Chapter 8). These tracings are extensions of the movement and take place with the teeth parted but they are reproducible and represent an extreme or border movement limited by ligaments. One wonders what Sir Norman Bennett would have thought of it all.

The mandibular ligaments

Muscles move and ligaments limit. In forming part of the attachment of the mandible to the skull, the ligaments provide the borders of the circumductory mandibular movements.

The fibrous capsules of the joints (see Figure 2.2b, c) constitute the chief ligaments, particularly the outer thickened portions which form the *temporomandibular* ligaments. The capsules are thin, fibrous structures attached to the temporal bone at the anterior, medial and lateral boundaries of the articular tubercles and fossae. They are inserted into the necks of the condyles and are continuous with the menisci and with the loose connective tissue behind the menisci. The thick, lateral portions of the capsules forming the temporomandibular ligaments arise from the zygomatic processes of the temporal bones and run down and backwards to narrow insertions at the condylar necks. These ligaments are thus fan-shaped and act to limit various movements of the mandible, particularly the retrusive, when the condyles are, as it were, cornered in their most retruded and superior relationships to the skull. It is in this relation that the mandible can be made to rotate on its retruded arc. These ligaments also serve to protect the posterior extensions of the menisci which are vascular and innervated and might otherwise be subject to damage by the condyles. There are nerve endings within the capsules which relay information on positions and movements of the condyles to the central nervous system.

The accessory ligaments are the *sphenomandibular* and *stylomandibular*; Sicher refers to them as 'so-called' since neither has any functional part to play in the mandibular articulation. The sphenomandibular ligament runs from the spine of the sphenoid bone and has a fan-like insertion into the lingula, the lower border of the mandibular foramen and up to the lower border of the mandibular neck. The stylomandibular ligament runs from the styloid process and stylohyoid ligament to the region of the angle of the mandible. The majority of its fibres continue into the fascia on the medial surface of the medial pterygoid muscle and would therefore seem to share in the activity of this muscle, perhaps by limiting its stretch.

Mention is made of a ligament attaching the malleus ossicle in the ear to the capsules of the mandibular joint. Pinto (1962) established the presence of a 'tiny ligament' connecting the malleus, the capsule of the joint and the meniscus. He described it as being inserted into the neck of the malleus immediately above the anterior process and spreading out cone-shaped, running forwards, downwards and laterally to be inserted into the medioposterosuperior part of the capsule and meniscus of the joint. Based on this article, Christensen (1969) suggested that, as spasm of the lateral pterygoid can interfere with the function of the meniscus, it could interfere with the action of the malleus. He suggested that the malleus would be prevented from vibrating normally, resulting in a loss of hearing. This requires confirmation by anatomists and embryologists but it would seem unlikely that the malleus, which vibrates in one plane, would be inhibited by a tiny ligament which is attached at right angles to this plane.

The temporomandibular ligaments play a passive part in mandibular movements and are of value when transferring jaw positions and movements to an articulator.

The mandibular joints

The joints have been said to permit movement and, whereas they do not promote it, they guide it from the information of nerve receptors within the capsule and from the shape of the bones comprising the joints. The joint tissues provide for smooth movement of the condyles and menisci but they are subject to disease and dysfunction, as are other joints. Cineradiographic films of these joints in function demonstrate the speed with which the condyles move and it is obvious that proprioception and lubrication are properties which the joints possess in good measure. This is not the text for detailed descriptions of the joints but some of their features and significances will be mentioned and discussed.

Since his paper in 1948, Sicher has taught and written about the tissues and functions of the mandibular joint to the benefit of the dental profession and has provided information, guidance and caution on deductions made from clinical observations. Rees (1954) described the structure and function of these joints in a paper which has become a standard source of information and is quoted in many books and articles on this subject. From these sources and others, the following relevant features are presented.

Anatomy of the condyles

The elongated shape of the condyles and their angled relationship to each other (Figure 2.4) make mechanical analogies misleading. The analysis of mandibular

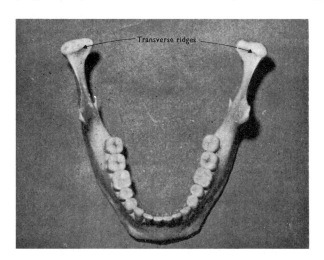

Figure 2.4 Mandible. Angled relationship of condyles and transverse ridges

movements into centres of rotation is acceptable only if it is assumed that the movements are reproducible, made by healthy muscles and limited by taut ligaments. Each condyle presents a transverse ridge in front of its summit, with the posterior slope from the summit longer than the anterior one. It is this ridge which may become temporarily jammed against the meniscus when the phenomenon of click occurs. The lateral and medial poles of the condyles present bony tubercles, just below the articular surfaces, to which the capsules and menisci are attached. The anterior surfaces of the necks of the condyles are roughened, indicating the tendinous insertions of the lateral pterygoid muscles.

The glenoid fossae and eminentiae

The hollow fossae (Figure 2.2a) permit a freedom of movement for the condyles but this movement is cushioned by the menisci which fill the spaces and provide continuous contact between the menisci and condyles in all movements. The convex eminentiae are continuous with the fossae and provide a path for the condyles in forward and lateral movements. During these movements, the condyles are in unstable relations to the eminentiae and any alteration to the established pattern may result in click or even muscle spasm, which is the phenomenon of locking. The shapes of condyles and eminentiae vary between individuals and steep or shallow paths have led to their association with various classifications of malocclusion. This, however, has not received sufficient investigation for proof. In addition, a flat eminentia has been claimed to be a cause of condyle dislocations but this, too, is more likely to be attributable to muscle spasm. The translatory condylar movements can be shown to be reproducible by pantographic tracings and, while these are made with the teeth parted (Chapter 8) and at a fixed level of jaw separation, it would seem to demonstrate that the path of the condyle may be determined by the slope of the eminentia.

The articular cartilage of the condyles and fossae provide resistance to tensile forces. This mechanical property depends on the combination of a collagen network impregnated with proteoglycans and the water content of the matrix. The cartilage can be said to function as a water cushion that resists compressive forces; it is described in histological detail by Christensen and Ziebert (1986) in a series on the effects of experimental tooth loss on the intra-articular temporomandibular joint tissues in a number of experimental animals. They reported that loss of teeth, with consequent abnormal loading, resulted in histomorphological and pathological changes in the articular cartilages and menisci, the synovial membranes and the bony articular components of the joints.

The interarticular menisci

The division of these fibrous sheets into four ellipsoidal zones (Figure 2.5a, b) makes them flexible and allows them to adapt in shape from concave below, when the mandible is in intercuspal position, to convex below, as the condyles glide forwards (Figure 2.5c, d, e). The *anterior band* is thick but narrow from before backwards; the *intermediate zone* is thin and narrow and provides the flexible element; the *posterior band* is thicker and wider than the anterior band and provides the filler for the condyle–fossa space at IP; the *bilaminar zone* is the distal extension and is attached to the posterior wall of the glenoid fossa and to the squamotympanic suture by its upper stratum and to the neck of the condyle by its lower stratum. The tissue of the meniscus is chiefly dense fibrous tissue with occasional cells suggestive of cartilage. The upper stratum of the bilaminar zone is composed of loose fibroelastic tissue and contains blood vessels and nerves, while the lower stratum is mostly fibrous tissue without elastic fibres. This latter differentiation of tissue suggests that the upper stratum is more freely mobile than the lower and moves forward to take the place of the condyle as it moves forwards, while the lower stratum travels with the condyle (Figure 2.5). The tissues of these zones permit contact between condyle and meniscus without pressure being borne. The menisci are continuous with the capsules and receive muscle insertions anteriorly, laterally and medially. Translatory and rotary movements are permitted by the flexibility of this tissue, the elastic fibres of which consist largely of the insoluble and amorphous elastin (Christensen and Ziebert, 1986). In one of the experimental animals, an island of elastic cartilage appeared in the distal section of the meniscus following unilateral loss of teeth. It appears that abnormal loading of

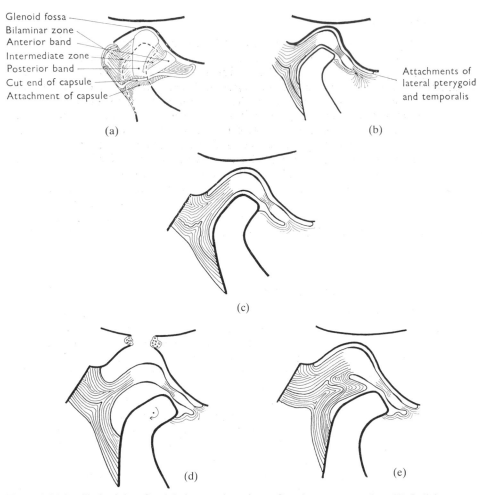

Glenoid fossa
Bilaminar zone
Anterior band
Intermediate zone
Posterior band
Cut end of capsule
Attachment of capsule

Attachments of
lateral pterygoid
and temporalis

(a)

(b)

(c)

(d)

(e)

Figure 2.5 Mandibular joint. Condyle fossa and meniscus. Opening movement from IP. In living person meniscus in contact with fossa and condyle. No air enters the joint. (a) Parts named. (b) IP. Posterior band is in deepest part of fossa. (c) Retruded rotary opening phase. (d) Protrusive opening phase. (e) Beginning of closing phase. Condyles rotate backwards on bicondylar axis. (After Rees, 1954)

the meniscus results in metaplasia and ectopic calcifications (Christensen, 1975; Ramfjord and Blankenship, 1981).

Muscle insertions

Fibres of the lateral pterygoid merge with the anterior and medial aspects of the meniscus and form a true insertion by tendinous fibres, while fibres from the masseter and temporalis muscles, running mostly at right angles to the main fibres of the muscles, are inserted laterally and anteriorly into the meniscus. These muscle insertions suggest the possibilities of distracting pulls on the meniscus during sudden reflex movements and provide further causes for click as the condyle moves forward with the meniscus position altered (see p. 242). There are no muscle insertions posteriorly into the meniscus.

The synovial membrane

This vascular layer of connective tissue lines all structures of the articulation that are not involved in the gliding condylar movements and is found chiefly in the posteriorly placed bilaminar zone. The synovial secretion lubricates the rapid three-dimensional movements of the condyles and menisci. The viscosity of this fluid is probably under the control of the autonomic nervous system and is therefore subject to alteration. Any reduction in viscosity of this secretion will lead to frictional resistance within the capsule, thus providing a further cause of joint noise (crepitus), inflammatory response and dysfunction. The factual and hypothetical details of this aspect of joint function were explained by Toller (1961).

Once again, Christensen and Ziebert (1986) report on animals inoculated with mycobacteria, causing polyarthritic changes. If the molar teeth are then removed, the incidence and severity of temporomandibular joint arthritis increases. In addition to synovitis with infiltrations of round cells, there is villous hypertrophy of the condylar fibrous connective tissue and surfaces of the menisci. This paper repays further study.

Movements of the condyles and menisci

The observations of Rees (1954), albeit on dissected cadavers, revealed the possibilities of movement up to a distance of 8 mm between condyle and meniscus from retruded to full opening. During the forward movement to partial opening, the transverse ridge of the condyle moved across the posterior band of the disc. On full opening of the mandible the condyle ridge crossed the anterior band and came to rest in front of it (Figure 2.5e). It was calculated that the total forward condyle movement from retruded to full opening was at least 15 mm and that, consequently, the meniscus would move forwards at least 7 mm on the temporal bone. In other words, the movement of the condyle is greater than that of the meniscus. Another observation made by Rees was that the space vacated by the condyle in its forward movement is occupied by the soft bilaminar zone tissue, since there is no air space in the joint cavity. This supports Sicher's (1964) assertion of articulating bones being kept in 'sharp contact' during movement. Finally, the condyles can move in an arc due to their being separated from the temporal bones in retrusion by the thickest parts of the menisci and by the thinnest parts when they move on to the eminentiae. They do not have to follow the contours of the eminentiae.

The flexibility of the condylar movements and the fact that there are two condyles makes for a three-dimensional space in which any one point of the mandible can move with considerable freedom. It can move from one limit (or border position) to another without going through a central or median position such as the rest position. The presence of teeth, however, provides restrictions to these *circumductory* movements and when this inhibitory effect is associated with parafunctional habits or deflective tooth contacts the muscle activity can itself be disturbed by injury. The joint tissues can suffer through persistent low-grade injury (click and crepitus), through inflammatory or degenerative processes and through severe injury resulting in fracture or effusion into the joint. But in function generally, and for the majority of people, the mandibular joints permit various and versatile movements throughout the average life span.

The relation between occlusal function and the movements of the mandibular condyles is one of interdependence. The teeth determine the various occlusal positions of the mandible; the joints provide a guide to the movements of the mandible to, from, and between these positions. It could be said that the teeth perform and the joints permit occlusal function and that the comfort and efficiency of this function depend on the neuromuscular control of the movements and the occlusal shapes of the teeth. It is desirable that these shapes conform to the stable patterns of joint and jaw activity and that the joints are not called upon to perform movements to which they cannot adapt.

The occlusal surfaces of the teeth

Neuromusclar activity causes the mandible to move towards the maxilla, stimulated by impulses from the masticatory system or the higher centres of the brain. If the objective or result of this movement is tooth contact, the shapes of the occlusal surfaces of the maxillary and mandibular teeth will determine the position of the mandible during occlusion. Since the occlusion and articulation of the teeth have an effect on the behaviour of the muscles, it is necessary to have a knowledge of the shapes (or anatomy) of their occlusal surfaces and to know how they can most efficiently occlude in order to provide occlusal function.

Normal occlusion

Tooth surfaces and relationships will be described as applying to what is generally accepted as normal occlusion. Figure 2.6 shows the labial and buccal segments in class I (Angle) relationship to their opposing segments where the key teeth are the first molars. The mesiobuccal cusp of the mandibular first molar occludes between the maxillary first molar and second premolar. The maxillary and mandibular incisors occlude at an oblique angle to each other which is constant within certain limits and provides an index for assessing the need for correction. 'Normal occlusion' as a term is of less importance than the need to have an objective for efficient and comfortable occlusal function. A further criticism of the term is that it

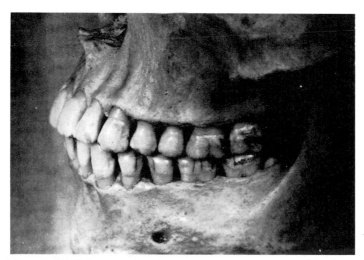

Figure 2.6 Skull. Intercuspal position of mandible

implies a static relationship between the teeth that seldom exists in function. It is an incident in the swallow, as is contact with the ball in a golf swing but, as in the golf swing, it must be efficient to be effective and preventive of harm. Normal occlusion is therefore a term of reference related to muscle and joint function, to skeletal relationships, and to the effect it produces on the masticatory system.

The incisor teeth

The development of the incisor teeth usually results in occlusion between maxillary and mandibular incisors at an angle of between 130° and 135° in the skeletal class I relation (Figure 2.7). This angle will vary with the angle between the mandibular plane and one of the fixed planes of the skull, say, the Frankfort plane (see Figure 4.1). The angle is important, however, since a pleasing appearance is provided when the angle of the maxillary incisors to the Frankfort plane is about 108°. Secondly, it allows a gliding contact between the maxillary and mandibular incisors in protrusion, separating the buccal teeth. Variations in this angle will be discussed in Chapters 5 and 11.

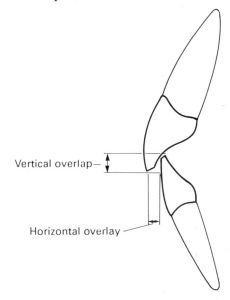

Vertical overlap—

Horizontal overlay —

Figure 2.7 Vertical and horizontal overlap in incisors

When the incisor teeth occlude in IP the resultant of force will be forwards, tending to displace the maxillary incisors forwards. This force is balanced by the lip muscles which not only balance the occlusal forces but those of the tongue muscles in function. It should not be forgotten, however, that in intercuspal occlusion the posterior teeth will be sharing the occlusal forces generated. The incisor teeth are thus stabilized in occlusion, in the functions of speech and facial expression and, not least, in the rest position of the mandible.

Horizontal and vertical overlap and incisal guidance

The incisal edges of the mandibular incisors contact the lingual surfaces of the maxillary on their cingula at intercuspal occlusion. The vertical distance between the incisal edges at this occlusion is called the *vertical overlap*. The horizontal distance between the incisal edges is called the *horizontal overlap* (Figure 2.7). When the mandible protrudes in articulation, the lingual slopes of the maxillary incisors determine the path which the mandible will follow and the influence on protrusive movement created by the inclination of this slope is called the *incisal guidance*. Together with the variable angles mentioned above, these three features of incisor occlusion have some significance when analysing occlusal function and when planning reconstruction or complete dentures. When to these features of incisor relationships is added the variables of lip and tongue muscle activity, it is understandable that orthodontists and prosthodontists find occasional difficulties and disappointments in their treatment procedures.

The canine teeth

In addition to their characteristic labial appearance the maxillary canine teeth have a well marked lingual ridge and cingulum which divide the lingual surface into two slopes. These slopes have significance in occlusion and may provide guidance during articulation with the opposing mandibular teeth. The distal cusp ridge of the mandibular canine occludes on the mesial of these two slopes; the mesial cusp ridge of the mandibular first premolar occludes on the distal slope (see Figure 2.11). The lingual ridge of the maxillary canine also provides guidance for the articular movement of the buccal and mesial cusp ridge of the mandibular first premolar in protrusion of the mandible and for the cusp of the mandibular canine in lateral movement to its side. This articular movement has clinical significance in the development of canine guidance (see Chapter 5). The lingual ridge and cingulum are not so well marked in the mandibular canines and this emphasizes their function in the maxillary arch. This is to divide the occlusion between mandibular canine and first premolar and to provide guidance for their articular movements.

The buccal segments

The posterior or buccal segments will be treated as groups of four teeth although they comprise two different forms of teeth, namely, the premolars and molars. Their occlusion and articulation conform to patterns as a group, however, and this justifies their consideration as segments. Drawings of the four maxillary and four mandibular posterior teeth can be seen in Figure 2.8. Each posterior tooth has a varying number of cusps, ridges and grooves and each cusp is at the summit of three ridges and a buccal or lingual surface. There is a mesial and distal cusp ridge descending from each cusp, and a triangular ridge descends towards a central fossa and fissure. The buccal and lingual cusp ridges either join adjacent cusp ridges or continue as mesial and distal marginal ridges.

Characteristics (Figure 2.8)

Each premolar and molar has its own characteristics and the significance of each is by no means certain. The third molars are not included since they appear in many variable forms. The *maxillary first premolar* has an angular shape while the *second premolar* is more rounded; both have well-marked cusps. The *maxillary first molar* has a dominant mesiolingual cusp which gives a triangular ridge to the central fossa and a supplemental (or oblique) ridge which joins the triangular ridge of the

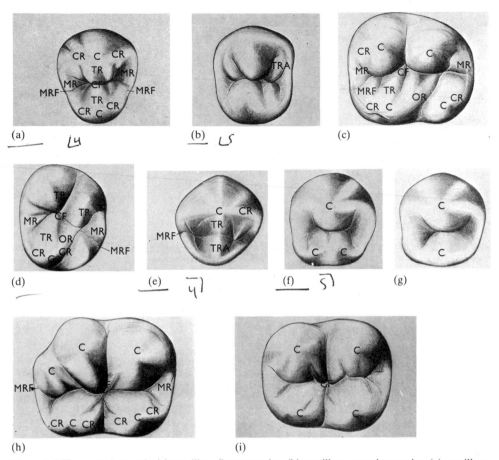

Figure 2.8 The posterior teeth: (a) maxillary first premolar; (b) maxillary second premolar; (c) maxillary first molar; (d) maxillary second molar; (e) mandibular first premolar; (f) mandibular second premolar; three cusps; (g) mandibular second premolar; two cusps; (h) mandibular first molar; (i) mandibular second molar. C, cusp; CR, cusp ridge; MR, marginal ridge; TR, triangular ridge; TRA, transverse ridge; OR, oblique ridge; CF, central fossa; MRF, marginal ridge fissure

distobuccal cusp across the central fissure. This molar usually has a diminutive extra cusp lingual to the mesiolingual cusp and this distinguishes it from the *second molar* to which it is otherwise similar. The *mandibular first premolar* has a small lingual cusp which does not have any occlusal function and this is sometimes blamed for creating adverse forces on the maxillary first premolar. The ridge running from the lingual cusp to the central fissure is called a 'transverse ridge'. The *mandibular second premolar* has three forms, two of them giving it two lingual cusps. The *mandibular first molar* has a characteristic pentagonal shape with three buccal cusps while the *second molar* is more rectangular and only occasionally has the third buccal cusp.

Each posterior tooth has central, transverse and supplemental fissures and the central fissure usually has mesial and distal extensions which cross the marginal ridges. Their direction varies but usually they run towards the lingual embrasures. They are thought to provide channels for directing food away from the contact areas and are valuable for this reason when carved on restorations. The lingular and buccal fissures provide this function and the supplemental fissures aid the milling function of the occlusal surfaces.

The triangular and oblique ridges are separated by central fissures and they provide the central fossae for opposing cusps and ridges to occlude. The area between the buccal and lingual cusps is also known as the occlusal table.

Supporting and guiding cusps

In order to understand the functions of posterior teeth their cusps are classified into two groups: those which provide the main support for intercuspal occlusion and those which guide the teeth towards intercuspal occlusion. Thus the terms 'supporting' and 'guiding' cusps are used. They were introduced by Kraus, Jordan and Abrams (1969) in their book on dental anatomy and occlusion, which is recommended reading on this subject. They were also used by Beyron (1969) in his observations on optimal occlusion which repay careful study.

Supporting cusps

These are the buccal mandibular and lingual maxillary cusps and they occlude wholly within the opposing occlusal table and thus support the occlusal vertical relation of the mandible in its intercuspal position. They are more rounded in shape than the guiding cusps and are more centrally placed. Ideally they occlude on three sides with opposing ridges leaving a space between the cusp itself and the opposing fossa (Figure 2.9). The contact area between the inner facing ridges is larger than between the outer facing ridge and opposing ridge. Together with a third contact this constitutes a stable tripod contact and should be a feature of all restorations

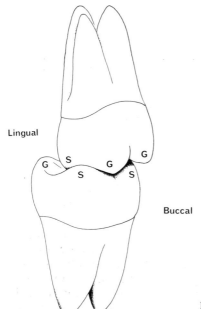

Figure 2.9 Supporting (S) and guiding (G) cusps

involving cusp–fossa relations. The outer facing surface of the supporting cusp is known as its functional outer aspect. One further significant feature is that only two maxillary and two mandibular supporting cusps occlude in opposing central fossae. These are the mesiolingual cusps of the maxillary first and second molars and the distobuccal cusps of the mandibular first and second molars. The remaining supporting cusps occlude in the opposing marginal ridge areas (Figure 2.10). Being rounded, however, this does not imply that they are acting as plunger cusps, although this is a feature which has to be carefully watched in assessing food stagnation between teeth.

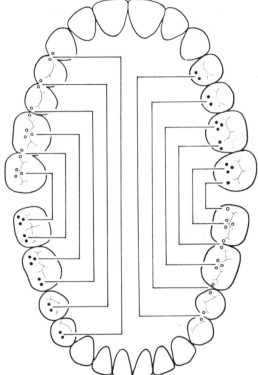

Figure 2.10 Tripod contact sites in cusp–ridge IO. Distobuccal cusp ridges of mandibular first and second molars in opposing fossae. Mesiolingual cusp ridges of maxillary first and second molars in opposing fossae. Otherwise, cusp–ridge. ●, Supporting cusps; ○, contacts

Guiding cusps

These are the lingual mandibular and buccal maxillary cusps and they occlude lightly with their inner facing triangular ridges against the functional outer aspects of the opposing supporting cusps in intercuspal occlusion (see Figure 2.9). Thus they occlude outside the opposing occlusal table. The outer aspects of guiding cusps have no opposing tooth contacts. Guiding cusps are sharper and more outwardly placed on the tooth than the supporting cusps and exhibit vertical and horizontal overlap over (or under) their opposing supporting cusps. This feature provides protection against tongue and cheek biting as the mandible closes into intercuspal position. Guiding cusps overlap the opposing embrasure areas and may provide a cause of food stagnation if the marginal ridges are incorrectly restored.

Cusp–ridge occlusion

The contacts described and illustrated (Figure 2.10) constitute cusp–ridge intercuspal occlusion and represent normal occlusion in class I jaw relation. Deviations are common and may result in unstable cusp relations with consequent tendencies to deflexions of individual teeth or of the mandible on closure. One clinical application of the relative shapes and positions of supporting and guiding cusps is the expectation of opposing tooth contact when making restorations on teeth in the mouth which involve marginal or cusp ridges. Cusp–ridge occlusion accounts for many broken restored marginal ridges. This is common when caries or wear has destroyed a marginal ridge which has remained untreated. There is a tendency for the opposing tooth to tilt and permit the supporting cusp to occupy the ridge area. There is little space left to restore the ridge to its original shape and attempts to do so often lead to breakages.

During incoming or outgoing lateral chewing movements, the guiding cusp ridges may make contact with the opposing supporting cusp ridges on the side being used (working contacts). This contact is often prevented, however, by canine contact which separates the posterior teeth. On the opposite side there may be contact between the triangular ridges of the opposing supporting cusps (non-working contacts). During the protrusive movements, the mesial cusp ridges of the mandibular supporting cusps may make contact with the distal cusp ridges of the maxillary guiding cups. The inclines of these cusps determine the articular paths followed, thereby justifying the term 'guiding cusps'. These contacts are potential because the articular guidance provided by the maxillary incisors and canines should cause a separation of the posterior teeth, thus demonstrating the phenomenon of *disclusion* (Chapter 5).

Cusp relations in occlusion and articulation will be discussed further in Chapter 5 when assessing the existence of occlusal forces on the teeth and articular contacts between them.

Wear, caries and change

The occlusal surfaces of the teeth are subject to wear by function and parafunction and loss of surface by caries with consequent changes in the contours of ridges and fossae, of cusps and fissures. Therefore, the occlusal relations are continually changing and the cycle of adaptation, repair and further change, is the often unrecognized story of occlusion. Occasionally, in the hands of skilled operators occlusal contours are adjusted or created in such a way that their relations are not so subject to wear and change. Therefore, it is helpful to have a clear picture of the teeth as they should be before attempting to restore them.

The roots of the teeth

Root shape and size, the number of roots per tooth and their direction are usually specific. The size and direction of the roots have a direct relation with crown size, although this can vary. When correct, this feature provides stability for the crowns in function. Surrounding each root is the periodontal membrane which permits movement of the roots within the membrane space in a limited but omnidirectional manner. The function of the roots cannot be considered without their membranes since all forces on them are received by the membranes which act as resilient cushions between the roots and alveolar bone. This membrane is often referred to as a ligament since the principal collagen fibres in it seem to run from bone to root surface in an apical direction and act as a stay to the apical movement of the root. Recently is has been suggested that no fibres have been seen to cross the membrane space from bone to tooth and consequently the function of the tissue between root and bone acts more as a membrane than as a ligament. Further, since few forces are directed axially on to a tooth, the function of the membrane is to be displaced within its bony socket when a force is applied to the tooth and to recover when the force is removed. Forces in excess of those which can be accepted by this membrane are directed to the alveolar bone which then responds by the phenomenon of resorption. Such forces can also be excessive in an apical direction and cause strangulation of the vessels as they enter the tooth, with potential death of pulp.

The periodontal membranes contain nerve receptors which act proprioceptively to give information about position and movement to the central nervous system. As a result of forces on the teeth, stimuli are transmitted from these receptors and this results in reflex activity of the masticatory muscles (Chapter 3).

The size and direction of roots are subject to developmental alterations from those established as normal. These take the form of short and narrow roots relative to crown size and this can predispose to a tendency to tooth movement, especially where adjacent teeth thave been lost. Also, twisted roots will provide less stability against occlusal forces. It is possible to determine, using study casts and radiographs, the centre of resistance of a tooth against these forces and the closer this is to the apex the less stable the tooth will be. There are four factors which will help in assessing this resistance value: the crown:root ratios of the teeth, the height

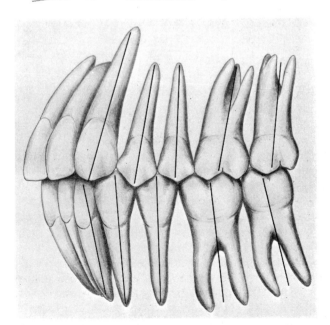

Figure 2.11 Intercuspal occlusion. Relationship between maxillary and mandibular canine, premolar and molar cusp ridges. Incisor relationships. Crown and root inclinations of canines, premolars and molars. (After Kraus, Jordan and Abrams, 1969)

of alveolar bone, the resultant of force following intercuspal occlusion, and the health of the gingival and periodontal tissues.

Axial stress

It has always been asserted that the most favourable stresses for the supporting tissues of the roots to receive are those in an axial direction. This can seldom be expected in view of the lines of forces suggested by the diagram in Figure 2.11. The second premolars come closest to this ideal but all occlusal forces depend on cusp–fossa and cusp–ridge relations and these are subject to variation in both direction and force. There are many teeth in good periodontal health performing adequate function whose roots are not receiving axial forces in occlusion or mastication. The variable factors providing stability for such teeth will be discussed in Chapter 5.

Comment

The integration of muscles, joints and teeth to provide comfortable and efficient occlusion is a proposition which depends on the health of these tissues and on healthy responses to the demands made on them. In order to understand the various disturbances which can threaten the function and health of these tissues it is necessary to examine the poistions and movements of the mandible in relation to the maxilla and the neuromuscular function which controls them. These features will be the objectives of the next two chapters.

References

Bennett, N. G. (1908) A contribution to the study of the movements of the mandible. *Transactions of the Odontological Section of the Royal Society of Medicine,* **1**, 79

Beyron, H. (1969) Optimal occlusion. *Dental Clinics of North America,* **13**, 537

Christensen, F. G. (1969) Some anatomical concepts associated with the temporomandibular joint. *Annals of the Australian College of Dental Surgery,* **2**, 39

Christensen, L. V. (1975) Elastic tissue in the temporomandibular disc of miniature swine. *Journal of Oral Rehabilitation* **2**, 373

Christensen, L. V. and Ziebert, G. J. (1986) Effects of experimental loss of teeth on the temporomandibular joint. *Journal of Oral Rehabilitation,* **13**, 587

Kraus, B. S., Jordan, R. E. and Abrams, L. (1969) *Dental Anatomy and Occlusion,* Williams & Wilkins, Baltimore

Last, R. J. (1966) *Anatomy Regional and Applied,* 4th edn, Churchill, London, p. 576

Pinto, O. F. (1962) A new structure related to the temporomandibular joint and middle ear. *Journal of Prosthetic Dentistry,* **12**, 95

Porter, M. R. (1970) Attachment of lateral pterygoid to meniscus. *Journal of Prosthetic Dentistry,* **24**, 555

Ramfjord, S. P. and Blankenship, J. R. (1981) Increased occlusal vertical dimension in adult monkeys. *Journal of Prosthetic Dentistry,* **45**, 74

Rees, L. A. (1954) Structure and function of the mandibular joint. *British Dental Journal,* **96**, 125

Sicher, H. (1948) Temporomandibular articulation in mandibular overclosure. *Journal of the American Dental Association Dental Cosmos,* **36**, 131

Sicher, H. (1964) Functional anatomy of the temporomandibular joints. In *The Temporomandibular Joint,* (ed. B. G. Sarnat), Thomas, Springfield IL, pp. 34–37

Sicher, H. (1965) *Oral Anatomy,* 4th edn, Mosby, St Louis

Toller, P. A. (1961) Synovial apparatus and temporomandibular function. *British Dental Journal,* **111**, 356

Chapter 3

Neuromuscular function

The masticatory system receives its full share of mechanical analogies when attempts are made to describe its functions. These are justified when jaw positions and movements are transferred to a mechanical mandible and maxilla with varying degrees of accuracy. On the laboratory bench, however, the movements depend on hinges and tracks and the power derives from the technician's hand. However necessary it may be to make these transfers for the diagnosis and treatment of occlusal problems, it should be realized that in the live system mechanical analogies tend to oversimplify these movements and to be misleading. The limitations of mechanical analogies and transfers are best appreciated by a knowledge of the neuromuscular control of posture and movement.

In this chapter an attempt will be made to describe the neuromuscular function which provides mandibular movement and briefly to apply some of its principles. The chapter will include some notes on muscular function and observations on spasm, fatigue, injury and pain in muscles. All the information comes from standard sources and it is hoped that the selection and pruning will not have excluded any essential facts and that the observations made are no more speculative than most authors agree are still a feature of this subject. It is also hoped that the practitioner and student alike will appreciate that the complex nature of muscle activity is slowly reaching comprehension.

Skeletal muscle has sensory and motor innervation. The sensory (afferent) endings give rise either to sensations of discomfort and pain, as when a muscle is fatigued and protection is required to control overactivity, or to the transmission of information about the state of contraction (shortening) or relaxation (lengthening) of the muscle fibres to the central nervous system at both spinal and higher levels. The motor (efferent) nerves receive this information and use it to make adjustments to the discharge of impulses which are transmitted along the motoneurones and result in contraction or relaxation of the muscle fibres.

Muscle contraction

Skeletal muscle has intrinsic abilities to contract and relax. This is achieved when an impulse is transmitted along the motoneurone and reaches a group of muscle fibres. At the junction of neurone and muscle fibres are to be found the motor end-plates which liberate minute amounts of acetylcholine when stimulated by the impulse. This initiates a depolarization which spreads across the muscle and tension is developed. This, in turn, causes the fibres supplied by the neurone to contract.

Innervation ratio

The basic unit of the neuromuscular system is the motor unit, which transmits efferent impulses to a varying number of muscle fibres by means of the motoneurone (the cell). The ratio of fibres to neurone depends on the movement required: the more refined the movement the lower is the ratio. One motoneurone may supply two or three fibres when adjusting the lens of the eye while many hundreds of fibres are supplied by one motoneurone in the more massive task of raising the back. A smaller but equally significant difference exists between the innervation ratio of the lateral pterygoid muscles. These provide the fine adjustments required for the various horizontal mandibular positions and of the masseters which provide the forceful closing movement into a bolus of food against gravity.

Muscle fibres

Skeletal muscle consists of two types of muscle fibre. These are the *extrafusal* fibres which are contractile and make up the bulk of the muscle and the *intrafusal* fibres which are minutely contractile and are found in the muscle spindles. Contraction of the extrafusal fibres shortens the muscle. Contraction of the intrafusal fibres in the spindle provides information about the state of the muscle. In this respect the muscle spindle acts as a stretch receptor.

Muscle spindles

These consist of elongated bundles of intrafusal muscle fibres bound together by their own connective tissue sheaths. They extend beyond the poles of the spindle and are attached to the connective tissue structure of the muscle. They are called 'spindles' because they lie near the middle of the length of the whole muscle and may appear as a small swelling (Figure 3.1). In length the spindles vary between 4 and 7 mm and in breadth between 80 and 200 μm. There are two types of intrafusal muscle fibres in the spindles, namely 'nuclear bag' and 'nuclear chain' fibres; the difference lies in the position of the nucleus in the muscle fibre. Each is provided with a nerve receptor, a primary receptor arising from the nuclear bag fibres and a secondary receptor from the nuclear chain fibres (Figure 3.1).

Innervation of the muscle spindles

Afferent fibres arise from the primary and secondary receptors and carry impulses to the relevant nuclei in the central nervous system. They are given numerical group numbers Ia and II and are classified according to size. The larger fibres conduct their impulses at higher speeds and possess a lower threshold to electrical stimulation. The motor nerve supply to the intrafusal fibres is by fusimotor nerve fibres. These are given the alphabetical classification of gamma (γ) fibres or *gamma efferents* to distinguish them from the *alpha* (α) nerve fibres which supply the extrafusal fibres (Figure 3.1). A single fusimotor axon may run to intrafusal muscle fibres in several different spindles all lying within the same muscle. Thus, whereas each extrafusal muscle fibre or group of fibres receives impulses from only one (α) motoneurone, there may be several (γ) motor axons running to each of the intrafusal muscle fibres. A single spindle may receive from 7 to 25 motor axons (Roberts, 1966).

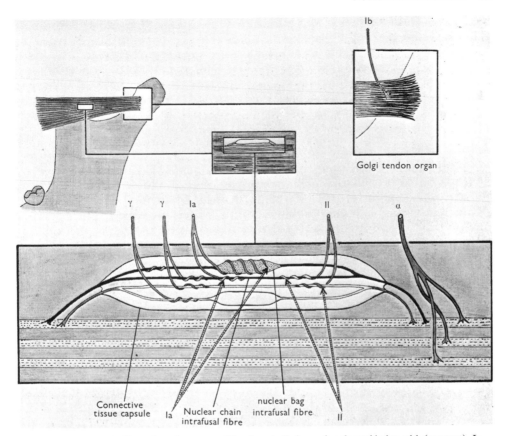

Figure 3.1 Muscle spindle and tendon organ. Muscle spindle is much enlarged in breadth (see text). Ia, Primary afferent path to central nervous system where synapse with α motoneurones. Ib, Afferent path to central nervous system from tendon organ. II, Secondary afferent path to central nervous system (impulses transmitted at lower speed). α, Efferent motoneurones to extrafusal muscle fibres for contraction of muscle. γ, Slower conducting efferent motoneurones to intrafusal muscle fibres which alter bias of spindle and cause afferent impulses. Stretch reflex arc. (Adapted from Bell, Davidson and Emslie-Smith, 1972)

Golgi tendon organs

A complex spray of branching nerve fibres are embedded in the connective tissue of the tendons that attach the muscle fibres to the bone. These are the Golgi tendon organs and they discharge afferent impulses in response to tension or contraction within the whole muscle. They are the group Ib afferents that transmit stimuli and occupy a place between groups Ia and II afferents from the spindles in terms of conduction velocity and threshold of electrical stimulation (Figure 3.1).

Spindle action

The forces created by skeletal muscles are the function of the extrafusal fibres, while those created by the intrafusal fibres are immeasurably small. The function of intrafusal fibre contraction is to signal information about the state of the muscle as a whole. The interaction between intra- and extrafusal fibres depends on various conditions. The following is an abstract from Bell, Davidson and Emslie-Smith (1972) on this topic.

In a passively extended muscle the spindles are stretched. If the extrafusal fibres contract but the intrafusal fibres remain relaxed, the spindle shortens passively and the sensory discharge declines or stops. If the intrafusal and extrafusal fibres are stimulated simultaneously the spindle discharge varies according to the resistance to shortening experienced by the extrafusal fibres. If the muscle meets little resistance to shortening (isotonic contraction) it brings together the two ends of the spindle and the tension applied to the equatorial zone is slight. There is little afferent discharge. If the extrafusal contraction is resisted (isometric), the intrafusal contraction is concentrated on the equatorial zone and a vigorous discharge from the sensory endings results. Thus if the motor centres send simultaneous impulses to the intra- and extrafusal fibres the response from the spindle endings will indicate how much shortening has occurred in the extrafusal fibres. The spindle discharge of impulses is relayed back to the motoneurones of the extrafusal fibres and, if the muscle meets resistance during contraction, extra contractile force is supplied by spindle activity. This provides for correction of errors by co-activation.

One further aspect of muscle spindles that should be mentioned is their variation in density; this applies to the tendon organs as well. Their greatest densities are found in muscles requiring the most delicate movements. The occurrence of muscle spindles in the lateral pterygoid muscles has been demonstrated by Honée (1966, 1970) who states that the relatively few but highly differentiated spindles in this muscle have the same function as the relatively high number of less complex spindles in the other masticatory muscles.

Control of muscle activity

The significance of the foregoing information on neuromuscular function is that of control. How this is performed is not clear but it has been suggested (Wright, 1961) that the γ efferent system is permanently active, though it does not necessarily set up movement, and that the γ discharge keeps the α cells reflexly in preparation for the reception of impulses arriving from the cortex or for the receipt of afferent impulses from the spindles. It is possible that all but the fastest voluntary movements are controlled by the link between the γ efferents, the spindle afferents and the α motoneurones. This combined output produces the required contraction or inhibition of the muscles, with the neuromuscular system keeping, as it were, a check on itself. Thus, impulses initiated in the motor cortex signalling voluntary movement synapse with the γ motoneurone. They travel to the spindle (Figure 3.2) and become integrated with the afferent output from the spindle receptors. The combined output passes back to the α motoneurone and thence to the extrafusal fibres when the relevant muscle contraction takes place. If the afferent fibres returning from the spindle are cut, the muscle fails to contract but the γ motoneurones continue to fire at an increased rate. Therefore, the spindle afferents exert an inhibitory action on the γ motoneurones but remain excitatory to the α motoneurones. This concept was developed by Eldred, Granit and Merton (1953) and applied to the masticatory system by Newton (1969). When a sudden impulse for contraction is sent out it is thought that the direct α motoneurone pathway is used. The resultant abrupt onset of contraction may cause damage to muscle fibres (pulled muscle) or may institute painful spasm (or cramp).

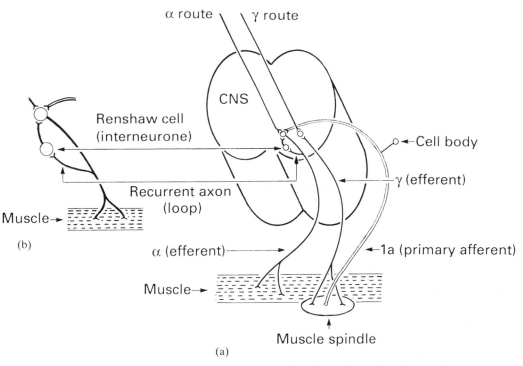

α route   γ route

CNS

Renshaw cell
(interneurone)

Cell body

Recurrent axon
(loop)

γ (efferent)

Muscle→

(b)

α (efferent)————→   ←1a (primary afferent)

Muscle→

Muscle spindle

(a)

Figure 3.2 (a) Muscle spindle and central nervous system (CNS). In afferent fibres in synaptic connections with α motoneurones, γ efferent fibres supply contractile poles of spindle. Muscle contracts either by impulses from higher centres (α route) or by impulses through γ route which activates muscle indirectly via stretch reflex arc. (b) Renshaw recurrent inhibitory loop. (Adapted from Bell, Davidson and Emslie-Smith, 1972; see text for note on modification to diagram by Yemm)

Another aspect of control concerns the Renshaw recurrent inhibitory loop (Figure 3.2). If the stretch applied to a muscle is more prolonged or intense than that which typically elicits the tendon-jerk impulses are passed through this loop before emerging in the α motoneurone. Impulses in this loop cause a reduction in excitability of the anterior horn cells which has an inhibitory effect on the reflex movement. This pathway exerts a stabilizing action on the large (α) motoneurones (Buller, 1961). Thus, if the force applied to elicit the knee or jaw tendon-jerk is applied slowly and forcefully the reflex response will be inhibited. However, R. Yemm (personal communication, 1989) has pointed out that the corresponding diagram in the 1975 edition of *Occlusion* (Figure 13, p. 37) lacks the separate cell necessary to produce this effect (see Figure 3.2b) which is activated by a recurrent axon from the α motoneurone. A further correction is necessary in the γ motoneurone where the cell body should be part of the neurone (Figure 3.2a). Finally, a cell body has been added to the Ia primary afferent from the spindle and this afferent neurone is redrawn to indicate more clearly the anatomical arrangement in the spinal cord. If impulses pass from the spindle via this afferent path the α motoneurone will be stimulated reflexly to provide contraction of the muscle fibres or to increase the activity if the muscle is already contracting as a consequence of direct α-route drive.

Protection of teeth

A further observation concerns the protection of the dentition during mastication. When muscles contract, afferent impulses are discharged to the neuraxis from the spindles, causing activation of the protagonist muscles and inhibition of the antagonists. Information is also sent to the central nervous system about the degree of contraction or relaxation of the muscles involved and what precautions may have to be taken. Thus, the vigorous closing movements of the mandible during mastication can be halted as the teeth approach occlusion, so preventing jarring contacts between the opposing teeth. This feature supports the advice given throughout this text that the teeth need not and should not occlude during mastication.

Thus, if a movement is as expected, the spindle afferents play little part. If, on the other hand, the main muscle fibres produce less than the expected result then the spindles fire and correct the movement. If the movement is excessive the spindle action reduces the force of the movement. This is known as parallel activation and protects the muscles against overactivity at a reflex level. This can, however, be overruled by voluntary impulses from the cortex.

It will be appreciated that these observations on neuromuscular function apply to skeletal muscle activity at all levels supplied by the 12 pairs of cranial nerves giving off the upper motoneurones and the 31 pairs of spinal nerves arising from the anterior horn cells and comprising the lower motoneurones. This activity is the result of sensory (afferent) impluses received by the cortex, brain-stem and spinal cord.

The neuromuscular function of the masticatory system is transmitted largely by the trigeminal nerve which contains sensory and motor fibres. The nerve cells receive afferent impulses from the periodontal membranes of the teeth, from receptors within the capsules of the mandibular joints and from the muscle spindles. They lie within the brain-stem in the mesencephalic nucleus of this nerve. There is a complex distribution of sensory impulses to higher levels in the brain but the reflex control of jaw movements is carried out between the mesencephalic nucleus and the trigeminal motor nucleus according to the principles already stated. Ramfjord and Ash (1972) report that, in additon to the type of afferent nuerones from the spindles, two other types of neurones reach the mesencephalic nucleus: (1) a neurone which conveys impulses from the periodontal membranes of several teeth and adjacent gingival and oral mucosa; and (2) a neurone transmitting impulses from the periodontal membrane of a single tooth.

The activities of the tongue are controlled by the hypoglossal nerve whose nucleus receives fibres from the trigeminal, glossopharyngeal and vagus nerve.

There are several features of muscle activity which should be understood and which derive from these principles. These are: reflex action, reciprocal innervation, muscle tone, conscious control, stable patterns and irrelevant muscle activity.

Reflex action

This is usually defined as the response resulting from a stimulus which passes as an impulse along an afferent neuron to a posterior nerve root, or its cranial equivalent, where it is transmitted to an efferent neurone via the anterior horn cell or motor cranial nucleus to the skeletal muscle. The response is independent of the will and can be facilitatory or inhibitory. The pathway is called a monosynaptic relex arc.

The stretch (myotatic) reflex which causes a muscle to contract when stretched provides an example and is to be found when the chin is suddenly pulled downwards (jaw-jerk). Afferent stimuli may arise from varying sources to provide the same action and these sources include the higher centres of the brain. Impulses reach the same efferent motoneurone through interconnecting facilitatory neurones. These are polysynaptic reflex arcs and, in the masticatory system, include such responses as yawning, laughing and the clenching of the teeth.

Reciprocal innervation

This feature of muscle activity ensures that when a stimulus for muscle activity is received the muscles that are to provide the movement (the protagonists) contract, while the muscles which would normally oppose the movement (the antagonists) are inhibited from contraction. Thus, smoothness is imparted to the movement. If, during the movement, an interfering stimulus is received (the unexpected encounter with a sharp piece of food during mastication), a reflex opening is intitiated by an α motoneurone impulse.

Muscle tone

Muscle tone is the reflex contraction of skeletal muscle concerned with maintaining posture. It is probably due to a slow, asynchronous discharge of impulses from the anterior horn cells producing a partial tetanus. Tonic muscle gives a steady uniform pull because groups of fibres contract and then relax as other groups contract. Muscles in tonic contraction permit the blood supply to provide full metabolic requirements and fatigue is prevented indefinitely. By contrast, muscles in full tetanic contraction fatigue rapidly because it is not possible for the circulation to cope with the increased metabolic demands. Muscle tone can be further defined as a maintained resistance to stretch in healthy skeletal muscle subject to passive displacement.

In the case of the mandible this accounts for the phenomenon of rest position (see also p. 50) and the resistance to stretch may be provided by tissue elasticity. From experiments on anaesthetized rats, Yemm and Nordstrom (1974) suggested that forces produced by tissue elasticity are capable of maintaining jaw posture in the absence of muscle activity. They found that a force tending to close the mouth of the anaesthetized animal remained essentially constant for some time after death, indicating that there was no tonic muscle contraction contributing to the force. It was concluded that there was a justifiable support for the hypothesis that mandibular rest position is governed by tissue elasticity and that the asynchronous activity and gravity play only a minor role.

At the same time, Wyke (1974) was making extensive studies of the neuromuscular mechanisms influencing mandibular posture following his investigations on the mechanoreceptor reflex innervation of the mandibular joints with Greenfield and Klineberg (Greenfield, Klineberg and Wyke, 1970). Wyke (1974) claimed that the tissue elasticity explanation of the rest position was 'incomprehensible to a neurologist' and that this was borne out by the fact that the mandible will tend to fall open when an individual falls asleep in sitting posture; and he gives further examples. However, he does acknowledge that there are three factors contributing to the maintenance of muscle tone: (1) the static elastic properties of the connective tissue components of muscles; (2) the static elastic properties of the fibrillary muscle protein within the muscle fibres; and (3) the number, size and frequency of firing of the active motor units in the muscles. Wyke concludes that the rest position is not an immutable posture of the mandible but that it represents a state of equilibrium determined by continuous low-grade motor activity in the supramandibular muscles, by the static elastic forces of the supra- and inframandibular musculature, and by gravity.

It is accepted, however, that mandibular rest position can be maintained indefinitely without fatigue provided that the health and length of the muscles remain constant. This assumption has considerable significance in analysing problems of occlusion.

Factors affecting muscle tone

Muscle tone is affected by the number of motoneurones firing at the time, and the rate at which they are firing. Facilitation and inhibition are also affected by the level in the neuraxis at which the impulses originate, i.e. either segmentally in a horizontal reflex arc, intersegmentally in a vertical path of impulses, or supersegmentally downwards from the higher centres. All receptors affect muscle tone and activity to some extent through the segmental mechanism, but some more so than others. For example, the receptors in the mandibular joints are found mostly in the fibrous pericapsular ligament, some in the synovial membrane but none in the meniscus. Stretching the joint capsule stimulates the afferents which run in the mandibular division of the fifth cranial nerve to its sensory ganglion. Even when the mandible is at rest, some of the receptors are firing at 15–20 impulses per second and this is thought to maintain muscle tone in the elevator muscles. Evidence of this is seen when local anaesthetic is injected into the joints, whereupon the mandible will drop open. So there are two sets of factors involved: tissue elasticity and the muscle activity. On the other hand, pain receptors are found only in the surfaces of the joint capsules; there are none in the meniscus or synovial membrane. Thus, stretching the capsule fibres is the only way that pain can be produced traumatically in the mandibular joints.

The neurological researches on the control of mandibular posture are reviewed by Wyke (1974) and his observations on this topic are of value to clinicians; in particular, to those concerned with the replacement of teeth.

Conscious control

All voluntary muscle action is predominantly under conscious control and is the result of excitatory and inhibitory impulses. This can be replaced by reflex action when an emergency arises. On the other hand, reflex control can be overruled by impulses from the cortex via interconnecting facilitatory neurones using the same muscle patterns. The mandible may be moved from its rest position by thinking to move it. Any learned movement subsequently performed can be altered by conscious control. This is achieved by the supersegmental mechanism, referred to in the previous section, and operates downwards only and in the neuraxis. It has three divisions: the pontomedullary from the lower centres; the mesencephalic from the midbrain; and the cortical by voluntary control (F. Nally, personal communication).

1. *The pontomedullary control* embodies impulses from three nuclei in the pons and medulla: the vestibular nucleus and lateral reticular system, which are

facilitatory, and the medial reticular system which is inhibitory. The vestibular system is constantly receiving impulses from the internal ear and therefore contributes to the maintenance of muscle tone and posture. The lateral reticular nucleus descends in the lateral reticular tract through the brain-stem and cord. It is facilitatory and sends a constant discharge of γ motor efferents to the muscle spindle involved. The medial reticular system is inhibitory and receives impulses from the cerebral cortex to provide indirect cerebral inhibition.

2. *The mesencephalic nuclei* influence muscle tone in two ways: from the tectospinal nucleus (facilitatory) and from the red nucleus (inhibitory). The cells of the tectospinal tract lie in the quadreminal region and their tracts descend on both sides of the neuraxis. The impulses derive from the eyes and ears and increase muscle tone in the whole body. From the red nucleus the rubrospinal tracts inhibit motoneurone activity.

3. *The cortical mechanism* controls muscle tone in two ways:

(a) By indirect cortical projection whereby fibres arise in all areas of the cortex and descend to the two reticular nuclei, finishing in the lateral and medial reticular mechanisms. They have both facilitatory (lateral) and inhibitory (medial) influences on muscle tone.

(b) By direct cortical projections, down the pyramidal tracts; they are both facilitatory and inhibitory.

The neuromuscular control of posture, tone and movement would, therefore, seem to be complex and likely to suffer disturbance and consequent disorder. However, the stability of the system has been maintained through countless species and human generations for two million years and nothing short of disease and congenital disorders is likely to alter this stability. In the section that follows it will be asserted that muscle activity conforms to stable patterns that are themselves innate and that when the activity becomes irrelevant problems may arise.

Stable patterns of muscle activity

These are organized movements which provide for the functions of useful movements and are said to be endogenously determined. Several are present at birth and include respiration and the ability to suckle. As growth proceeds, other endogenous activities become apparent, such as those which cause a limb to move or a face to smile. These and other stable movements are then organized at a higher level of brain development to provide such activities as walking and mastication. At a still higher level they become further organized to produce such complex behaviour patterns as speech, mating and providing shelter. This is known as the hierarchical concept of behaviour organization and was outlined by Weiss (1950). It emphasizes the stability of endogenous patterns of muscle behaviour. Gesell (1942) expressed this by saying that just as bones and teeth have characteristic forms, so do patterns of behaviour. They account for all movements which provide natural function and make it possible to distinguish someone by his gait, smile or the way he eats. These patterns are organized within the nervous system and are performed without conscious thought. As was suggested in the previous section, they can be altered but when the conscious stimulus to change has been withdrawn the stable patterns return.

In addition to the conscious stimuli which may alter these patterns, disease or disturbance may cause a change. Thus a painful ankle causes a limp and a tooth in supracontact alters the masticatory movements of the mandible. When the disturbing stimulus is removed the endogenous or established movement will be restored. A missing tooth may restrict mastication to one side and the altered movements will be composed from the existing coordinated patterns. These are usually performed within the limits of injury and fatigue. However, tolerance to these habitual movements is not unlimited and pathological responses may develop in the affected muscles. The application of these principles of muscle activity to the posture and movements of the mandible was outlined by Ballard (1955) and is recommended for further study.

Adjustment to disturbances is achieved, first at reflex level, and secondly, if the disturbance is maintained, by a more permanent change in muscle patterns. But the γ system serves to provide the muscles with a controlled feedback system to deal with conflicting α and γ impulses, such as may happen when stepping unexpectedly off the pavement. In this context it is referred to as a *servomechanism* and provides optimal muscle function in both normal and abnormal conditions.

Irrelevant muscle activity

This is the term given to muscle contraction which does not participate in the execution of a particular movement. It is commonly experienced during the performance of a task which requires mental as well as physical effort and is manifest as an involuntary increase in muscle activity unconnected with the job in hand. Thus, one can observe or experience pursing of the lips while threading a needle. These activities may be explained in part by the secretions of the hormones adrenaline and noradrenaline in preparation for a task where there is no opportunity to fight or fly. Thus, the public speaker paces the rostrum or makes excessive use of his hands.

The stimuli which produce these tensions are thought to arise from various excitatory and inhibitory foci believed to be a part of the reticular system in the central part of the brain-stem. The reticular system is not a morphological unit but consists of many nuclei of different nervous structures and has the function of modifying motoneurone activity (Bell, Davidson and Emslie-Smith, 1972). In this respect it is thought to exert a correlation between sensory and motor signals from the higher centres. For example, strong stimulation from the reticular system facilitates the contraction of the masseter muscles and inhibits that of the digastrics, thus promoting irrelevant closure of the mandible while the hands are extracting a mandibular molar tooth.

Irrelevant muscle activity may also derive from anxiety states and can occur during sleep. The tossing and turning experienced while trying to sleep are well known, although the body is supposedly in its most resting posture. The anxiety which causes or is caused by insomnia provides an explanation for this irrelevant muscle activity and, when asleep, the movements usually subside. But movements while asleep are equally well known and these include hyperactivity of the masticatory muscles. An introduction to the possible functions of the limbic system may be helpful in understanding these phenomena.

The cortex and the limbic system

Whereas the reticular system was said to modify motoneurone activity it can act as a relay station for transmitting sensory stimuli to the cortex. These stimuli generate a response from the cortex which are either passed back to the reticular system or proceed directly as motor impulses to various parts of the body. The function of the cortex appears to be one of evaluation and decision and has been likened to a computer. It provides the direction of the impulses. This function can, however, be modified by various emotional states which provide the quality of intensity to the impulses. This quality arises from the functions of the limbic system. This system consists of a group of structures in the brain which include the amygdala, the hippocampus and the septum. Stimulation of the amygdala produces the varying responses of fear, panic, aggression and anxiety, depending on the intensity of stimulation and the area stimulated. The septum and hippocampus control these emotions but produce anger if stimulated. Stimuli from the limbic system combine with those from the cortex and decide the action which the brain takes in terms of direction and intensity. The parts of the body affected by these stimuli must be prepared for the appropriate level of physical exertion and this is the function of the hypothalamus. Acting through the autonomic nervous system, the hypothalamus organizes the physical resources of the body. Both the hypothalamus and the amygdala are thought to have connections in such activities as physical effort resulting from anxiety (*Nobrium*, 1971).

Much of this information is speculative but, in summary, it can be said that impulses from the higher centres of the brain are the result of interaction between the various centres involved and that sometimes the intensity of impulse exceeds the direction. The result may take the form of irrelevant muscle activity and provide an explanation for the parafunctional movements of the mandible in both the waking and sleeping states. At such times the directive control of the cortex is overruled by the activity of some of its parts.

Silent periods

This phenomenon, whereby electrical activity in the masseter muscles ceases shortly after tooth contact, has been investigated by several workers and there are many theories to account for it. Schaerer, Stallard and Zander (1967), Brennan, Black and Coslet (1968), Ahlgren (1969) and Griffen and Monro (1969) attributed the silent period to an inhibition following feedback from the periodontal receptors, but Matthews and Yemm (1970) and Owall and Elmqvist (1975) found silent periods in masseter activity on artificial tooth contacts in edentulous subjects. Watt and colleagues (1976) investigated silent periods during percussion of the bony structures of the head during occlusion of the teeth on surfaces of varying hardness and during the chewing of different foods. More silent periods were observed during hard food chewing and more were observed at the beginning of chewing sequences than towards the end. Differences in latency and duration of silent periods were also observed in relation to artificial changes in the occlusion. Silent periods may become a useful diagnostic tool when observing and analysing occlusal function but no explanation for them has so far been claimed.

Summary

Skeletal muscle possesses an intrinsic ability to contract and relax. The provision of the γ system of motoneurone supply to the muscle spindles controls the α motoneurone impulses which cause the muscles to contract. This permits the control of excitatory and inhibitory functions by reciprocal innervation and leads to the coordination of groups of muscles to provide effective movment. Sudden contraction of the muscles generally bypasses the γ system and proceeds directly by the α motoneurone route. Conscious impulses to contract muscles overrule the reflex control but the latter is always present to maintain muscle tone and posture. The activities of the limbic system may provide an explanation of the phenomenon of irrelevant muscle activity which is manifest as parafunctional movements in the masticatory system.

Muscular function and dysfunction

As a postscript to this discussion on neuromuscular function some notes will be given on the metabolism of muscle function followed by descriptions of three muscle disturbances, namely, fatigue, spasm and intramuscular injury. This will provide a prescript to the discussions on the mandibular dysfunction syndrome to which references will be made throughout the book.

Metabolism of muscle contraction

The metabolic changes which take place when muscle fibres contract will serve to emphasize the complexity of this function and to indicate the numerous possibilities for dysfunction.

The arrival of a neural impulse at the neuromuscular junction, resulting in the release of acetylcholine, produces a change in the permeability of the membrane surrounding the muscle fibres. This permits a flow of potassium ions out of the fibre cells and a flow of sodium ions into the cells. This exchange is accompanied by a depolarization of the membrane, and contraction of the fibres follows.

Under the light microscope the sarcolemmas of the muscle fibres consist of numerous nuclei, mitochondria, undifferentiated cytoplasm (sarcoplasm) and cross-striated material. The electron microscope reveals these cross-striations to consist of sarcomeres, which are the smallest contractile units of the muscle fibre. Each sarcomere consists of a regular arrangement of thick and thin filaments. These filaments are thought to consist of myosin and actin respectively, both of which are proteins essential to the process of contraction. Myosin has enzyme properties and in resting muscle the tendency to form actomyosin is prevented by the presence of adenosine triphosphate (ATP). When the muscle is stimulated, the ATP is hydrolysed to adenosine diphosphate (ADP) and actomyosin is formed. In this reaction phosphoric acid is produced. Shortening is then brought about by the thin filaments sliding between the thick ones. This reaction is also governed by the presence in the sarcoplasm of a high concentration of calcium ions which are discharged. When the calcium ions are reduced the chemical interaction between actin and myosin ceases and the muscle relaxes.

Three other reactions going on at the same time provide and produce the energy necessary for muscular contraction. Firstly, the glycolytic utilization of glycogen is brought about by the action of the enzymes phosphorylase and phosphofructokinase giving off pyruvic and lactic acids. Secondly, creatininic phosphate is reduced to creatinine and phosphoric acid. Thirdly, there is the supply of oxygen which governs these biochemical reactions and the removal of carbon dioxide, which in turn plays its part in the control of respiration necessary for the supply of oxygen.

It will be obvious that an arterial blood supply and venous return is necessary to supply these biochemical elements and to remove the metabolic by-products. These by-products include the acids already mentioned and the salts subsequently formed; they are potentially irritant to sensory nerve endings in the muscles if allowed to remain. There are, therefore, many requirements for effective function and many possibilities for dysfunction, including fatigue, spasm and injury.

Fatigue

The detailed processes which produce muscular fatigue are unknown. Bell, Davidson and Emslie-Smith (1972) suggest that the reduction in contractility may be due to failure at a number of different places, including the central synapses, the motor end-plates and the contractile processes, but that the cause is probably in the muscle fibres themselves. Horrobin (1968) states that fatigue is not due to a failure of the neuromuscular transmission and that experimental evidence suggests that it is due to a failure of the blood to supply an essential metabolic element or to remove some waste product or to a combination of both. A lack of oxygen and an accumulation of acid metabolites are probably involved. Also involved is the voluntary response to fatigue by the higher centres which may lead to tiredness or to further effort, both of which can disturb efficient function. There is also a psychological component in fatigue in that it depends largely on motivation. There is also the phenomenon of the hypnotized subject who can maintain postures and tensions for long periods without fatigue. The influences of the higher centres on normal actions and disease processes is well known, if not fully understood, and may explain why some people succumb to the mandibular dysfunction syndrome and others do not, although they demonstrate similar clinical features.

Another uncertainty is that fatigue may cause pain. It has been suggested that the metabolities of muscular function are potentially irritant to the sensory nerve endings within the muscles. The responses to such a stimulant may be interpreted as pain which will subside when the muscle recovers. Pain, however, is a separate entity and is not simply due to an excessive stimulation of nerve endings, thus presenting the diagnostician with his biggest problem. The muscle may also respond by spasm or, if further effort is required by the higher centres, by injury of the muscle fibres involved.

Spasm

Skeletal muscle spasm is broadly defined as an abnormal involuntary contraction of skeletal muscle. However, Buller (1961) adds to such a definition, 'with a subject so vague in definition, and so little studied in detail, ideas may prove as important at this stage as the few available facts'. Travell (1960) says that when muscles are subject to mechanical, emotional, infectious, metabolic or nutritional noxious stimuli they react in one way – *they develop spasm and shorten*.

The clinician is thus presented with a combination of doubt as to cause and dogma as to effect. This becomes a problem when treating spasm since the cause must be discovered if the effect is to be prevented. There are four levels or zones where excessive excitatory or diminished inhibitory influences may arise. Firstly, there is the muscle spindle where the intrafusal fibres may suddenly shorten, causing a prolonged γ efferent discharge resulting in spasm. Secondly, at the supraspinal level, there is the possibility of an abnormal pattern of descending impulses which might upset the balance of spinal excitation and inhibition. This may result in an abnormal discharge of impulses along the α motoneurone and cause spasm. Thirdly, a severe cutaneous stimulus will provide a sudden barrage of impulses which can reach the α motoneurones. The phenomenon of spasm following pain provides an example. Finally, there is the metabolic irritant within the muscle which, as has been suggested, can provide the noxious stimulus to the sensory nerves within the muscle and cause spasm.

Muscle spasm has to be differentiated from contracture, which may be indistinguishable from spasm but which is caused by an 'artificial' stimulus, such as the prick of a needle or the effects of certain drugs, e.g. acetylcholine, noradrenaline and caffeine. In addition, the condition of spasticity has to be differentiated and this is a pathological response to a lesion of the nervous pathways.

The commonly held view that spasm is antalgic and protective is discounted by Capener (1961) who gives several reasons, including that of the pain which it provokes. This can sometimes be so intense as to affect the whole constitutional state of the individual, but when relieved may still leave the cause untreated. A personal view is expressed here that the pain of trigeminal neuralgia could be simulated by a severe spasm of one of the masticatory muscles. According to Ritchie (1961), local intramuscular spasm serves no purpose except to establish the ischaemic background for later fibrous change.

Intramuscular spasm perhaps provides the most significant cause of pain in the mandibular syndrome. Here, groups of fibres can be in spasm without immobilizing the whole muscle and provide a cause of intermittent pain which is relieved by gentle stretching but which recurs if the cause (? cusp interference) is not removed. A further speculation is the possibility that intermittent spasm results in an excessive discharge of calcium ions which, in the connective tissue surrounds of the fibres, could build up calcification of this tissue and cause a more permanent limitation of movement.

Referred pain. Travell (1960) refers to trigger areas in muscles in spasm which are small hypersensitive zones. They have a lowered pain threshold to stimulation by pressure and cause pain some distance from the zone. The areas to which the pain can be referred have been plotted and the muscle in spasm can be named by the site of referred pain.

No discussion on the clinical aspects of spasm would be complete without mention of its incidence during sleep. True spasm is rarely psychogenic (Layzer and Rowland, 1971) and one must look to the vascular changes and maintained postures to explain spasm during sleep. Exercise of untrained muscles is often followed by nocturnal spasm and this can be explained by increased permeability of the blood vessel walls during sleep and the increased presence of metabolites acting as irritants. Spasm can also be induced by forcible stretching or sudden movements on waking which suggests the presence of irritants ready to be effective. With regard to posture, the forced retraction of the toes or feet by tight sheets can have a prolonged stretching effect on the calf muscles, with consequent spasm. The mandible can be deflected during sleep and its muscles stretched for long periods by the head posture on the pillow and lead to spasm. This is a common symptom of the mandibular dysfunction syndrome but this posture theory does not provide the only explanation. Mandibular spasm and consequent grinding of the teeth while asleep are so common, especially in children, that a psychogenic cause, as from the limbic system, must be suspected. Such a cause has been described for irrelevant muscle activity which, if prolonged, could presumably lead to spasm.

Cramp. A more recent aspect of this topic is presented by Joekes (1982) in a review of cramp, which may be defined as muscle spasm with pain. It is the term more often used by patients. Joekes describes cramp as voluntary, irrational and painful contractions of voluntary muscle and compares it to tetany, which is involuntary but not painful and is due to lowered plasma concentrations such as hypocalcaemia. Joekes describes four groups of cramp: (1) as caused by effort and perhaps not manifest until resting some hours later; (2) while asleep, often affecting the elderly and may be caused by loss of upper motor neurones; (3) secondary to disease, as following profuse loss of fluid or from tetanus infection where the toxin reaches the spinal cord and causes severe spasm; and (4) following diuretic treatment with loss of fluid. Treatment measures in tabulated form are provided and these include sodium replacement, quinine, muscle relaxants and salicylates. Joekes concludes that there may be no adequate theoretical explanation for most forms of cramp but that there are clear causal associations and, in some cases, effective empirical treatment.

In conclusion, systemic causes of spasm are to be found in pregnancy, dehydration, salt depletion, hypothyroidism and uraemia.

Intramuscular injury

In addition to spasm, sudden impulses to contract can result in torn muscle fibres and consequent replacement by connective (scar) tissue. Christensen and Moesmann (1967) describe muscular hyperfunction as causing a primary mechanical lesion of the interfibrillar connective tissue since it cannot provide the necessary tension without damage. Their histopathological examinations reveal inflammation of the connective tissue with oedema and a fibrinous exudate, together with degeneration of the muscle fibres. The degenerated muscle fibres are replaced by scar tissue or newly formed fibres. These findings may cause a revision of the 'torn muscle' diagnosis but the possible effect of producing resistant scar tissue is the same. This will cause a persistent localized stiffness or pain in muscles.

Another intramuscular condition which resists effective movement concerns the elasticity of the interfibrillar connective tissue. Prolonged contraction of muscles, as in so-called 'body building' exercises or in the isometric contraction when the teeth are being clenched (or ground), leads to abnormal contraction of the connective tissue. The elasticity of this tissue is less than that of the muscle fibres and it tends to resist relaxation of the muscle fibres. If these movements continue, the connective tissue resistance increases due to its relative inelasticity and a 'muscle bound' condition results. This will account for stiffness and a resistance to refined movements required in many functions, including those of mastication. This condition was given the name 'cumulative strain' by McLurg Anderson (1951) and can account for many disturbances of muscle function. These include excessive, irrelevant or unbalanced movements such as the parafunctional habits and unilateral chewing in the masticatory system.

General disorders of muscles

Horrobin (1968) lists five disorders of muscle which should be borne in mind when assessing disturbances of the masticatory muscles.

1. *Motoneurone disorders* in which trauma or disease (as in poliomyelitis) destroys the motoneurones. The muscle fibres atrophy and the contractile tissues are largely replaced by fat.

2. *Neuromuscular transmission* is blocked by a failure to release acetylcholine. This can occur in rare cases of food poisoning by the botulinum toxin and in myasthenia gravis.

3. *Ionic disorders,* such as a low calcium level, render the motoneurones abnormally excitable and the irregular contractions of tetany may result.

4. *Myotonia,* where muscles become contracted for an abnormal length of time in response to a normal stimulus.

5. *Muscular dystrophies,* where the muscle fibres atrophy without obvious cause.

Summary

A brief account has been given of the metabolic changes which take place when a muscle is stimulated to contract. These involve the presence of myosin and actin in the sarcomeres, which are the smallest contractile units of muscle fibres. The energy necessary for muscular contraction is provided by the utilization of glycogen, the reduction of creatininic phosphate and the supply of oxygen from arterial blood. The by-products of these reactions are potentially irritant to the sensory nerve endings in muscle if not removed by venous return. Functional disorders of muscle activity consist of fatigue, intramuscular injury, stiffness and spasm. These may result from two main causes: a stimulus causing a rapid change of the established pattern of movement and prolonged isometric contraction. These can result in the conditions known as sprained ankle, housemaid's knee, aching back, tennis elbow, frozen shoulder, crick in the neck and the mandibular dysfunction syndrome.

Comment

The chief requirements of healthy muscles are to respond effectively to impulses and to return smoothly to their starting length or resting posture.

References

Ahlgren, J. (1969) The silent period in the EMG of jaw muscles during mastication and its relationship to tooth contact. *Acta Odontologica Scandinavica,* **27**, 219

Ballard, C. F. (1955) A consideration of the physiological background of mandibular posture and movement. *Dental Practitioner and Dental Record* **6**, 80

Bell, G. H., Davidson, J. N. and Emslie-Smith, D. (1972) *Physiology and Biochemistry.* Churchill Livingstone, Edinburgh, p. 826

Brennan H. S., Black, M. A. and Coslet, J. G. (1968) Inter-relationship between the electromyographic silent period and dental occlusion. *Journal of Dental Research,* **45**, 502 (abstract)

Buller, A. J. (1961) *Symposium on Skeletal Muscle Spasm* (ed. W. Ritchie-Russell), British Medical Association, London

Capener, N. (1961) *Symposium on Skeletal Muscle Spasm* (ed. W. Ritchie-Russell), British Medical Association, London

Christensen, V. and Moesmann, G. (1967) On the etiology, pathophysiology and pathology of muscular fibrositis due to hyperfunction (in Danish with summary in English). *Tandlaegebladet,* **71**, 230

Eldred, E., Granit, R. and Merton, P. A. (1953) Supraspinal control of muscle spindles and its significance. *Journal of Physiology,* **112**, 498

Gesell, A. (1942) Morphologies of mouth and mouth behaviour. *American Journal of Orthodontics,* **29**, 297

Greenfield, B. E., Klineberg, I. J. and Wyke, B. D. (1970) Contributions to the reflex control of mastication in the TMJ. *Dental Practitioner and Dental Record*, **21**, 73

Griffen, G.J. and Munro, R. R. (1969) Electromyography of the jaw closing muscles in the open–close–clench cycle in man. *Archives of Oral Biology*, **14**, 141

Honée, G. L. J. M. (1966) An investigation on the presence of muscle spindles in the human lateral pterygoid muscle. *Netherlands Dental Journal*, **73** (supplement)

Honée G. L. J. M. (1970) *De musculus pterygoideus lateralis*, Academisch Proefschrift, University of Amsterdam. (Summary in English, p. 126)

Horrobin, D. F. (1968) *Medical Physiology and Biochemistry*, Arnold, London

Joekes, A. M. (1982) Cramp: a review. *Journal of the Royal Society of Medicine*, **75**, 546

Layzer, R. B. and Rowland, L. P. (1971) Cramps. *New England Journal of Medicine*, **285**, 31

McLurg Anderson, T. (1951) *Human Kinetics*, Heinemann Medical, London

Matthews, B and Yemm, R (1970) A silent period in the masseter electromyogram following tooth contact in subjects wearing full dentures. *Archives of Oral Biology*, **15**, 531

Newton, A. V. (1969) Predisposing causes for temporomandibular joint dysfunction. *Journal of Prosthetic Dentistry*, **22**, 647

Nobrium (1971) Publication by Roche Products Ltd., London.

Owall, B. and Elmqvist, D. (1975) Motor pauses in EMG activity during chewing and biting. *Odontolgisk Revy*, **26**, 17

Ramfjord, S. P. and Ash, M. (1972) *Occlusion*, 2nd edn, Saunders, Philadelphia, p. 41

Ritchie, A.E. (1961) *Symposium on Skeletal Muscle Spasm* (ed. W. Ritchie-Russell), British Medical Association, London

Roberts, T. D. M. (1966) *Basic Ideas in Neurophysiology*, Butterworth, London

Schaerer P., Stallard, R. E. and Zander, H. A. (1967) Occlusal interferences and mastication: an electromyography study. *Journal of Prosthetic Dentistry*, **17**, 438.

Travell, J. (1960) Temporomandibular joint pain referred from muscles of the head and neck. *Journal of Prosthetic Dentistry*, **10**, 745

Watt, D. M., Turnbull, J. R., Saberi, M. *et al.* (1976) The influence of percussion, occlusion and mastication on the occurrence of silent periods in masseter muscle activity. *Journal of Oral Rehabilitation*, **3**, 371

Weiss, P. (1950) Experimental analysis of co-ordination. *Symposia of the Society of Experimental Biology*, **4**, 92

Wright, S. (1961) *Applied Physiology*, Oxford University Press, London

Wyke B. D. (1974) Neuromuscular mechanisms influencing mandibular posture: a neurologist's view of current concepts. *Journal of Dentistry*, **2**, 111

Yemm, R. and Nordstrom, S. H. (1974) Tissue elasticity determining mandibular posture. *Archives of Oral Biology*, **19**, 347

Chapter 4

Positions and movements

If the term 'occlusion' in dentistry implies the comprehensive and complex pattern of mandibular movements and contacts between the maxillary and mandibular teeth, the fact remains that the word itself means 'contact'. Therefore, an understanding of mandibular positions during contact is as important as the movements which lead to them.

It has been asserted that the muscles, joints and contours of the teeth provide occlusal function. Muscle activity results in various occlusal positions and, in natural function, these are momentary. Apart from sleeping and various resting postures, the maintenance of bodily positions causes fatigue. The guardsmen at attention and the immobile young ladies who used to adorn the Windmill Theatre are highly trained for inspection but their efforts cannot be considered as natural, however pleasing. Fear can freeze and practice will sustain the stationary trunk and limbs, but in healthy natural function, with the exceptions mentioned, to remain still is to tire.

In this chapter the positions of the mandible at rest and in various occlusal positions will be considered. These occlusal (contact) positions are momentary and generally serve as a stimulus to movement and other positions. Otherwise, as has been suggested, the muscles will tire. The movements described will be those between the various occlusal positions and this will include a description of deflective (premature and initial) contacts. The border movements, the Bennett movement and the condyle positions and movements will then be described and discussed in relation to the functions they perform. Articular movements will be described in Chapter 5 under patterns of articulation, and masticatory movements in Chapter 6, when considering functions of the masticatory system.

Rest position

The rest position of the mandible is the posture that the mandible adopts when the muscles attaching it to the maxilla are in minimal contraction. It can be maintained indefinitely, without fatigue, by the intermittent contraction and relaxation of groups of fibres within the muscles. It represents a reflexly-maintained resistance to stretch of the muscles by the force of gravity acting on the mandible. It assumes that no other stimuli are being received which might cause movement or other posture. The teeth are parted and the distance between them is usually about 3 mm. This position of the mandible is said to be endogenously developed (Ballard, 1967) and is determined by the length and direction of the muscles which run between mandible and cranium. It constitutes a stable pattern of minimal activity and the position is constant provided that the muscles remain healthy. It is said to be unaffected by the posture of the head or body and is therefore controlled by the higher centres of the brain as well as by the resting length of the muscles. In this posture of the mandible the face is in its *rest vertical relation* (RVR).

Much of the foregoing is assumed from clinical observations, and few of the statements have withstood the test of scientific investigation. Berry (1960) observed that registration of the vertical relation 'is no more scientific today than a hundred years ago'. Watkinson (1987), quoting this statement and discussing the rest position as a suitable subject for electroymographic investigation, said that uncertainty about its exact location still remains. This may be accounted for in part by difficulties associated with inducing the mandible to assume the rest position with any degree of consistency and in part by imprecision in the methods used to measure and record the vertical relation (Tryde, McMillan and Christensen, 1976). In his studies of the electromyographical investigations, Watkinson points out that, whereas the objective is to establish a position at which the activity of the masticatory muscles is minimal, the methods in clinical use may not elicit a position which is coincident with the lowest level of muscle activity as determined by electromyographic methods. This article repays study and opens the door to further studies, both present and past. Reference is again made to the explanation by Yemm and Nordstrom (1974) (see p. 39) on tissue elasticity.

Skeletal relations at rest position

The horizontal relation between the dental bases of the resting mandible and the maxilla is of clinical significance when assessing the intercuspal position of the mandible. The dental bases are those regions of the mandible and maxilla which lie below and above the apices of the mandibular and maxillary teeth respectively. They are not subject to change so long as the teeth are present. One method of occlusal analysis (Chapter 9) is to observe the path of closure from rest position to intercuspal position and to assess any interfering tooth contacts.

The vertical relationship between the dental bases of maxilla and mandible at rest provides a reference plane for assessing the correct vertical level of occlusion, which should be 3 mm above the rest vertical level. The clinical application of this principle will be repeated many times. It is of value, therefore, to be able to classify the dental base relationship at rest position in order to assess optimal expectation of tooth relations.

Tracings made from lateral skull radiographs provide information about the skull, mandible and teeth in relation to each other. For assessing dental base relations, the angles SNA and SNB allow the classification into skeletal classes I, II and III to be made (Figure 4.1a). S is the centre of the sella turcica and N is point nasion or the anterior end of the nasofrontal suture. Point A is the deepest midline point on the premaxilla and point B is the deepest midline point on the mandible. The difference between SNA and SNB is 3° in class I skeletal relation. It is greater than 3° in class II and less than 3° in class III. These are also referred to as *normal*, *postnormal* and *prenormal* relations. This classification corresponds to Angle's molar relationship classification. The variability of the incisor relations which correspond to these skeletal relations depends on the angle between the Frankfort or maxillary planes and the mandibular plane (Figure 4.1b) and on the forces

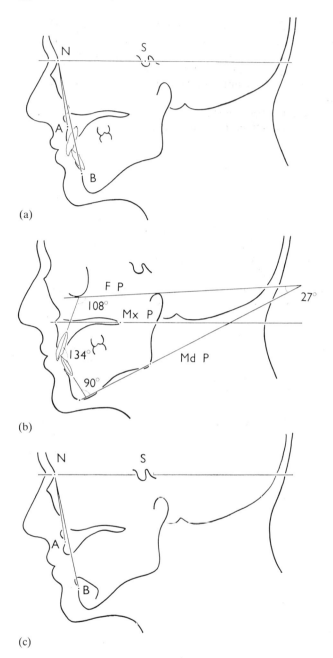

(a)

(b)

(c)

Figure 4.1 (a) Tracing of lateral skull radiograph to illustrate class I jaw relation. S, sella turcica; N, nasion; A, deepest midline point on premaxilla; B, deepest midline point on mandible. SNA gives relation between cranial base and face. SNA and SNB give relation of maxillary to mandibular base. Normal SNA is 81° and SNB is 78°. (b) Tracing of lateral skull radiograph to illustrate normal angle between Frankfort and mandibular planes (27°) and normal angles between the incisors and both the Frankfort and maxillary planes. These angles produce favourable incisor relations and a pleasing appearance. (c) Tracing of lateral edentulous skull radiograph. Mandible at rest position in class I jaw relation where the angle SNA − SNB is 3°

exerted by the orofacial muscles labially and the tongue muscles lingually. These variables make the assessment of optimal tooth positions and their occlusion a complex study, as orthodontists will agree, but the skeletal classification at rest position is a useful aid towards the expectation of Angle's molar relation. This is particularly true in the edentulous mouth when determining tooth positions for complete dentures (Figure 4.1c).

Rest position is a reference plane for assessing intercuspal position and is usually assumed to be the position from which all mandibular movements begin and to which they return after function.

Habitual posture

While rest position is endogenously developed and maintained, it is subject to reflex adaptation. In patients where there is a class II dental base relation and where the incisors do not permit a comfortable seal between the lips, the mandible may move anteriorly in order to attain this seal at rest. This is clinically recognized as habitual posture. At the new position of the mandible the muscles are no longer minimally contracted but the posture can be maintained for purposes of mouth comfort and good appearance for varying periods. Lip seal keeps the mouth moist and preserves a closed-mouth appearance, but the habitual effort required to maintain it is no longer minimal and may result in muscle fatigue. Also, there is a tendency to shift between the two positions and this can result in changes in the paths of closure, such as when saliva is being swallowed. Variations in intercuspal positions may follow and this can lead to premature contacts, especially if there are missing teeth. If the cause of this reflex adoption of habitual posture is removed, the endogenous rest position will be resumed.

The clinical significance of habitual posture is that it is often adopted by patients in the belief that they are in the rest position and this can lead to a mistaken diagnosis of premature contacts. Alternatively, some patients like it to be thought that their lip seal is natural although it requires a habitual posture to provide it. Difficulty in making an analysis of occlusion from rest or habitual rest position can be solved by a test which will be described in Chapter 9 when discussing functional analysis.

Intercuspal position

IP is reached by an upwards and slightly forwards movement from rest position that ends with intercuspal occlusion, at which moment the mandible is in intercuspal position. The distance travelled by the mandible in this movement is between 2 and 4 mm and intercuspal occlusion is reached by simultaneous contact between both arches from rest position. This is a physiological requirement for comfort, stability and efficiency in the mouth. At this level the closing muscles are in optimal contraction. Any further movement upwards (as when teeth are lost), or laterally (as when teeth are tipped and cause displacement), or if the movement is cut short by restorations or prostheses, can result in discomfort, fatigue or even injury in the muscles. The *occlusal vertical relation* (OVR) of the face is seen when the mandible is in intercuspal position and the difference in height between rest and occlusal vertical relation is referred to as the *interocclusal distance* (IOD) or freeway space.

Thus RVR − OVR = 3 mm in the normal or average facial development. Intercuspal position from rest position is reached many times throughout the day as saliva is swallowed from the empty mouth.

IP is also one of the positions reached when the teeth meet in parafunctional contact. Here the occlusion may be prolonged and cause fatigue of the muscles and discomfort in the periodontal tissues.

The movement from rest position is endogenously determined, as is the posture from which it began. It is as characteristic of the individual as is the blink of the eyelids or a sudden smile. If an interference prevents any of these natural (endogenous) movements, the muscles will often adapt and produce a new movement. When the cause of interference is removed the natural movement will be restored.

Deflected occlusion

When the positon of a tooth and its cuspal relation with an opposing tooth is altered, the mandible may not be able to reach intercuspal position without deflexion or repositioning of the teeth. When the mandible is reflexly deflected the muscles perform a *displacing activity*. The mandible is displaced until a new intercuspal position is achieved, implying altered cusp contacts. This represents a series of reflex adaptive movements and the term *habitual intercuspal position* is given to the new occlusal position of the mandible. In the adolescent, when the dentition is developing, displacing activities are continuously taking place as teeth erupt and move into their permanent positions. It is questionable whether any tooth position is permanent in view of the ease with which they can move at any age. Thus it is claimed that all intercuspal positions are habitual. The exception to this is the rare occasion when intercuspal occlusion takes place on the retruded arc when, as was explained in Chapter 1, the term *retruded intercuspal position* is used.

Premature and initial contacts

In order to clarify the confusion that often exists between altering habitual intercuspal positions and repositioning of the teeth, the terms *premature* and *initial* contacts were introduced by Thompson (1954) and were restated by him in a symposium on the temporomandibular joint (Thompson, 1964). These constitute momentary positions of the mandible. *Premature contacts* between teeth may occur within the interocclusal distance (freeway space) and the teeth are displaced prior to intercuspal occlusion. There is no alteration in intercuspal position nor in the interocclusal distance. *Initial contact* is the momentary occlusion that takes place at the summit of the IOD, following which the mandible is deflected horizontally or vertically until IP is reached. On closing from various open positions the mandible goes directly to its habitual IP. On closing from rest position it will usually encounter the initial contact. This displacing activity is also referred to as a mandibular displacement (Figure 4.2). As Thompson pointed out, the distinction between premature and initial contact is more a matter of judgement than of measurement. It is an important distinction, however, when treatment is being planned. Teeth in premature contact may be tender or mobile. Initial contact followed by displacement may produce muscle pain and restricted movement. Both conditions may require treatment. A vertical extension of mandibular displacement

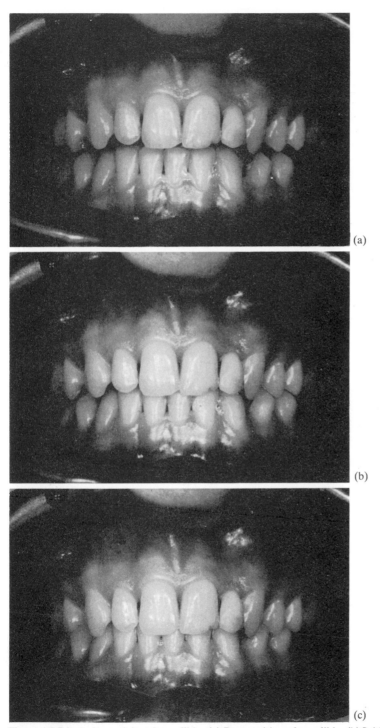

(a)

(b)

(c)

Figure 4.2 Displacing activity of mandible. (a) Rest position of mandible. (b) Initial contact between mandibular and maxillary left premolars. (c) IP following displacing activity to right side

where the IOD is in excess of 4 mm is referred to as *mandibular overclosure*. A further description of these disturbances will be given in Chapter 7 and treatment described in Chapters 12 and 14. For the present, it is important to be able to recognize rest position (as opposed to habitual posture), to visualize intercuspal position and clinically to diagnose any deflexion in the path of closure.

Intercuspal occlusion can therefore occur in many positons of the mandible as a result of changing surfaces and positions of the teeth. So long as the maximum number of teeth in opposing arches are in contact, intercuspal position is achieved.

Ligamentous, tooth and muscular positions

Brill and colleagues (1959) introduced these terms to define three horizontal mandibular positions in the sagittal plane in order to clarify functional movements of the mandible as distinct from extreme or artificially induced movements. The *ligamentous* position is defined as an extreme position and corresponds to the retruded relation of the mandible. 'It is limited by the lateral ligaments of the joints.' The *tooth* position corresponds to the habitual intercuspal position and can be estimated as a vertical or horizontal component of the mandibular position. The *muscular* position is 'the contact position of the mandible defined by the reflex muscle pattern acting as the mandible closes from rest position'. The authors suggest that the coincidence of tooth and muscular positions constitutes a physiological condition and that, when they do not coincide, a potentially pathological condition results. 'In a very few patients' the three positions coincide, corresponding to retruded intercuspal position.

Criticism of these terms is threefold. First, all positions are reached by muscle activity and confusion may be caused in assessing the difference between the tooth and muscular positions. However, this confusion can be cleared if it is understood that tooth position may follow a premature or initial contact on closure from rest position. Secondly, all border positions (and movements) are ligamentous (presumably meaning limited by ligaments) and are often functional. Thirdly, tooth (occlusal) positions include lateral, protruded and retruded occlusions in addition to intercuspal position. These may be pedantic criticisms and they are offered to emphasize that mandibular positions and movements are under neuromuscular control and are, therefore, continuously subject to adaptation by the contours of the teeth. Definitions which are confined to the use of one tissue are therefore limited and could be misleading. The term 'intercuspal' is, admittedly, limited, in that it only describes an occlusal position which takes place between cusps. One has to imply that this means the greatest number of cusps and opposing surfaces in contact.

Other occlusal positions

The mandible can voluntarily close into several occlusal positions. There is usually only one such position preferred in each horizontal direction. Thus there is the retruded occlusal position (or retruded contact) on the retruded arc, the left and right lateral, and the protruded occlusal positions. The mandible can hold these positions but usually they are avoided in mastication when the bolus acts as a buffer. Occlusion, if any, is light and acts as a guide to IP. They cannot be called deflective contacts. However, these occlusions can cause premature contacts and deflected mandibular movements. The effects of these contacts will be discussed in the next section and again in Chapter 7.

Border movements

Functional movements of the mandible conform to a pattern when the dentition is complete; this applies to speech and other activities as well as to mastication. When teeth are lost or their shapes altered by disease, wear and restorations, the patterns of movements will adapt to the changing environment. The neuromuscular function will ensure optimal efficiency and comfort within the limits of muscle, joint and tooth tolerance. Excluding tooth contacts, however, the mandible is capable of a wide range of *circumductory* movements limited by the ligaments of the joints, as described in Chapter 2. These movements are more simply called *border* movements and they are reproducible if the muscles are in good function. For the purposes of this study of occlusion, border movements also include those limited by the teeth in the vertical upwards and lateral directions (Figures 4.3 and 4.4).

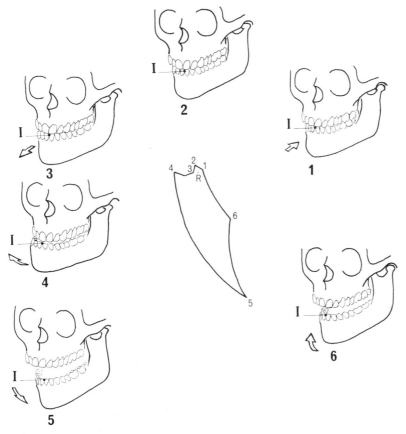

Figure 4.3 The median vertical envelope of motion traced by point I. 1, Retruded occlusion. 2, IP. 3, Protruded occlusion. 4, Full protrusion. 5, Full opening. 6, Opening at lower extent of retruded arc. R, Rest position (see text, p.58)

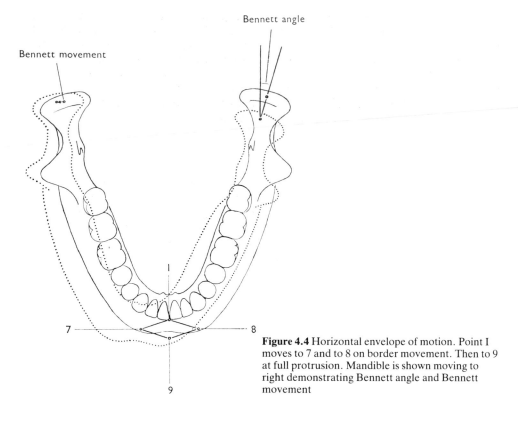

Bennett angle

Bennett movement

7

8

9

Figure 4.4 Horizontal envelope of motion. Point I moves to 7 and to 8 on border movement. Then to 9 at full protrusion. Mandible is shown moving to right demonstrating Bennett angle and Bennett movement

Border movements are those limited by ligaments and teeth against the maximal effort of the muscles. They form a characteristic, reproducible shape and can be demonstrated in vertical and horizontal planes. Where tooth contacts provide the limits, the shape will vary according to the varying number and occlusal surfaces of the teeth. If the mandible is prevented from closing by the insertion of a central bearing screw and plate, so that lateral movements are possible without tooth contacts, the characteristic Gothic arch tracing can be scribed on the plate. If the complete range of horizontal movements is performed, a reproducible diamond shape is achieved.

The median vertical envelope

Figure 4.3 shows a series of diagrams of jaw positions during the vertical border movements. In the centre is the plane covered by a point I between the two mandibular incisors during the movement. Beginning at the retruded occlusal position (1), the mandible moves upwards to intercuspal position (2); thence to the protruded occlusal position (3); and full protrusion or reverse vertical overlap (4). The line 1–4 constitutes the upper limit of the border movement determined by tooth contact. The mandible then swings to full opening (5) with the chin forwards, following which the chin is pulled back to begin closure. As the condyles reach their retruded positions in the fossae (6), the closure on the retruded condyle axis begins. The line 6–1 is the retruded arc and is the arc of a circle with the retruded condyle axis as centre. It can measure up to 20 mm on point I. Point R represents the rest position which exists 3 mm below IP (2) but in front of and slightly below the retruded occlusal position (1). The vertical component of all mandibular movements takes place within this envelope and its chief significance is its reproducibility, particularly the retruded arc (6–1). As tooth positions change, so will 1–4 change, but this can be under the control of the dentist.

This basis for the foregoing observations on the median vertical envelope is Posselt's (1952) studies on the mobility of the mandible.

The horizontal envelope

Figure 4.4 shows the mandible from above and the same point I making left and right lateral movements at a precontact level determined by the central bearing screw and plate. The border limits of these movements are shown in the diamond shape I–7–9–8. The lines I–7 and I–8 represent the Gothic arch. The horizontal diamond shape can be repeated at all levels of jaw separation, although it will become smaller as the opening increases (Figure 4.5).

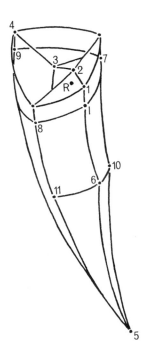

Figure 4.5 Space parcel. Combination of median vertical envelope and series of horizontal envelopes. Numbers refer to positions indicated in the text. R, rest position

The three-dimensional (or space) parcel

As the mandible moves laterally and protrusively while the teeth are in contact, the shape of the border movements will be modified by the occlusal surfaces of the teeth. These movements can be followed in Figure 4.5, which is a diagram of the completed three-dimensional parcel.

Explanations and comments

1. The retruded occlusal position can vary in height with tooth loss and wear but it remains on the retruded arc. The arc does not vary unless the muscles are inhibited in function by injury or fatigue, or the joint by derangement or disease. Ideally, intercuspal position should be a little higher on the arc at the horizontal level of the habitual IP (Figure 4.6). This is the level on the arc at which IP is optimal in reconstruction procedures and in complete dentures. Expressed by initials this reads: IP on RA above RP.

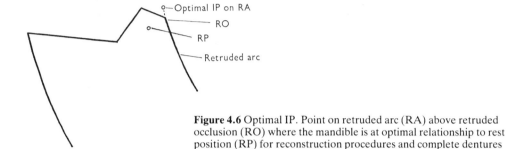

Figure 4.6 Optimal IP. Point on retruded arc (RA) above retruded occlusion (RO) where the mandible is at optimal relationship to rest position (RP) for reconstruction procedures and complete dentures

2. The path 1–2 (Figures 4.3 and 4.5) is the upward articular movement to IP from retruded occlusal position and represents a bilateral sliding contact between one or more mandibular supporting cusps and maxillary distal cusp ridges (inner surfaces). If this articulation is not bilateral a deflexion to an altered IP takes place and a muscle disability may result.
3. The articular movement to the protruded occlusal position from IP (2–3) represents the incisal guidance and should be a straight line. If it wavers to one side or the other there may be tooth interferences combined with a minor joint derangement.
4. The opening path 4–5 should also be seen as a straight movement, viewed from the front, otherwise a joint derangement may be suspected. It represents rotation and translation of both condyles.
5. The first phase of the closing movement (5–6) represents the condyles moving back along both eminentiae as they rotate and this, too, should be a straight vertical movement until both condyles reach the glenoid fossae, when they begin to rotate.
6. The closing (and opening) retruded arc movement (6–1) is fundamental to all studies and analyses of occlusion and its main feature is the reproducibility of the retruded condyle axis.
7. The rest position (RP) lies within the parcel of movement. Its significance is the constancy of its vertical and horizontal relations to the maxilla and its value is as a reference position for the OVR and for the interocclusal distance between OVR and RVR.
8. The Gothic arch movements I–7 and I–8 are flattened arcs, since the centres of rotation of both movements are moving (Bennett movement). Similar arcs of movement can take place at 6–10 and 6–11 while the mandible is still on the retruded arc. The significance of these movements is that during lateral articulations (beginning or ending at point 2) the same flattened arcs of movements are caused by each cusp opposing each fossa, depending on the

articular contacts between incisors and canines. Ideally, the mandible should be able to move along these borders during articulation without cusp interferences.

9. All mandibular movements take place within this space and seldom reach a border, except perhaps in retruded occlusion which is sometimes used in forceful closure and parafunctional movements. However, if cusp interference prevents movement towards a border position, disorders may result in the musculature. Further, if a joint derangement (such as click) exists, border movements may be prevented and, again, the musculature may suffer.

10. The practical application of the border movements is the possiblity for transferring the vertical retruded arc and the horizontal (Gothic arch) movements to an articulator (Chapter 8). This application provides the basis for gnathology and the fully adjustable articulators. In the diagnosis and treatment of occlusal disturbances the accurate transfer of the border movements to such an articulator is of great assistance, since all occlusal positions and articular movements made in the mouth can be seen on the articulator.

A study of the parcel of mandibular movement, therefore, has more than academic interest and reference to it will be made in subsequent chapters.

Bennett movement

There should now be some familiarity with this movement and emphasis is now on the lateral shift that takes place in lateral masticatory movements in both incoming and outgoing phases where the teeth meet lightly, if at all. Any alteration to cusp height or shape, particularly in guiding cusps, may cause premature contacts and consequent disturbances. In parafunctional grinding movements, too, the Bennett movement dominates the initial outgoing phase from IP and obstructions to this movement can be equally, if not more, harmful. The Bennett movement is composed of two distinct phases: an immediate translation which takes place before the rotation, and a progressive translation which accompanies the rotation. Tracings of these movements can be seen in the transfer of these movements to a fully adjustable articulator (see Chapter 8).

In a study of 30 dental students, Preiskel (1972), using ultrasonic measurements, observed that the amount of Bennett shift varies between individuals but that the movements could be repeated in the same individuals. He also observed that there is a graduated increase in the movement when the occlusal vertical dimension was increased. The clinical significance of this component of masticatory movement lies in the need to allow for this movement in making restorations involving the cusps, cusp ridges and triangular ridges.

Border movements are performed voluntarily for the most part but in the healthy system it is likely that they are used involuntarily when effort in function is required.

Condyle positions and movements

When considering the positions and movements of the mandibular condyles it is helpful to remember that there are two and that they move as if joined by an axle.

This axle is the retruded condyle axis and can be seen to rotate only when the mandible (and its condyles) is fully retruded and uninhibited by stiff, sore or resistant muscles.

Three-dimensional movements

In the Preface it was said that a three-dimensional approach was necessary for an understanding of mandibular movments. In Chapter 2 it was said that all the muscles of mastication are in function (either contracting or relaxing) in all movements of the mandible. A three-dimensional movement is, therefore, inevitable. In applying this principle, the movements of the mandible can be analysed into three centres of rotation in each condyle region (Figure 4.7). These are: the *horizontal-sagittal axis of rotation* (the retruded condyle axis) resulting in the vertical opening and closing of the mandible (Figure 4.7a); the *vertical axis of rotation* resulting in a horizontal arc of movement (Figure 4.7b); and the *horizontal-coronal axis* resulting in a vertical arc of movement in the coronal plane (Figure 4.7c). In visualizing these movements it may be helpful to refer to a diagram (Figure 4.8) of the three planes mentioned.

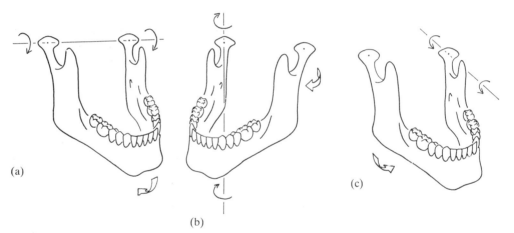

(a)

(b)

(c)

Figure 4.7 Mandibular centres of rotation. (a) Horizontal-sagittal (retruded condyle axis). (b) Vertical axis with horizontal rotation. (c) Horizontal-coronal axis. Permits descent of orbiting condyle

Rotation on the retruded condyle axis will produce a two-dimensional vertical arc of movement. All other movements are three-dimensional and represent movements of the same condyle axis when it is moved away from its retruded relation to the glenoid fossae. Thus the axis (both condyles) protrudes and, as tooth contacts are encountered, it rotates and tilts to accommodate the varying interruptions to a straight protrusive movement. During this movement the condyles maintain a 'sharp contact' with the menisci and the movement itself is reproducible. If the condyle path could be seen it would probably be slightly curved, but the rotations of the axis permit an uneven course for the teeth (and the mandible) to follow. If the movement is lateral the arc of the orbiting condyle will follow a steeper path and the axis will rotate while making this movement. At the same time the rotating (working) condyle will follow its Bennett shift. The path

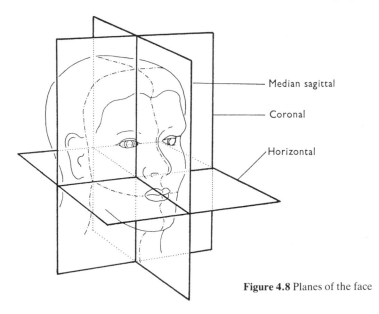

Median sagittal

Coronal

Horizontal

Figure 4.8 Planes of the face

followed by each mandibular cusp in relation to bolus or opposing tooth can therefore adapt to any encounter. The clinical application of this information is that, if the retruded condyle axis and both protrusive and lateral paths of condyle movements can be recorded and transferred to an articulator, all mandibular movements can be copied (see also Chapter 8).

Condyle positions

At rest position and intercuspal position the condyles occupy positions in their respective fossae which show a small change in outline between each position. The movement of the mandible is upwards and forwards for a distance of 2–3 mm and the condyle axis rotates fractionally and rises bodily upwards. The outline of one condyle traced from lateral skull radiographs taken at rest position (with the head held in a cephalostat) show little change in relationship to the fossa to one traced at IP (Figure 4.9b). Initial contacts and consequent displacements may show varying degrees of change in outline when compared with rest position.

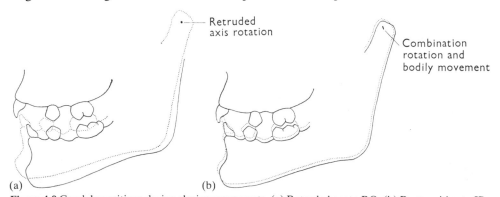

Retruded axis rotation

Combination rotation and bodily movement

(a)   (b)

Figure 4.9 Condyle positions during closing movements. (a) Retruded arc to RO. (b) Rest position to IP

On the retruded axis the condyle outline demonstrates rotation (Figure 4.9a). On protrusion and lateral movements the condyles move downwards and forwards at a measurable angle to the horizontal plane as the mandible makes protrusive and lateral gliding articulation movements. The angle of descent can be measured by inserting a wax wafer (or fast setting stone plaster) between the posterior teeth just prior to protruded occlusion and by transferring this record to casts mounted on an adjustable articulator. The angle of condyle descent can then be adjusted on the articulator when the cast teeth of both arches are seated in the record. When the mandible moves laterally to one side, the angle of the orbiting condyle is steeper than the angle seen in straight protrusion when both condyles move simultaneously. The transfer of condyle axis positions and movements to articulators will be described in Chapter 8.

Joint space

The 'spaces' (occupied fully by menisci) between the condyles and glenoid fossae at intercuspal and open positions, as seen on radiographs, have a characteristic shape; an example is shown in Figure 4.10. The spaces become narrowed in old age but can also be reduced in arthritic conditions (see Chapter 9). (These are, of course, radiographic spaces, there being none in the joints themselves which are filled with menisci.) Effusion into the joint cavity will increase this space and in the early stages of rheumatoid arthritis it is often increased due to the formation of the pannus. These differences in joint appearance can be seen between two joints in the same individual and this feature can be helpful in diagnosis.

Condyle displacement

As was suggested above, initial contact and subsequent displacement can result in a change between condyle outline at rest position and at intercuspal position. Lateral skull radiographs of the condyles at rest position are superimposed over those taken at IP, using the fossa outline and auditory canals as references. Differences between the two condyle outlines are indicative of mandibular displacement on closure (Figure 4.11).

Comment

There are three aspects of this study of positions and movements that deserve emphasis. The first is that occlusal positions are not voluntarily maintained for more than a fleeting contact during function. Intercuspal positon is used when swallowing but this, too, is an occlusion momentarily held. On the other hand, all occlusal positions are liable to be used during parafunctional habits and whether these are positions or movements the reflex response to contact is overcome by the muscle forces used.

Secondly, the reflex response to contact is so immediate that whether the contact is with an opposing tooth, food bolus or outside agency an alteration in the path of movement is inevitable. This makes the registration of a mandibular position in relation to the maxilla an operation uncertain of success. The proprioceptive response to any interocclusal substance, such as wax, plaster, resin or compound, is so sensitive that a change of position is likely to alter the resultant record. In addition, the operator's fingers on the patient's mouth are equally certain to cause a

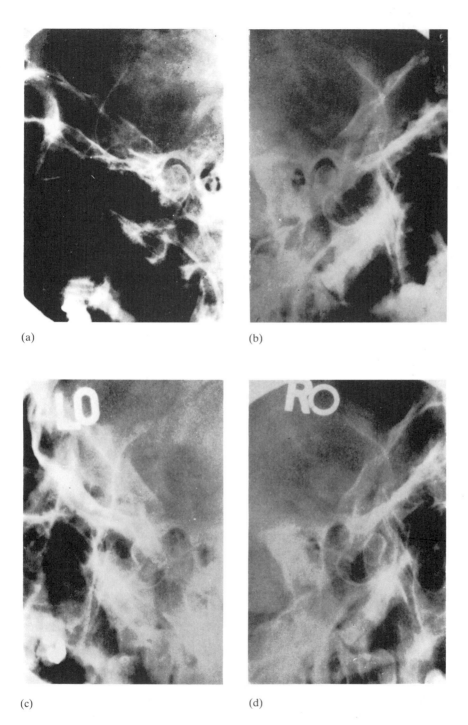

(a)

(b)

(c)

(d)

Figure 4.10 Radiographs of condyles open and closed. (a) and (b) Normal joint 'spaces' at IP. (c) and (d) Normal degrees of translation and rotation on opening. (By courtesy of Dr J. J. Prior, Eastman Dental Hospital)

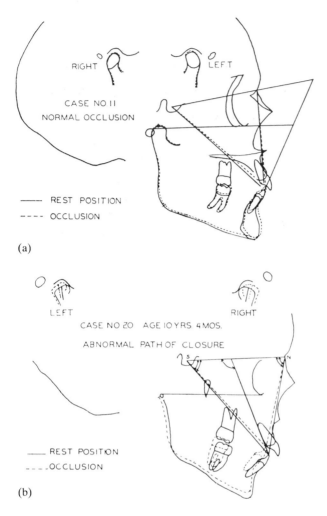

Figure 4.11 Tracing of lateral skull radiographs. Rest position superimposed on intercuspal position. (a) Normal and (b) abnormal paths of closure. (By courtesy of Dr J. R. Thompson)

reflex adaptive movement. The solution to this neuromuscular problem is to use the reproducible retruded arc on which a forcible closure into the registration substance is less likely to produce a reflex alteration of position or movement.

The third aspect for comment is the existence of reference positions and movements which are necessary for diagnosis, treatment and the transfer of dental arches to an articulator. The rest position is constant enough to be a vertical reference level in relation to intercuspal position but any attempt to register the relationship between mandible and maxilla at this position will fail for the reasons given in the previous paragraph. The reproducible retruded arc and the retruded occlusal position on it are the only reliable references for transfer. One must look to the borders of mandibular movement for reliable reproduction.

References

Ballard, C. F. (1967) Mandibular posture. *Dental Practitioner and Dental Record*, **17**, 377

Berry, D. C. (1960) The constancy of the rest positon of the mandible. *Dental Practitioner and Dental Record*, **10**, 129

Brill, N., Lammie, G. A., Osborne, J. and Perry, H. T. (1959) Mandibular position and mandibular movements. *British Dental Journal*, **106**, 391

Posselt, U. (1952) Studies in the mobility of the human mandible. *Acta Odontologica Scandinavica*, **10** (supplement 10)

Preiskel, H. (1972) The canine teeth related to Bennett movement. *British Dental Journal*, **131**, 312

Thompson, J. R. (1954) Concepts regarding stomatognathic system. *Journal of the American Dental Association*, **48**, 626

Thompson, J. R. (1964) Temporomandibular disorders: diagnosis and dental treatment. In *The Temporomandibular Joint* (ed. B. G. Sarnat), Thomas, Springfield IL, p. 152

Tryde, G., McMillan, D. R. and Christensen, J. (1976) The fallacy of facial measurements of occlusal height in edentulous subjects. *Journal of Oral Rehabilitation*, **3**, 353

Watkinson, A. C. (1987) The mandibular rest positions and electromyognathy: a review. *Journal of Oral Rehabilitation*, **14**, 209

Chapter 5

Occlusion and articulation

The purpose in this chapter is to describe the forces that are received by the teeth in function and to relate the instantaneous moments of occlusion to the various patterns of articulation which constitute occlusal function.

The forces acting on the teeth

Forces and responses

The forces which act on the teeth and cause them to move within their periodontal tissues vary in magnitude, duration, frequency and direction. The responses by the teeth to these forces depend on such factors as the shape and length of the roots, the characteristics of the fluid content of the periodontal space, the composition and orientation of the periodontal fibres and the extent of alveolar bone (Lewin, 1970a, b). It is, therefore, difficult to assess what is a normal response to a force on a tooth and what is potentially harmful. Lewin (1970a, b) has reviewed the literature on this subject and has devised methods of measuring the omnidirectional displacements of a tooth when subject to forces causing mesial and distal translations, buccal and lingual translations, and rotations about its long axis. An omnidirectional transducer is used and the information which this supplies can be used to specify the displacement of the whole tooth or any point on the tooth. Other references on this topic are Picton (1962a, b), Mühlemann (1967) and Parfitt (1967). Lewin (1970a) divides the displacements which a tooth can make into translatory and rotational components. Each of these components can be subdivided into apical, mesial-distal and buccal-lingual translations and rotations. A tooth can be displaced in one or more of these six basic motions and the result is an omnidirectional movement in response to a force (Figure 5.1). The extent of this movement will depend on the variable forces caused by occlusion, food bolus or outside agency. It should be remembered that, in intercuspal occlusion, the forces are shared by the remaining teeth in contact. Therefore the forces produced on individual teeth will be opposed by adjacent tooth contact, where this exists.

Omnidirectional and unidirectional responses

These omnidirectional tiltings and rotations of a tooth when subject to a vertical or horizontal force reach a limit when the periodontal receptors cause a reflex stoppage of the force or when an equal opposing force is reached. When the force is

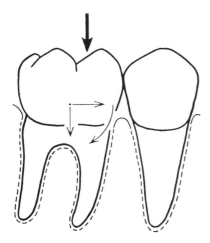

Figure 5.1 Omnidirectional movements in response to force on a tooth

removed the tooth will recover its position due to the elastic recovery of the compressed periodontal tissues. Each tooth has a centre of resistance (Fish, 1917) through which the forces pass and this can alter when alveolar bone is lost. Each tooth has adjacent tooth support, the loss of which may alter the elastic response. Each tooth has horizontal muscle support on its buccal and lingual surfaces and the forces created by them can be habitually altered. These three factors may result in a unidirectional movement of a tooth when subject to a force and this will result in repositioning of the tooth. A tooth will continue to move unidirectionally until it reaches a position of stability, where opposing forces are equal to the moving forces. These features of omnidirectional movement and elastic response and of repositioning of teeth are characteristic responses to forces.

The forces which act directly on the teeth are muscular, occlusal and extrinsic. Occlusal and extrinsic forces are generated by muscles but the contact is made by teeth and outside agencies respectively.

Muscle forces

The muscles of the tongue on one side of the teeth and those of the lips and cheeks on the other (the orofacial muscles) maintain a varying source of horizontal forces on the teeth. The activities of these muscles conform to a stable pattern throughout life and are responsible for the horizontal positions of the teeth as they develop vertically. Overcrowding of teeth may lead to alterations of these positions against the forces of the muscles. Various skeletal and muscular abnormalities may lead to inadequate muscle forces being directed on the teeth. The class III skeletal relation and the short upper lip are examples that may lead to an incompetent lip seal and to the tongue producing a forward force on the maxillary teeth. The forces between the opposing orofacial muscles usually result in a stable horizontal relationship of the teeth. The position which the teeth occupy in this relation is known as the *neutral zone*. This term does not satisfy the scientists but is helpful to the clinician in assessing possible causes of repositioning of the teeth. It is also helpful when deciding the horizontal positions of denture teeth. Artificial teeth set on one or other side of the neutral zone will always be subject to unfavourable muscular forces.

All activity by the orofacial muscles produces movement of the teeth. Provided that it is equally opposed, the movement will be omnidirectional and the teeth will be restored to their original positions. If not, they will be repositioned.

Occlusal forces

Intercuspal occlusion takes place between cusp ridges and opposing fossae (formed by triangular ridges) or between cusp ridges and opposing marginal ridge areas. The cusp ridges make a tripod of contact, leaving the cusp apex out of occlusion (see Figure 2.9). In the case of occlusion with marginal ridges it is the opposing cusp ridges which make contact and not the cusp itself. This feature provides stability of contact and distributes the forces produced on intercuspal occlusion. It also emphasizes the difficulty of seeing occlusal contacts in the mouth and the need to tilt the casts in order to see them (Figure 5.2). Even on casts it is difficult to see

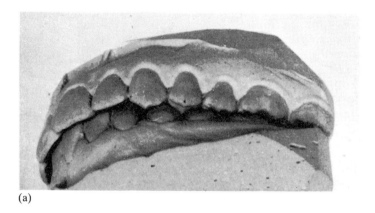

(a)

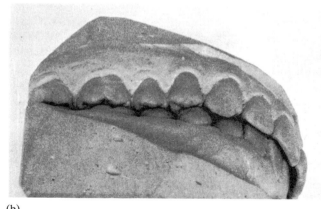

(b)

Figure 5.2 Casts of buccal quadrants. (a) Left. Cusp–ridge IO. (b) Right. Cusp–fossa IO

contacts from the lingual aspect without removing the lower lingual cusps. This feature also demonstrates the shortcomings of two-dimensional line drawings of teeth in occlusion. As was pointed out in Chapter 2, only two supporting cusps in each buccal segment contact an opposing fossa, the remainder making contact in the opposing ridge areas. In view of the majority of ridge contacts ι ιis is referred to as cusp–ridge occlusion and is illustrated in Figure 5.2a. The potential harm which may accrue from this occlusion is the action of the plunger cusp which may develop when proximal restorations are made with ill-defined ridge shapes or when adjacent teeth separate. It can be seen in Figure 5.2a that the mandibular first premolar has moved forwards into an unstable occlusion between the maxillary premolar and canine. This may lead to repositioning of the affected teeth and to interdental problems. The disturbance is not helped by the absence of the lingual (guiding) cusp on the mandibular premolar. When reconstruction procedures are being planned, efforts are made to provide cusp–fossa occlusion, wherever possible, in order to prevent (or cure) this disturbance. Figure 5.3 illustrates a mouth restored in this way by Dr P. K. Thomas. Figure 5.2 illustrates how it is

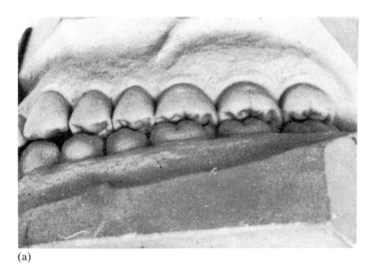

(a)

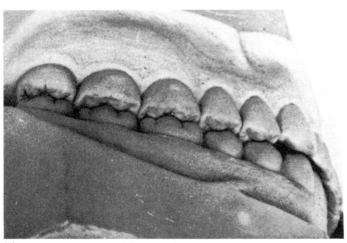

(b)

Figure 5.3 Casts of buccal quadrants of reconstructed dentition. (a) Left. Cusp–fossa IO. (b) Right. Cusp–fossa IO. (By courtesy of Dr P. K. Thomas)

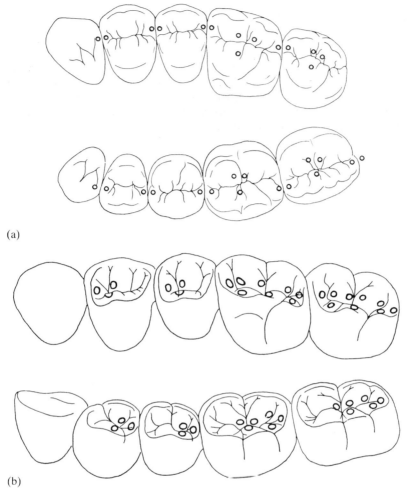

(a)

(b)

Figure 5.4 Sites of contact by supporting cusps. (a) Cusp–ridge IO. (b) Cusp–fossa IO. (After Lundeen, 1971)

possible to have cusp–ridge occlusion on one side (Figure 5.2a) and cusp–fossa on the other (Figure 5.2b) in the natural dentition. Figure 5.4 illustrates the location of the contacts in cusp–ridge and cusp–fossa occlusions.

As has been pointed out, the forces in empty mouth intercuspal occlusion (when swallowing) are shared between all the teeth present. If tripod contact exists between all posterior tooth contacts and if two complete arches are present, all teeth will return to their original positions when the teeth part. Parafunctional closures, however, may lead to wear of the interproximal contact areas and a forward drift of all teeth may be the result. As a preventive measure against these and all other closures of the teeth in the empty mouth, all patients (and people) wherever and whenever possible, should be advised to maintain the posture of lips together and teeth apart.

Antagonistic occlusal forces

These can occur when two teeth in the same segment, either adjacent or separated by other teeth, are receiving occlusal forces in opposing directions. This is illustrated in Figure 5.5 where the mandibular second molar is producing a forward force and the mandibular first premolar a backward force in intercuspal occlusion. These opposing forces have the adverse effect on the maxillary second premolar of aiding its extrusion and the possibility of compressing its periodontal tissues. This is a missing tooth problem and is often associated with a periodontal disturbance of the affected teeth.

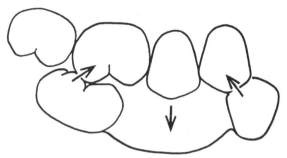

Figure 5.5 Antagonistic occlusal forces (see text and also Figure 9.1)

Healthy responses

A healthy response to occlusal forces depends on six factors. These are: stable intercuspal occlusion; stable contact points; healthy periodontal tissues; competent orofacial muscle activity; favourable crown–root ratio and root direction; and occlusion of limited magnitude and duration. The direction of the occlusal forces is of less significance than the health and function of the tissues involved.

Two phases of occlusion

A phenomenon of tooth contact provided by the periodontal membranes is the two phases or levels of occlusion. The first contact between the arches is followed by the omnidirectional movement of each tooth within its membrane. The combination of maxillary and mandibular tooth movements results in a difference in level of occlusion which, though not measurable, has some clinical significance. It will include any premature contact and movement of the affected teeth and can confuse the clinician on the occlusion reached between two plaster casts of the teeth. When casts of both arches are placed together the occlusion recorded is that of the first and lightest contact, since there are no periodontal membranes in plaster of Paris. This feature may account for errors in transfers of occlusal relationships and in diagnosis and treatment (see also p. 177).

Other occlusal forces

The contact forces between the teeth mentioned so far have related to those in intercuspal occlusion. However, the principles apply to protruded, retruded and lateral occlusions. These are generally articular forces and take place as guiding contacts during mastication or as parafunctional contacts to and from intercuspal position. In the case of the former, the forces are light and easily reciprocated except perhaps in the unexpected non-working side contact when the muscles suffer more than the teeth; in the case of the latter, the forces are likely to be heavier, although they can vary between light sliding and gnashing of the teeth. A sustained force between two canines can be a cause of wear facets as seen in many adolescents. Between two centrals it can be a cause of pulp death in adults (see Disorders, Chapter 7).

Extrinsic forces

These are the forces caused by biting on pencils, pipes, finger-nails and other outside agencies. These represent parafunctional activities of the muscles but the force on the teeth is created by the object. The cause may be prolonged enough to cause reposition of the affected teeth (Figure 5.6). The proprioceptive response to an occlusal masticatory force is to part the teeth but this is overruled by the voluntary impulse to contract the muscles and may constitute an irrelevant muscle activity (p. 42).

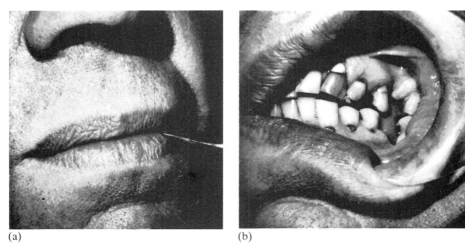

(a)   (b)

Figure 5.6 Effect of holding pipe. (a) Pipe in habitual position. (b) Reposition (depression) of affected teeth. Remaining teeth in IO

If the forces on the teeth could be limited to those exerted by the bolus in mastication, and by light closure into intercuspal position while swallowing, there would be few disorders of occlusion to diagnose and barely a need to write this book. However, dysfunction can lead to disorders of the masticatory system and these may include harmful occlusal and articular forces acting on the teeth, and should be considered before making diagnoses and planning treatment.

Articulation

In most people, the endogenously determined stable patterns of mandibular movement are efficiently related to the articular contacts between the teeth. The occlusal forces acting either through a layer of food or directly between the teeth are seen as moments of contact making up the patterns of articulation. The patterns vary but the objective is the same, and what is natural or normal for one individual has to be seen in relation to the efficiency of the mastication and other oral functions.

The topic of articulation between the teeth was first brought to the attention of dentists by Bonwill (1887) who was 'fully persuaded that of all that constitutes dentistry proper the mechanical forms the basis'. This view still dominates much of restorative and prosthetic dentistry although, in the past forty years, the physiological basis for the study and functions of the masticatory system has provided a balance to the mechanistic approach. None the less, Bonwill's contribution is a milestone and his influence on other celebrated names in dentistry is undoubted. In particular are those of Gysi (1910) and Schuyler (1935), whose works are still standard on the subject of articulation of the teeth.

Bonwill introduced the term 'articulation' for the teeth as 'a word of action throughout' while occlusion 'answers to the mere act of closing the teeth and lips'. In a stirring phrase from the lectern he cried; 'We must impart action to those otherwise whited sepulchres'. He is perhaps better known for his observation that in the mandible an equilateral triangle exists bounded by the two condyles and the contact point between the mandibular central incisors. The sides of this triangle measure 4 inches (10 cm) in the average mandible, and this forms the basis for his articulator which will be described in Chapter 8. However, Bonwill's claim that 'nature's triangle' with the double joint permitted 'the largest number of teeth to antagonize at every movement' provided an objective for articulation that is still an objective for successful complete dentures today. It was inevitable, perhaps, that he should refer to the occlusal surfaces of the teeth as the grinding surfaces, thus giving emphasis to the habit of parafunction in the empty mouth almost as a desirable objective in the natural as well as in the artificial dentition.

Joint articulation. It should not be forgotten that the term 'articulation' applies to the contact that exists between bones with their respective cartilages and opposing bones. In the masticatory system it applies to the mandibular condyles, as well as to the teeth, and the term 'articulator' derives from this application.

Patterns of articulation

Before proceeding to a description of articular patterns, attention is drawn to the glossary of terms where balanced and free articulation are defined in additon to articulation itself. It is pointed out that these terms refer to tooth contact in the empty mouth. This infers that articulation between the teeth in the empty mouth is a natural function of the masticatory system, but the reverse is true. It was stated in Chapter 1 that occlusion (including articulation) is not necessary for efficient mastication and that the more efficient the occlusion (and articulation) the less the teeth need touch each other. One of the causes of empty mouth (parafunctional) contacts is cusp interferences and when they occur there is a tendency to glide on them. This habit is self-perpetuating and potentially harmful. The analogy of the itch is mentioned to emphasize the point. One is unaware of healthy skin but an itch will induce scratching, and the habit can hurt. It is therefore necessary to assess a mouth for the efficiency and comfort of its articular movements in the empty mouth. Mastication introduces the bolus between the teeth and articulation can only be observed with difficulty. It can be assumed, however, that if cusp interferences exist in the empty mouth they are likely to exist similarly in the masticating mouth. This assumption is based on another: namely, that articulation occurs during mastication. Experimental evidence suggests that it does and this will be discussed in Chapter 6.

Patterns of articulation are individual and, when free from interferences, are contacts of which most people are unaware. The need to analyse and classify them arises when interferences arise and cause disturbances and when restorations and replacements have to be made. The classifications may seem to be largely theoretical and not related to natural function but they will serve to provide a yardstick of what is possible, what is desirable and what is potentially harmful. Nairn (1973) has drawn attention to certain fallacies in the assessment of articulation. He disputes the conventional views that a 'deep overbite' (steep incisal guidance) constitutes a 'locked bite' and that protrusive articulation balanced by posterior tooth contacts is necessarily a requirement for either the natural or artificial dentitions. He points out the error, firmly established by many authorities, that working side articular movements result in mandibular cusps gliding down maxillary triangular ridges (Figure 5.7c). In support of this criticism he refers to

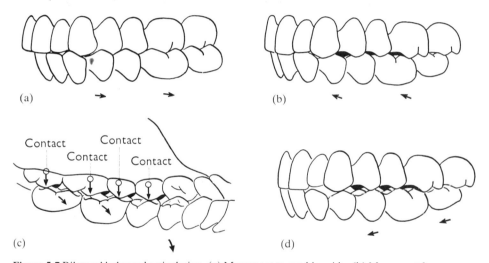

Figure 5.7 Bilateral balanced articulation. (a) Movement to working side. (b) Movement from non-working side. (c) Movement from non-working side viewed from lingual. (d) Movement to protrusion

Gysi (1910, 1913) who stated that in working side occlusion (and, therefore, articulation) 'cusp does not climb cusp'. Nairn's recommendations for providing free articulation in the setting of artificial teeth are threefold. First, even interdigitation of cusps on the working side with an unobstructed articular movement to IP. Secondly, avoidance of premature contacts on the non-working side. Thirdly, protrusive articular balance should not be achieved at the expense of unstable tooth positions with consequent disturbed function or appearance. Thus, bilateral balance may be helpful towards maintaining stability for complete dentures but only if tooth positions permit. Articulation protected by anterior guidance is more favourable for the natural dentition. This causes disclusion of the buccal teeth as the mandible slides forwards or laterally and the mandibular incisors and canines maintain contact with the lingual surfaces of the maxillary incisors and canines. After D'Amico (1961) examined primitive skulls in California he suggested that the wear on the teeth of these skulls causing reverse curves and edge-to-edge incisor occlusions was arrested with the advent of refined food during the past two centuries. It was deduced that the canines and incisors were necessary to protect the posterior teeth against such wear. Thus began the practice, still much in vogue, of the canine rise, the mutually protected occlusion and articulation and anterior guidance.

Reference will be made later in the chapter to the anatomical features which influence the patterns of articulation and these have to considered when providing free articulation for complete dentures. It should not be forgotten, however, that the lateral and protrusive movements of the mandible are governed not only by incisal guidance but also by the rotation of the condyle axis. Therefore, any lateral or protrusive movement can be modified by an opening or closing component. This permits the phenomenon of reflex adaptation, to which many references are made throughout the text.

The patterns of articulation that follow will be described as occurring in the empty mouth for the natural dentition. This will be followed by some comments on their application to the artificial dentition where their requirements are more practical. These can be seen by asking the patient to move his mandible from side to side, backwards and forwards, while keeping the teeth together. The paths of movement will generally be those which offer the least resistance to free articulation. The contacts vary between single opposing teeth and groups of teeth and between one or more opposing segments. The patterns will be described, firstly, according to the movements made and, secondly, according to the contacts observed.

Movements of articulation

There are four articular movements: retrusive, protrusive, left and right lateral retrusive movements.

Retrusive

This takes place from retruded to intercuspal occlusion and is usually confined at first contact to the cusps and cusp ridges of two opposing molar teeth on each side of the mouth (see Figure 4.3). During the forward and upward movement the cusp ridges of the mandibular teeth progressively engage the maxillary triangular ridges until they glide into intercuspal occlusion. When these articular contacts are not bilaterally balanced and the resultant movement is deflected to right or left, disturbances may result in the musculature.

Arstad (1956) referred to wear facets on the teeth between intercuspal position and retruded occlusal position and described this as lack of harmony between the two positions which could result in an anterior displacement.

Protrusive

This takes place from protruded to intercuspal occlusion and, in mouths where class I jaw and tooth relations exist, there is usually group contact between maxillary and mandibular incisors at the beginning of the movement. This may continue to intercuspal occlusion and be combined with balanced articulation between labial and buccal segments. In class II mouths this will not be possible if the horizontal overlap does not permit it (division 1) or if the vertical overlap causes disclusion between the buccal segments in protrusion (division 2). This movement is often reversed (from intercuspal to protruded occlusion) during parafunctional articulation.

Right lateral retrusive

This takes place as the mandible moves in from the right side when contact may begin between the opposing canines. Group contact between the opposing buccal cusp ridges on the right side may then take place as the mandible glides into intercuspal position. When this articulation is accompanied by contact between the opposing lingual cusp ridges on the right side there exists *cross tooth balance* on the working side. When, in addition, there is contact between left mandibular buccal cusps (their occlusal facing triangular ridges) and their opposing maxillary lingual cusps (their occlusal facing triangular ridges) there exists *cross arch balance*. This is also known as 'bilateral balanced articulation'. This movement can also take place in reverse, from intercuspal position outwards during parafunctional articulation.

Left lateral retrusive

This is the reverse of the right lateral articular movement.

In the natural dentition these movements are usually confined to one pathway in each of the four directions. In many mouths only one or at most two are used and this restriction is dictated by cusp interferences. These movements can often be recognized by facets of wear on the teeth that are usually an indication of articulation in the empty mouth. Facets of wear can, however, be caused by abrasive foods or by outside agencies. In a lifetime of function and parafunction, almost any contact will cause wear if it continues for long enough. And once a facet always a facet; often, more of a facet.

Contacts during articulation

There are three recognized categories into which articular contacts can be classified: bilateral balanced, unilateral balanced and anterior guidance (also referred to as disclusion with canine rise, or mutually protected occlusion).

Bilateral balanced articulation

During lateral movement

Working side.   The mandibular buccal cusp ridges make articular contact with the maxillary buccal cusp ridges as the mandibular lingual cusp ridges are making contact with the maxillary lingual cusp ridges. The maxillary and mandibular cusps pass each other with minimal lift or change in the occlusal vertical relation on the working side during this movement (Figures 5.7a and 5.8b).

Non-working side.   The mandibular buccal cusps and their occlusal facing triangular ridges make articular contact with maxillary lingual cusps and their

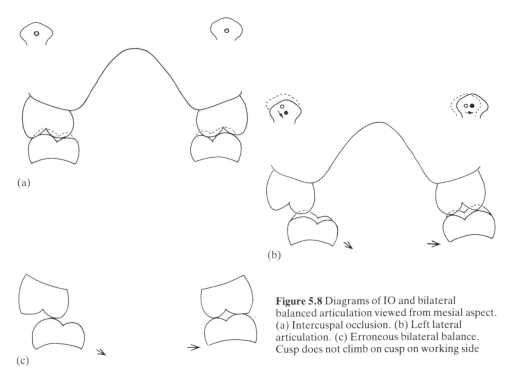

(a)

(b)

(c)

Figure 5.8 Diagrams of IO and bilateral balanced articulation viewed from mesial aspect. (a) Intercuspal occlusion. (b) Left lateral articulation. (c) Erroneous bilateral balance. Cusp does not climb on cusp on working side

occlusal facing triangular ridges. The path of this movement causes a separation between the opposing non-working segments, determined jointly by the slopes of the ridges involved and the downwards and inwards path followed by the orbiting side condyle (Figures 5.7b, c and 5.8b).

Each working and non-working path made by a cusp on the opposing tooth traces a miniature Gothic arch (Figure 5.9). This can sometimes be seen when lateral articular movements are made on a newly packed amalgam or direct wax pattern for an inlay or crown. The apex of this arch does not represent the retruded relation since the mandible is in habitual IP. The apex is, therefore, blunted.

Anterior segment. The mandibular canine cusp and mesial cusp ridge glides along the distal–lingual surface of the maxillary canine on the working side and passes between the canine and first premolar cusp ridges. The working side lateral and central incisors maintain contact. On the non-working side contact is lost.

During protrusive movement

Anterior segments. The incisal edges of the mandibular incisors and canines make articular contact with the lingual surfaces of the maxillary incisors and canines (see Figure 5.7d).

Posterior segments. The mesial buccal and lingual cusp ridges of the mandibular teeth make articular contact with the distal buccal and lingual cusp ridges of the maxillary teeth (Figure 5.7d).

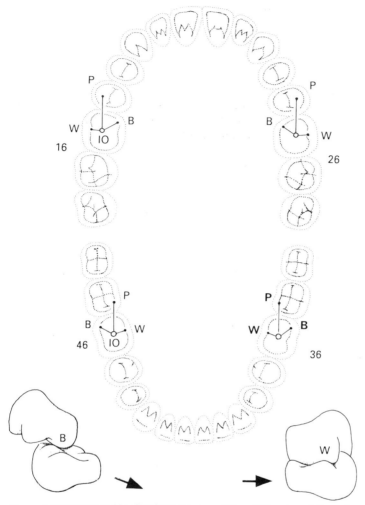

Figure 5.9 Paths traced by distobuccal cusps of 46 and 36 and mesiolingual cusps of 16 and 26 against opposing fossae. IO, intercuspal occlusion; W, working; B, balancing (non-working); P, protrusive

This is the prosthodontic concept of balanced articulation and has been advocated for the past eighty years as an aid to stability for complete dentures.

Unilateral balanced articulation

During lateral movement

Working side.   The articular contacts are as for bilateral balanced articulation.

Non-working side.   No articular contacts.

During protrusive movement

Anterior segment.   As for bilateral balanced articulation.

Non-working side.   No articular contacts.

Anterior guidance articulation (disclusion with canine rise)

During lateral movements

Working side.   Usually the only articular contact is between the canines as the mandibular cusp glides along the distal facing lingual surface of the maxillary canine. This articulation separates all the remaining teeth and as the mandible moves into intercuspal position it acts as a guide (Figure 5.10a).

Non-working side.   No articular contacts.

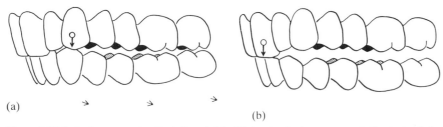

(a)   (b)

Figure 5.10 Anterior segment articulation. (a) Left lateral articular movement. Contact only between opposing canines. (b) Protrusive articular movement. Contact only between opposing incisors

During protrusive movement

Anterior segment.   Articular contacts are as in bilateral and unilateral balanced articulation (Figure 5.10b).

Posterior segments.   There is no articulation. However, it is not unusual for lateral excursions in this dentition to involve contact between lateral incisors, canines and the buccal inner aspects of the buccal cusp ridges of the first premolars. This constitutes a modified form of group function.

Anterior segment articulation (anterior guidance) is also referred to as *mutually protected occlusion* and it exists in many natural dentitions. An example is illustrated in Figure 5.11. It is the objective in many reconstruction procedures, where it is combined with retruded intercuspal occlusion. From this retruded IP, all articular movements cause disclusion of the posterior teeth.

Articulation in the natural dentition

There can be no dogma about what is considered normal articulation in the natural dentition. It exists as it evolves and it changes according to loss and wear of teeth. Variations are numerous and changes are continually taking place. Further, adaptation to these variables and changes is favourable in the majority of mouths, by tooth movement or by jaw movement. This favourable response is not unlimited, however, and the disturbances which may result will be described in Chapter 7.

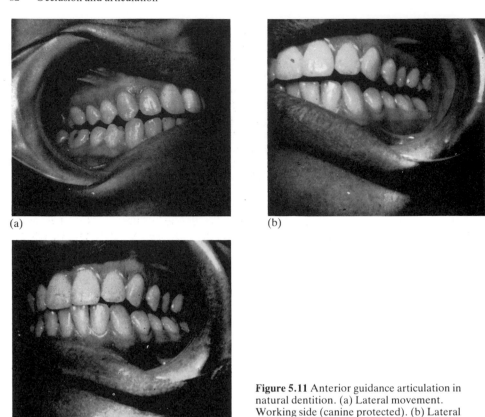

(a)

(b)

(c)

Figure 5.11 Anterior guidance articulation in natural dentition. (a) Lateral movement. Working side (canine protected). (b) Lateral movement. Non-working side (no contact). (c) Protrusive movement. Incisor contact

Two aspects of articulation in the natural dentition are worth restating. First, all articular movements take place within the parcel of motion and in three dimensions. Any cuspal interference which prevents a movement towards the border of the parcel may result in disturbance. Secondly, articular movements are often envisaged as starting from intercuspal position with the mandible moving back, laterally or forwards as previously mentioned. This may occur in empty mouth parafunctional movements, but in mastication these contact movements take place from the open position of the mandible and finish momentarily at intercuspal position prior to beginning the cycle of chewing again. It is not certain whether the paths travelled by the mandibular cusps along the maxillary teeth in the closing articular movements are the reverse of those taking place from intercuspal occlusion outwards. When adjustment or reconstruction of the articulation is planned, they are regarded as being the same.

Articulation in the artificial dentition

Articulation in the artificial dentition is planned and created by dentist and technician. Artificial articulation has to be developed so as to conform to the four articular movements and a choice of articular contact scheme has to be made from one of the three schemes outlined in the previous section. Having registered a chosen intercuspal position and transferred this to an articulator, a protruded registration is transferred and the condyle guidance on the articulator is adjusted to copy this position. It is then assumed that the articulator path between the intercuspal and protruded positions will copy those in the mouth (see Chapter 8). The dentist has to decide whether to incorporate bilateral or unilateral balanced articulation or disclusion in the reconstructed dentition. The success of articulation in the artificial dentition depends on the accuracy of the transfer of jaw positions and movements to an articulator and on the planning and skill of the dentist and technician in adjusting the occlusal surfaces of the teeth in order to provide the same articulation in the mouth as was developed on the articulator.

The choice of articulation scheme for the artificial dentition depends on whether complete or partial dentures are being made or if the natural dentition is being artificially reconstructed. It will also depend on the pre-existing jaw and tooth relations if records are available.

For *complete dentures*, one of the chief requirements is stability: this is the property which causes denture bases to resist displacement when subject to vertical and horizontal forces. The forces include those caused by occlusion and articulation. It is therefore desirable, in the empty mouth, that an occlusal force on one segment of a denture should be balanced by a similar force on one or both of the other two segments in order to prevent tilting of the denture bases. This requirement applies equally to articular forces while the mandible moves. If an occlusal force causes a denture base to tilt, the wearer will tend to persist in applying this force. The base will lose retention, the supporting tissues of the residual ridges will become bruised and the denture will often be discarded. When food is being chewed the confidence and comfort achieved by balanced articulation will help to stabilize the dentures. Further, cross-arch balance will still apply. As the bolus is chewed on one side, the balancing cusps will come close to or will contact on the other. The dictum 'enter bolus, exit balance' need not apply. Better still, the patient should be advised to divide the bolus in two and chew on both sides, simultaneously.

The occlusal and articular requirements for complete dentures are therefore: (1) intercuspal occlusion at a reproducible intercuspal position; and (2) balanced occlusions and free articulation achieved by the objective of bilateral balanced articulation where the skeletal jaw relation permits.

Balanced articulation may have to be modified in mouths where certain malocclusions and abnormal tooth inclinations have pre-existed in the natural dentition. This is particularly true of the class II, division 2 malocclusion where the vertical overlap has to copied for reasons of lip competence. Such an overlap will confine articulation to the anterior segment only. The application of these principles will be made in Chapter 12.

For *partial dentures*, articulation requirements for mouths where partial dentures are planned will depend on the existing articulation between the remaining natural teeth. Where there are bounded saddles and the occlusion and articulation have proved satisfactory in function it is advisable to leave well alone. However, where there are free-ending saddles opposing edentulous segments, where cusp interferences can be diagnosed or where overerupted natural teeth may have a disturbing effect on the prostheses, alterations may be necessary to the existing natural teeth. Bilateral or unilateral balanced occlusion and articulation may be desirable in order to preserve stability of the partial dentures in these cases. It is emphasized, however, that the decision has to be made when planning the denture.

For *reconstruction of the natural dentition*, articulation requirements are those which will reduce parafunctional articulation to a minimum. Disclusion by anterior guidance gives this protection but each case must be planned according to its pre-existing tooth positions and occlusal scheme. In addition, emphasis is laid on the desirability of a reproducible intercuspal position at which intercuspal occlusion is developed with stable contact relationships. These factors will be discussed further in Chapter 11.

Pros and cons of balanced articulation

By way of review, some aspects of this topic will be discussed. The three categories of articulation have to be seen as objectives in treatment rather than as diagnosable features of the existing natural dentition. Ideal occlusion and articulation is seen by some as incorporating one or other of these articulation schemes but seldom does one see any of these categories of articulation in an untreated mouth. The most desirable feature of articulation in the natural dentition is freedom from deflective cusp interferences, which will reduce to a minimum the adaptive jaw movements that may result from such interferences. Bilateral balanced articulation may promote non-working side interferences during mastication or parafunctional grinding; and even cross-tooth balance may provide a stimulus for such grinding. As an objective in treatment of the natural dentition, either by occlusal adjustment or by reconstruction, it may be necessary to adopt one or other of the schemes, and for this reason the classification serves a useful purpose.

In complete dentures, bilateral balanced articulation has few disadvantages. They will be more stable in the empty mouth where parafunctional grinding is inevitable at the outset of wearing the dentures. This awareness of stability promotes confidence in mastication and reduces tipping forces by cross-arch balance. There are two possible disadvantages of bilateral balanced articulation. First, it may tend to encourage lateral and protrusive grinding, although this habit may be confined to those people who are subject to irrelevant muscle activity. Secondly, it is difficult to achieve in mouths where an increased vertical incisor overlap is indicated, and it is better to retain the vertical overlap (as for a pre-existing class II, division 2 dentition) than to sacrifice it in order to achieve articular balance.

Features which influence articulation

An aspect of articulation which may help in the analysis of occlusal disturbances and in the planning of fixed or removable reconstruction procedures is that of the five anatomical features of the masticatory system that control the articulation. These are the guidances provided by the condyle movements, by the inclination of the lingual surfaces of the maxillary incisor and canine teeth, and by the height and shape of the posterior teeth cusps, together with the effect on these guidances of the inclination of the occlusal plane and the shape of the occlusal curve (Figure 5.12).

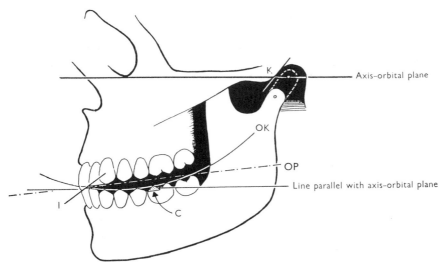

Figure 5.12 Articulation features. Protruded occlusion (by anterior guidance). K, Inclination of condyle path; I, inclination of labial surfaces of incisor teeth; C, inclination of posterior cusp ridges; OP, inclination of occlusal plane; OK, curvature of occlusal curve. (Adapted from Posselt, 1962)

Condyle guidance (K)

This is the inclination of the paths which the condyles follow when making protrusive or lateral protrusive movements. It represents the angle of downward and forward movement of the condyles relative to the axis–orbital plane. The angle of lateral protrusion (of the orbiting condyle) is slightly steeper than that made when both condyles move in forward protrusion. The governing factors of these movements are a combination of the directions of muscle pull and the shape of the articular eminences. These guidances are estimated as being independent of the effects of tooth contact. During articulation of the teeth, they are interdependent. It should also be remembered that there is a rotation of the condyle axis while these movements are taking place. Registration of this guidance, independent of tooth contact, should be made before teeth are prepared or, in the case of complete dentures, before teeth are set on bases. It can then be said to be an unalterable factor.

Incisal guidance (I)

This is the angle which the lingual surfaces of the maxillary incisor teeth make with the axis–orbital plane. It influences the protrusive articular movement and is interdependent with the condylar guidances. The canines exert a similar influence when the lateral protrusive movements are performed. In denture and reconstruction procedures these guidances can be altered.

Christensen's phenomenon
When the mandible moves in protrusion without the influence of incisor guidance, a separation occurs between the posterior teeth which has a characteristic shape.

This is known as Christensen's phenomemon (Christensen, 1905), and is best demonstrated when the maxillary and mandibular occlusal planes are replaced by flat occlusal rims, as used when making a jaw registration for complete dentures (Figure 5.13). Compensation for this phenomenon in the provision of balanced articulation may be made by adjustment of the features, except condyle guidance.

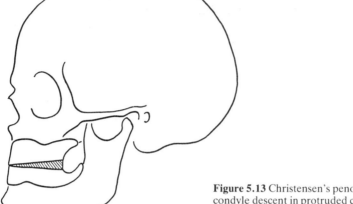

Figure 5.13 Christensen's penomenon. The gap created by condyle descent in protruded contact of occlusal rims

Resultant effect of condyle and incisal guidances

The constancy of the condyle movements is debatable since they are determined by muscles and are therefore subject to adaptation. When freed from tooth contacts, it is likely that they move in reproducible paths and this can be shown to be so in the border movements. It should also be remembered that the condyles are in contact with the menisci in all movements and the menisci are in contact with the fossae and articular eminences. Articular tooth contacts guide the movements and the condyles will usually adapt. None the less, it is worth making some theoretical observations on the relationships between the two guidances that have a bearing on setting the teeth for complete dentures. There are four possibilities.

1. When no incisal guidance exists, the mandible in protrusion will follow a curved path (with the convexity of the arc facing upwards), as in the Christensen phenomenon. This will occur with edge-to-edge incisor relation or with a marked horizontal overlap.
2. When the incisal and condylar guidances are the same, the mandible will move on a straight path.
3. When the incisal guidance is greater than that of the condyle, the mandible will move on a curved path with the arc facing downwards.
4. When the incisal guidance is less than that of the condyle, the mandible will move on a curved path with the arc facing upwards.

The practical significance of these theoretical considerations lies in the effect the curved path will have on the cusp relations of the posterior teeth while they are in articular contact.

Cusp height and inclinations (C)

These factors are interdependent with the condyle and incisal guidances during protrusive and lateral articular movements. They can be altered in denture and reconstruction procedures, but there are limits to these alterations.

The inclination of the occlusal plane (OP)

This is the inclination of an imaginary plane touching the incisal edges of the mandibular incisors and/or canines and the distobuccal cusps of the mandibular second molars. This is also called the plane of orientation and has considerable influence in the setting of lower teeth for complete dentures.

The curvature of the occlusal surfaces (OK)

This is an imaginary curve joining the mandibular buccal and canine cusps in the sagittal plane. A maxillary occlusal curve also exists and when the teeth are in intercuspal occlusion the maxillary curve is below the mandibular curve. Both are subject to correction in the natural and artificial dentitions.

Interdependence

The interdependence of the five articulation features was first described by Hanau in his curiously named Quint (Schlosser and Gehl, 1953). Thielemann subsequently simplified Hanau's factors by expressing them in the formula for balanced articulation: $(K \times I)/(OP \times C \times OK)$. This formula is of value when setting the teeth for complete dentures and where bilateral balanced articulation is planned. If, for example, the first setting of the teeth results in the separation of the posterior teeth on protrusion, balance between the posterior teeth can be achieved by raising the occlusal plane (OP), increasing the cusp heights (C) or deepening the occlusal curve (OK). Since the occlusal plane is determined largely by considerations of the tongue position, and the cusp height by the manufacturers of artificial teeth, the alteration made is usually that of the occlusal curve. Alternatively, the incisal guidance can be reduced or removed by advancing the incisors but the position and inclination of the incisors is determined by the factors of lip and tongue posture and activity and that of appearance.

Bilateral balance in lateral protrusive movements is also influenced by an imaginary occlusal curve in the coronal and sagittal planes, sometimes referred to as Monson's curve, with the convexity facing upwards (Figure 5.14). This curve determines the coronal and sagittal inclinations of the posterior teeth. In the lateral movements, it helps to establish the non-working side contacts while the working side mandibular cusps slide through the maxillary marginal ridge gaps. Thus, the non-working path of movement is curved while the working path is more horizontal, as determined by the lateral (or Bennett) shift of the working side condyle.

In certain natural dentitions where occlusal wear is excessive this curve becomes reversed and the convexity faces downwards. This may be the effect of wear by a fibrous or sand-containing diet which acts more forcefully on the supporting cusps. Where the consistency of the diet is not a factor in the wear of the teeth, however, the coronal curve generally retains its upwards facing convexity.

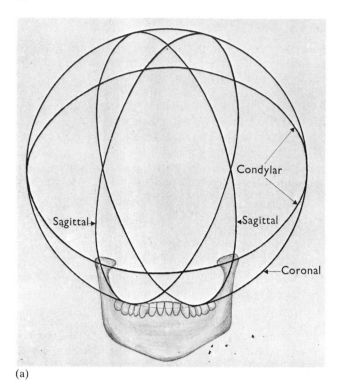

(a)

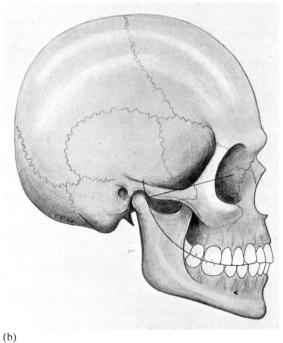

(b)

Figure 5.14 (a) Monson's curves. (b) Monson's sagittal curve with estimated 4-inch (10-cm) radius

Monson's spherical theory of occlusion

Monson (1932) proposed the theory that the centre of a sphere with a radius of approximately 4 inches (10 cm) is equidistant from the occlusal surfaces of the posterior teeth and from the centres of the condyles. He claimed that the long axes of the posterior teeth form extensions of radii from the centre of this sphere (Figure 5.14b). This is an extension of Bonwill's 'triangle' observations and the theory was applied by Wadsworth (1925), Mann and Pankey (1960) and others, in order to find the occlusal curve of the posterior teeth in complete dentures and reconstruction procedures. The application of this mechanistic approach has proved successful in many hands but the principle should be used warily in practice. The variations in bone and tooth size and in the relations which exist between maxillary and mandibular bones make it unrealistic to expect that all occlusal curves will perform natural functions if set on an arc of a circle whose radius is the distance between one condyle and the median contact point of the mandibular incisors. But the principle should not be discarded for this reason alone. In practice, errors will be reduced if the other factors in the analysis of form, relations and function are borne in mind.

Further references

The relations between the angles of condylar movements and those of the teeth (both anterior and posterior) have been a preoccupation of mathematically minded dentists for over a century. Bonwill's triangle has already been mentioned and Balkwill (1886) has left his mark in this field by describing the angle between the occlusal plane and Bonwill's triangle. This angle was said to have an effect on the setting of the artificial teeth and Balkwill's observations have been repeated (and criticized) by Kohler (1929), Hart (1939) and Bergström (1950). A mathematical study on the variations of Balkwill's angle and how these variations might influence cusp angles was made by Christensen (1960). This study refers to the Christensen angle (Christensen, 1958), which is that between the two flat occlusal planes in Christensen's phenomenon. There would seem to be an interdependence between this angle and the difference between the condyle guidance and Balkwill's angle. Christensen (1959) also concluded that cusp angles in complete dentures should be inversely proportional to the height of Bonwill's triangle. Such studies are not, perhaps, for the average student but they provide information which has been deduced from observations of human mandibles and their articulator copies. They should not be discounted because they are difficult to understand. Bergström's (1950) monograph on the reproduction of dental articulation is a classic of its kind and is required reading for those seriously interested in articulators. Weinberg (1959) made a study of the 'guidance system' of the mandible and its influence on the occlusal plane and cusp angles in the protrusive movement. He was careful to point out that only the mesiodistal cusp inclines were observed and suggested that the protrusive movement could be copied on an articulator provided that certain shortcomings of transfer methods were corrected.

Comment

These anatomical features and their geometrical applications are developmental in origin and only the incisal guidance can be altered (by the orthodontist) without removing or reshaping the tooth surfaces. In the stable adult dentition these features may seem to have a limiting effect on the articulation and, when replacements by artificial teeth have to be made, care should be taken before making any alteration to them. Sometimes the enemy of good is better. Stability of replacements depends partly on mechanical balance during articular movements but also on an accurate copy of the natural predecessors so that the orofacial musculature can maintain its endogenous activity without interferences from altered incisal guidances, cusp heights and the levels and curves of the occlusal plane.

Comfort and efficiency in the occlusion and articulation of natural teeth is the rule rather than the exception. Most people are unaware of their chewing ability, of the position where their teeth meet or if they meet. When changes come and losses have to be made good, it is not always easy to restore the natural positions and contours of the teeth and their functions with the means and materials available. Levels of occlusion, occlusal shapes and inclinations of the teeth do require accurate replacement, however, if patterns of articulation are to be retained. The empirical attempts at replacement, often made with the best intentions and in the most difficult of circumstances, do not always succeed in this objective and disturbances can result. It is therefore desirable to have a knowledge of these patterns so that in each patient good occlusal function can be maintained or restored.

References

Arstad, T. (1956) Capsular ligaments of the temporomandibular joint and retrusion facets of the dentition in relationship to the mandibular movements (Book review). *Journal of the American Dental Association Dental Cosmos*, **52**, 519

Balkwill, F. H. (1886) Form and arrangement of artificial teeth for mastication. *British Journal of Dental Science*, **9**, 278

Bergström, G. (1950) On the reproduction of the dental articulation by means of articulators. *Acta Odontologica Scandinavica*, **9** (supplement 4)

Bonwill, W. G. A. (1887) The geometrical and mechanical laws of the articulation of the human teeth–the anatomical articulator. *American System of Dentistry*, **3**, 486

Christensen, C. (1905) The problem of the bite. *Dental Cosmos*, 1184

Christensen, F. T. (1958) Cusp angulation for complete dentures. *Journal of Prosthetic Dentistry*, **8**, 910

Christensen, F. T. (1959) Effect of Bonwill's triangle on complete dentures. *Journal of Prosthetic Dentistry*, **9**, 791

Christensen, F. T. (1960) Balkwill's angle for complete dentures. *Journal of Prosthetic Dentistry*, **10**, 95

D'Amico, A. (1961) Functional occlusion of the natural teeth in man. *Journal of Prosthetic Dentistry*, **11**, 899

Fish, G. P. (1917) Some engineering principles of possible interest to orthodontists. *Dental Cosmos*, **59**, 881

Gysi, A. (1910) The problem of articulation. *Dental Cosmos*, **52**, 268

Gysi, A. (1913) The problem of dental articulators. *British Dental Journal*, **34**, (i) 213; (ii) 270; (iii) 367; (iv) 416; (v) 712

Hart, F. L. (1939) Full denture construction. *Journal of the American Dental Association Dental Cosmos*, **26**, 455.

Kohler, L. (1929) Die Volparthese. In *Handbuch der Zahnheilkunde* (eds Scheff and Pichler), Urban and Schwarzenberg, Berlin, Vol. IV, p. 286

Lewin, A. (1970a) The direction of tooth movement within the periodontal space. The omnidirectional transducer. *Journal of the Dental Association of South Africa*, **Sept.**, 308; **Oct.**, 333

Lewin, A. (1970b) The direction of tooth movement in response to masticatory forces. *Journal of Dental Research*, **49**, 699

Lundeen, H. C. (1971) Occlusal morphologic considerations for fixed restorations. *Dental Clinics of North America*, **15**, 649

Mann, A. W. and Pankey, L. D. (1960) Oral rehabilitation. Part I. Use of P-M instrument. *Journal of Prosthetic Dentistry*, **10**, 135; Part II. Reconstruction using functionally generated path. *Journal of Prosthetic Dentistry*, **10**, 151

Monson, G. S. (1932) Applied mechanics to the theory of mandibular movements. *Dental Cosmos*, **74**, 1039

Mühlmann, H. R. (1967) Tooth mobility. A review of clinical aspects and research findings. *Journal of Periodontology*, **38**, 686.

Nairn, R. I. (1973) Lateral and protrusive occlusions. *Journal of Dentistry*, **1**, 4

Parfitt, G. J. (1967) The physical analysis of the tooth-supporting structures. In *The Mechanisms of Tooth Support. A Symposium*, Wright, Bristol, p. 154

Picton, D. C. A. (1962a) Tilting movements of teeth during biting. *Journal of Dental Research*, **41**, 1252

Picton, D. C. A. (1962b) Vertical tooth mobility in man. *Dental Practitioner and Dental Record*, **12**, 406

Posselt, U. (1962) *Physiology of Occlusion and Rehabilitation*, Blackwell, Oxford

Schlosser, R. O. and Gehl, D. H. (1953) *Complete Denture Prosthesis*, Saunders, Philadelphia, p. 247

Schuyler, C. H. (1935) Fundamental principles in the correction of occlusal dysharmony, natural and artificial. *American Dental Association Journal*, **22**, 1193

Wadsworth, F. (1925) A practical system of denture prosthesis. *Dental Cosmos*, **67**, 670

Weinberg, L. A. (1959) Incisal and condylar guidance in relation to cuspal inclination in lateral excursions. *Journal of Prosthetic Dentistry*, **9**, 851

Chapter 6

Functions of the masticatory system

Functions of the masticatory system which involve the occlusion and articulation of the teeth are those of incision, mastication and swallowing. The teeth are also involved in the functions of respiration, the provision of a lip seal, speech and facial expression, although not necessarily in contact. Since these functions can affect or be affected by the occlusal and articular relations it is worth considering the movements which produce them and what happens when they are altered.

General

Most voluntary actions become involuntary with continued use but are subject to alteration by a response to stimuli either reflexly or by intention. The muscles providing the actions conform to an endogenously determined pattern initiated and sustained by both cerebral and reflex stimuli. The function of walking is generally considered as an involuntary action and the gait can be as characteristic of an individual as the features. If a stone gets into the shoe, a reflex protective limp is the immediate response to this noxious stimulus. If an unexpected drop in the ground is encountered, two adaptive possibilities may result: a stumble or a fall may occur and both can cause injury to muscle fibres almost anywhere from the neck to the ankle; alternatively, a bending of the knee, quickly performed, may restore normal gait and movement without harm, as the skilled footballer or skier knows. The gait can also be altered by a voluntary decision to do so, either, say, to slow down, to turn or even to affect a limp.

The involuntary gait is produced by the coordinated contraction and reciprocal relaxation of groups of muscles in a manner which produces the movement as efficiently and economically as possible. The minimum of effort is expended and the activity can be maintained almost indefinitely, depending on the health of the walker, of his individual muscles, and of the tissues covering his feet, either natural or artificial. This analogy can be applied to the masticatory system, the functions of which will now be discussed.

Incision

The incision of food is performed by a combination of rotary opening and protrusive movements of the mandible and the closing movement on the bolus is reflexly controlled by the consistency of the food and the relationship of the maxillary and mandibular incisor teeth. A smooth movement is the objective and contact between the teeth is either light and gliding or is avoided. If the incisor tooth positions and relationships are stable in relation to each other and to the orofacial muscles, the function of incision becomes involuntary, efficient and economical of effort. If the positions and relationships of the incisor teeth are not stable and premature contacts on incision take place, reflex adaptive movements will occur to avoid the uncomfortable contacts. Either these will succeed and the muscles may tire or the teeth will be traumatized. If these teeth are lost, the closing incisive movements will be inhibited and will have to be re-established when artificial teeth are replaced. The movement patterns of the mandible and the relationships of the teeth are therefore interdependent. Incisive parafunctional movements are common and these cause wear on the teeth or injury to the apical periodontal tissues (see Figure 7.6). They may also cause fatigue in the muscles.

Mastication

The act of chewing food prepares it for swallowing and involves the activities of the lips, cheeks and tongue, the mandibular joints, the palate, the secretions of the salivary glands, and the teeth with their supporting tissues. Coordinating these activities is the neuromuscular function which receives the stimuli of the bolus and responds by moving the mandible so that the teeth shred the food. Mastication is, and probably always has been, an enjoyment for the majority of people. It involves the five senses in turn. There is the call to food, the smell and the sight of it. There is the first touch and the taste of it. Then begins the neuromuscular activity which provides the complex, sensual and generally efficient function of preparing the food for digestion. The saliva having soaked the bolus, the tongue, lips and cheeks load the food on to the posterior segments of the mandibular teeth. The bolus is often divided into two portions, allowing bilateral chewing. During this function, stimuli from the bolus are being continuously received by the periodontal receptors and the reflex responses determine the amount and force of further mastication required. The value of two complete arches for the dentition in occlusion is not in doubt and in mastication this property provides the added advantage of containing the food bolus within the arches. Missing teeth can make mastication difficult by allowing food to pass through the arches into the vestibular regions where it has to be retrieved by the tongue. Also a more convenient platform for shredding has to be found. This entails further muscle activity which can lead to fatigue, to altered and to impaired function.

There are three main variables in mastication that make it difficult to determine what constitutes normal mastication. These are: first, the amount of mastication carried out per individual; secondly, the preference, if any, for one side or the other; and, thirdly, the contact, if any, between the teeth.

The amount of mastication

This can be observed by counting the number of jaw closures or, say, by watching a mark on the chin. The patient himself may be able to provide an answer and, if carefully phrased, information from groups of people can provide helpful data for this aspect of mastication, especially if related to numbers of teeth and efficiency of occlusions and articulations.

Side preferred

The side on which chewing is preferred, or whether both sides are used, can also be useful information to have when considering the cause of mandibular joint or facial pain. This variable is affected by the number and symmetry of the teeth present. However, Posselt (1961) made a study of side preference in mastication in people with complete natural dentitions and found that only 10 per cent chewed on both sides simultaneously and 12 per cent restricted themselves to one side. The remainder chewed alternatively left and right. There was no suggestion of any association with being right or left handed in the side preferred. Hildebrand's (1931) original work on this subject still provides a standard of investigation.

Studies by Hedegard, Lundberg and Wictorin (1968, 1969, 1971) on the position of the bolus and duration of the masticatory cycle, using cineradiography, are a helpful contribution to the understanding of this function.

Loss of teeth will affect the pattern of chewing, as will the side preferred, but it does not follow that the side with the greater number of opposing teeth is the side preferred. This can be explained by a well-established conditioned pattern of chewing being preferred to a greater number of opposing teeth. If mastication is unilateral, it is sometimes reported that contact seems to take place on the side not being used (the non-working side); if this contact is a sudden lateral occlusion as opposed to a sliding articulation, the point of occlusion will act as a fulcrum around which the mandible will momentarily rotate and the muscle adaptation required may be such as to cause torn fibres and pain. This can also happen when a hard piece of food is unexpectedly encountered on the side being used for chewing (the working side). These sudden tilts of the mandible in the coronal plane are potentially harmful. Simultaneous bilateral mastication performed without haste remains the more desirable method of function as a preventive against disturbance of the system.

Tooth contact

During mastication tooth contact remains a controversial variable. Studies on this subject using transmitting devices from teeth are a study in themselves and a bibliography can be found at the end of this chapter. They appear to establish that contacts do take place during mastication in both lateral and protrusive chewing movements as well as in intercuspal position. This may contradict the information from patients questioned on this aspect of masticatory function who are often unaware of the contacts. Further, it is doubtful if the presence of ingenious devices, however miniature, represents a mouth in natural function. It would seem desirable that contemporary diet be masticated by cusps and ridges passing close to fossae and fissures without their touching. Thus the food is shredded, not ground, and subsequently reduced to pulp by the addition of saliva. When ready for swallowing, the bolus is almost liquid and can often be swallowed without occlusion of the teeth. It is more usual, however, for intercuspal occlusion to take place prior to the swallow. Perhaps the sanest comment on this topic was made by H. Beyron (personal communication) who pointed out that even a thin layer of food between the teeth acts indirectly as a transmitting contact. This contact will vary in force and can act protectively against tooth contact.

Tooth contacts during mastication are acknowledged from patients, however, on working and non-working sides and usually take place following recent extractions when adjacent teeth have become repositioned. Their cusps then present targets for initial or premature contacts in function as well as in parafunction. Further causes of contact in mastication are the overcontoured restoration (supracontact) and the overerupted tooth, particularly the unopposed third molar. Contoured restorations may provide good intercuspal occlusion in the empty mouth but may offer initial contacts in lateral or protrusive mastication due to failure to allow for these movements on the articulator.

These contacts in habitual function are difficult to identify, since closing contacts in the empty mouth are not necessarily those which occur when food is present and it is in the empty mouth that the clinician has to make his observations and diagnosis. Removal of premature and initial contacts in the empty mouth movements, however, have often served to improve comfort and efficiency in function. Emphasis is placed on the need for accuracy in procedures concerned with adjusting the teeth and these will be discussed in Chapter 10.

The more efficient the occlusion and articulation between the teeth, the less they need touch in mastication. The analogy of a robin picking up seed from a stone path may illustrate this precept. Although the action is impressively fast there is no apparent contact between beak and path as the seed is grasped. We are not robins, it is true, and we do not peck our meals from stone paths, but the incidence in robins of beak wear, neck pain and joint disturbances would seem to be low and the example is good.

Incoming and outgoing articular movements

When the mandible moves during mastication the mandibular teeth move from the various open positions towards, but not reaching intercuspal position and thence to the opening movements. Contact may take place as intercuspal occlusion is approached and this articulation acts as a guide. Articulation may occur as the mandible moves away from intercuspal position but probably for no more than 2 mm before and after IP. On the other hand, parafunctional grinding habits may begin at IP and move outwards. These movements are similar to those made at the command of the dentist while investigating the articulation of the teeth. But they are not natural movements nor functions and this may explain the difficulty which many patients experience in performing lateral articular movements on request.

Condyle and cusp guidances

In spite of the limitations placed on condyle movements by the shape of the articular eminence and the close contact which the condyle maintains with the meniscus during all its movements, it would seem that the cusp inclinations direct the masticatory movements and the condyles adapt to them. It is easier for the condyles to alter their paths of movement than for the teeth to become repositioned. This is not to assert that the various angles of condyle movements have no significance. On the contrary, these movements have optimal directions and curves and the more accurately the articular relations between the teeth conform to these directions and curves the more harmonious will be the functions of the system. These guidances are interrelated and whereas the dictum 'teeth direct and muscles adapt' is justifiable, the primary response in all systems is adaptation.

Adaptation

This phenomenon of muscle activity is well known and when applied to mastication it refers to the reflex activity which takes place when changes in the consistency of the bolus are encountered and when occlusal contacts occur during mastication. The stretch reflex is produced when closure of the mandible encounters an unexpectedly hard object in the food and, less obviously, a premature contact is avoided in mastication. Neuromuscular adaptation also includes the responses made to missing posterior teeth. The responses by the tissues of the masticatory system to missing teeth, and whether to replace them, will be discussed in the section on partial dentures in Chapter 12. Mastication requirements are fulfilled by the tongue, lips and cheeks and by the postural masticatory muscles to provide chewing by the incisor teeth. Adaptation is a term that can also be applied to responses to injury, ageing and disease. Thus, all tissues in the masticatory system demonstrate adaptation. In addition to those mentioned, there are the responses of the pulp and cementum to loss of the occlusal surfaces by attritional wear, the responses of the periodontal tissues to toxins and to drift of the teeth, and the responses of the dentoalveolar tissues as a whole to the functionless tooth.

Adaptation and disorder

In the majority of adaptive movements or tissue changes the responses are well tolerated but there are occasions when a pathological response is induced. For example, pain can be experienced in abraded dentine, periodontal breakdown can lead to inflammatory responses, altered muscle activity can result in injured or fatigued muscles, and hyperactivity of muscles can result in grinding habits on interfering cusps. These unfavourable responses can all take place during mastication or in the empty mouth.

Associated muscular activities

The muscular activities of the system during mastication include those of maintaining posture of the head in relation to the shoulders and back and of the mandible in relation to the clavicle and sternum. In normal circumstances the head is kept relatively stationary during mastication but encounters with resistant food or uncomfortable occlusal contacts can lead to movements of the head which involve the neck, shoulder and even back muscles in adaptive movements. If these movements are sudden, especially if the back is unsupported, disturbances in any of the muscles from the sacrum to the sternum can be the result. Consequently, it is always advisable to suggest that the back be adequately supported while eating, the shoulders relaxed and the head maintained in comfortable posture. This supported posture is a good preventive measure against the sudden changes of muscle activity required from time to time during mastication.

Electrognathographics

The use of electronic methods for registering mandibular movements during various functions has been developed by Lewin (1985). He has constructed 'configurations of antennae' that are attached to the head and which establish planes of reference for relaying details of movement from a small magnet attached to the mandible. The device is known as a sirognathograph and the details of jaw movements recorded are electrognathographics; all this in the absence of intraoral clamps, clutches or wires. Patients from local practitioners, students, undergraduates and postgraduates have participated in research programmes at the dental school of Witwatersrand University in order to establish baselines for function and dysfunction. The result is a comparatively short book containing instructions for use (with clear diagrams), studies of border movement potential, of patterns of mandibular movement in both frontal and sagittal planes and the superimposition of one on the other. Anomalies in rhythm, pattern width, zones of mastication and speech, all with sample recordings are presented. The value of such a diagnostic instrument could be considerable.

Deglutition

The term 'deglutition' covers the four stages of swallowing, from the preparation of the bolus within the mouth, the passage of the bolus from the mouth to the pharynx, through the pharynx, to its subsequent descent through the pharyngeal sphincter into the oesophagus. This function is initiated voluntarily, by the bolus being placed on the tongue while the tip of the tongue is supported by the lingual surfaces of the incisor teeth and anterior surface of the hard palate. The second stage is also under voluntary control and consists of closure of the teeth into intercuspal occlusion, followed by contraction of the muscles at the tip of the tongue. Thirdly, the stability instituted by this contraction and by the mandible in intercuspal position allows the subsequent wave of muscle contractions in the tongue to take place reflexly and this forces the bolus into the pharynx. Finally, the subsequent movements and passage of the bolus into the oesophagus all take place reflexly and the phenomenon of peristalsis is set in motion. This continues until the food reaches the stomach.

The teeth in swallowing

The part played by the teeth is that of stabilizing the mandible in stage two; it is possible for the tongue to take over this function and to provide the dual function of holding the bolus and stabilizing the mandible. Here, the tongue is stabilized against the maxillary teeth or sides of the hard palate. This has been referred to as *infantile* (or *visceral*) swallowing and takes place before the teeth erupt and also when the mouth becomes edentulous and dentures are not worn. *Somatic* swallowing is the term given to a tooth-stabilized swallow.

Infantile swallowing takes place in dentulous mouths where it is uncomfortable to bring the teeth together, either for reasons of carious or sensitively abraded teeth or where initial contacts are markedly deflective. It is also used when swallowing liquids. This type of swallowing is also associated with an incompetent lip seal where the tongue is thrust forwards to contact the lips or tips of the incisor teeth in order to make the seal necessary for a closed mouth during deglutition. The adaptive movement required repeatedly by the mandible for this function can lead to discomfort in the muscles around the mandibular joints.

It is often claimed that the occlusion attempted for the act of swallowing is on the retruded axis and if intercuspal occlusion is not possible on this axis retruded contact is followed by a forward slide into the habitual intercuspal position. If this forward slide has a lateral component, the disharmony of activity produce lateral pterygoid muscles can produce pain in one or other of these muscl 'retrusion facets' on the posterior teeth observed by Arstad (1956), and to in many dentitions, could be caused by this slide between retruded and habitual occlusion during the swallow. It is likely that retrude' occlusion is attempted when an effort is required to stabilize the mandible, either when the food has been incompletely chewed prior to swallowing or when there is not enough to swallow. It is suggested that retruded intercuspal occlusion is the natural objective in the swallow but that alterations in cusp–fossa or cusp–ridge relations in the contemporary developing dentition rarely make it possible. Consequently, the mandible slides forwards or laterally until intercuspal occlusion is reached. It is true that when intercuspal occlusion occurs on the retruded axis it is both efficient and reproducible. It is also true that an element of effort is necessary to produce it. It may be that it is this effort which discourages parafunctional closure in this position. The observations of Reynolds (1970) on 50 caries-free complete dentitions indicated that facets of wear occurred least in mouths which demonstrated retruded intercuspal occlusion. He coupled this feature with disclusion by the incisors and canines in the lateral and protrusive articular movements.

It is only during the act of swallowing that teeth come together in functional intercuspal occlusion: all other intercuspal closures are parafunctional. It is therefore a function of considerable significance and the mandibular position at which it is achieved should be observed carefully in all analyses of masticatory function and re-established with care when prostheses are being made.

Respiration

Together with the heart beat and the circulation of the blood, the function of respiration is the first muscular activity that takes place after birth. The circulatory musculature has been active in embryo, although provided by a different kind of muscle. It cannot be brought under voluntary control. On the other hand, respiration can be voluntarily controlled and intercuspal occlusion may take place when difficulty in nasal breathing is encountered. This constitutes a parafunctional activity and may result in fatigue. During natural respiration the mandible is in rest position and the lips are together. Any obstruction to nasal breathing which results in mouth breathing does not necessarily alter the rest position. Competent lips can part without altering this position. Alternatively, incompetent lip posture does not necessarily imply oral breathing. Nasal breathing is generally adopted, if the airway is clear, irrespective of lip seal. An obvious exception to this is the oral breathing required during strenuous activity. If a race has to be won or an opponent tackled, a justifiable parafunction may be indulged. The association of pain around the joint with these activities is not uncommon.

Obstructions to nasal respiration will call for modifications to masticatory movements since breathing has to be performed through the mouth. The maintenance of a lip seal will be difficult if not impossible and the swallow may have to be infantile.

Lip seal

As has been said, the adoption of a lip seal is a physiological requirement for the comfort of a moist mouth. If this cannot be adopted because of tooth positions and relationships and it becomes necessary to place the mandible forwards in order to achieve the seal, an intermittent change of posture is the result. The change is between the mandible at rest position and at the habitual position required to achieve lip seal, that is, between the physiological needs for minimal activity and a comfortable interior to the mouth. This change can involve the postural muscles (the lateral pterygoids and temporales) in sudden changes of pattern which can cause pain. Articular contacts can take place in these changes of posture and cause deflective movements which, because they are sudden and unexpected, can add to the potentially harmful responses in the muscles mentioned.

Speech

The closest speaking space

One of the recognized methods of assessing the correct positions and relations of the incisor teeth is by noting how closely they come together in speech. In class I jaw relation cases with stable incisor relations, the tips of the maxillary and mandibular incisor teeth should approximate as closely as possible, without touching, when 's' sounds are spoken. This is known as the 'closest speaking space' and was introduced by Silverman (1953) as a method for assessing the vertical relation in the construction of complete dentures. In his book on *Occlusion* (1962), Silverman noted the variations in closest speaking space in the natural dentitions of 208 patients and this space varied between 0 and 10 mm, measured in the incisor regions. There was therefore no average space between individuals and the space varied in the same individual depending on the sounds used. It is, however, a valuable piece of information to have as a permanent record of the natural dentition and which should be duplicated in the artificial dentition if this becomes necessary. The closest speaking space is a measurement of the vertical dimension of the face (Figure 6.1).

The clinical application of the closest speaking space is twofold. Firstly, in functional analysis of occlusal contacts: the patient is asked to read a passage which includes 's', 'j', 'sh' and 'ch' sounds. These sounds bring the teeth closely together both anteriorly (s) and posteriorly (j, sh, ch). For example, 'The church by the

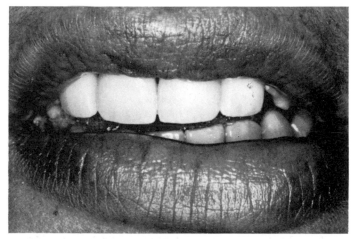

Figure 6.1 Closest-speaking space: 's' sound

Mississippi was judged to be the simplest on show' is read and the patient is asked if there were any tooth contacts while speaking. If so it is likely that premature contacts are present or, in the case of denture wearers, that the occlusal vertical dimension has been increased. Secondly, in the assessment of appearance the patient is asked to speak while watching himself in a mirror. Here it is preferable to have a large standing mirror at which both patient and dentist can look, standing side by side.

Speech tests are also of value in assessing the correct positions and alignment of the incisor teeth in relation to the lips and tongue. The 'f' and 'v' sounds produce contact between lower lip and maxillary teeth and the 't' and 'th' sounds are produced by the contact between the tip of the tongue and the lingual surfaces of the maxillary incisor teeth and anterior part of the hard palate. Two such sentences are given for these tests: 'The first victim was found visibly fainting' and 'The tip of the tongue, the lips, the teeth tell the sounds'. Careful listening is required to assess whether there is an excess of air escaping, or perhaps a blockage to the production of the sounds. In the natural dentition any malalignment of teeth will have produced muscle adaptation so as to make the sounds approximate those of the local dialect. In the artificial dentition these sounds can produce a useful guide for the alignment of the incisor teeth and the shape of the palate when there are no pre-extraction records.

Facial expression

The significance of the teeth in facial expression needs no emphasis. From the gnashing of teeth in youthful rage to the edentulous hollow of senility there is a lifetime of communication and expression. There are few better boosts to the morale than porcelain crowns for middle-aged incisors, and few sights more calculated to deflate it than the mirror's evidence of discoloration and disease.

Faulty occlusal relationships, particularly in the incisor segments, can affect facial expression. A loose or rotated tooth can cause interferences which will inhibit or alter the activities of the lip muscles playing their many parts in the function of communication. Other involvements of the occlusion in the manifestations of facial expressions are largely parafunctional but may require diagnosis and treatment.

There are, of course, many other functions performed by the tissues of the masticatory system and these include holding, cutting, carrying, breaking, licking, tasting, identifying and, if necessary, digging. The teeth can be used as weapons, the mouth for exchange of affection. A group of dentists and an invited anthropologist once listed thirty-four uses for these tissues and, whether they were parafunctional or atavistic, it was agreed that they were potentially harmful to the teeth, the muscles and the joints. In general, dentists are advised to miss no opportunity of warning their patients of the dangers to this system of abusing their teeth and advising them to avoid contact between the teeth except when preparing to swallow.

Criteria for occlusion

By way of revision, lists of criteria for good occlusion and occlusal function will be given. The adjective 'good' is preferred to 'normal' and 'ideal', which tend to emphasize the more static and structural relationships between the teeth.

The adjectives 'normal', 'ideal' or even 'natural' are not easy to define when applied to occlusion. Posselt (1962) emphasized the difficulty by separating 'normal' from 'no longer normal', since such changes as wear, loosening and loss of teeth are continuously taking place. He suggested that the word 'ideal' could be used to represent the specific, perhaps theoretical, requirements of optimal occlusal function. Ramfjord and Ash (1972) have elaborated on this theme in their book on *Occlusion* and have listed some requirements for ideal occlusion as a clinical objective for those patients who have a low tolerance to minor imperfections in occlusal contacts.

Thus, good occlusal function implies a range of acceptable contacts between the teeth during function, the absence of any disorders in the tissues of the masticatory system, and an adaptability to alterations as they occur. When this adaptability fails, and disorders result, it becomes necessary to recognize the disturbances causing the disorders and to correct them. A clinical objective of an occlusion designed to prevent all possible disturbances is then desirable and sometimes necessary. These criteria are based on the assumption of class I jaw and tooth relations but they apply equally to those dentitions where classes II(1) and (2) and III exist. Some further requirements will then be added for those mouths where a low degree of tolerance to developing changes and disturbances exists.

Criteria for good occlusion

1. Two complete arches of teeth with secure contact points and occlusal surface contours adequate for the functions required.
2. Root shape and alignment adequate to resist occlusal forces.
3. Rest position stable with adequate lip seal.
4. An interocclusal distance of 2–4 mm between rest position and intercuspal position.
5. Simultaneous and bilateral occlusion between all teeth of maxillary and mandibular arches at intercuspal position. No deflective contacts.
6. Simultaneous and bilateral occlusion on the retruded arc between one or more opposing posterior teeth.
7. Cusp–fossa and cusp–ridge occlusion having tripod contacts where possible.
8. Return of each tooth to its original position on removal of the occlusal force.
9. Articulation between retruded and intercuspal positions free from any interferences causing lateral deflexion.
10. Stable vertical and horizontal overlap.
11. Empty mouth articular movements free from deflective contacts.

Criteria for good occlusal function

1. Simultaneous bilateral mastication.
2. Light contact in intercuspal position while swallowing.
3. Incoming and outgoing chewing movements free from working or non-working side deflective contacts.
4. No adaptive chin or lip movements on swallowing.
5. No clenching or grinding (parafunctional) movements.
6. No joint noises in mastication or wide opening.
7. No deviation of mandible on wide opening.
8. No tooth contacts in speech or facial expression.
9. Pleasing appearance.

Further criteria for ideal occlusion

The adjective 'ideal' is used reluctantly and 'optimal' is equally unacceptable, since improvement on nature has nature to deal with. Alterations to natural function require acceptable adaptation. However, for mouths with a low tolerance to disturbances the following three criteria are suggested:

1. Intercuspal occlusion should take place on the retruded axis at a vertical level 2–4 mm above that of rest position.
2. All incoming articular movements to or outgoing movements from the retruded intercuspal occlusion should free all posterior tooth occlusion and should take place between the canines in lateral movements and between the incisors as a group in protrusive movements. This criterion implies that there are no sliding contacts between retruded and habitual occlusion. Thus, there is no habitual intercuspal occlusion; there is only retruded intercuspal occlusion.
3. All supporting cusps should occlude in opposing central fossae and each supporting cusp should have tripod contact with the opposing fossa. This criterion implies that there is no occlusion between cusps and opposing marginal ridges.

This is the concept of disclusion or mutually protected occlusion (see Chapter 5) and is currently believed to be the most protective for the function of the dentition. In order to produce it in the natural dentition, some degree of reconstruction or carefully planned occlusal adjustment is generally required. It seldom exists in the natural untreated dentition, although when it does, according to Reynolds (1970), much benefit accrues.

Considerable debate continues over the belief that this constitutes the ideal occlusal function. There are those who uphold the value of bilateral or unilateral balance in articular movements and of preserving a habitual intercuspal occlusion anterior to retruded intercuspal occlusion with free gliding movements between the two occlusions. This is the so-called *long centric* compromise for occlusal function, which serves to satisfy the ambivalently minded, but it promotes parafunctional movements in this long centric zone.

Comment

The majority of mouths examined in the course of dental practice show signs of occlusal disturbances but comparatively few require more than minor adjustments to improve and maintain good occlusal function. Nevertheless, it is desirable to have these criteria in mind so that treatment can be provided when disturbances result in disorders of the masticatory system.

References

Arstad, T. (1956) Retrusion facets (Book review). *Journal of the American Dental Association*, **52**, 519

Hedegard, B., Lundberg, M. and Wictorin, L. (1968) Masticatory function. A cineradiographic study. 1. Position of the bolus in denture cases. *Acta Odontologica Scandinavica*, **25**, 331

Hedegard, B., Lundberg, M. and Wictorin, L. (1969) Masticatory function. A cineradiographic study. 3. Position of the bolus in individuals with full complement natural teeth. *Acta Odontologica Scandinavica*, **26**, 213

Hedegard, B., Lundberg, M. and Wictorin, L. (1971) Masticatory function. A cineradiographic study. 4. Duration of the masticatory cycle. *Acta Odontologica Scandinavica*, **28**, 859

Hildebrand, G. Y. (1931) Studies in the masticatory movements of the human lower jaw. *Scandinavian Archives of Physiology*, 61

Lewin, A. (1985) *Electrognathographics*, Quintessence, Chicago

Posselt, U. (1961) Occlusal relationship in deglutition and mastication. *Transactions of the European Orthodontological Society*, **34**, 301

Posselt, U. (1962) *Physiology of Occlusion and Rehabilitation*, Blackwell, Oxford

Ramfjord, S. P. and Ash, M. (1972) *Occlusion*, 2nd edn, Saunders, Philadelphia

Reynolds, J. M. (1970) Occlusal wear facets. *Journal of Prosthetic Dentistry*, **24**, 367

Silverman, M. M. (1953) The speaking method in measuring vertical dimension. *Journal of Prosthetic Dentistry*, **3**, 193

Silverman, M. M. (1962) *Occlusion*, Mutual Publishing, Washington DC

Experimental tooth contacts in mastication

Adams, S. H. and Zander, H. A. (1964) Functional tooth contacts in lateral and centric occlusion. *Journal of the American Dental Association Dental Cosmos*, **69**, 465

Anderson, J. J. and Picton, D. C. A. (1957) Tooth contact during chewing. *Journal of Dental Research*, **36**, 21

Brewer, A. A. and Hudson, D. C. (1961) Application of miniaturised electronic devices to the study of tooth contact in complete dentures. *Journal of Prosthetic Dentistry*, **11**, 62

Gillings, B. R. D., Kohl, J. T. and Zander, H. A. (1963) Contact patterns using miniature radio transmitters. *Journal of Dental Research*, **42**, 177

Glickman, I., Pameijer, J. H. and Roeber, F. W. (1968) Intra-oral occlusal telemetry, 1. *Journal of Prosthetic Dentistry*, **19**, 60

Graf, H. and Zander, H. A. (1963) Tooth contact patterns in mastication. *Journal of Prosthetic Dentistry*, **13**, 1055

Jankelson, B., Hoffman, G. M. and Hendron, J. A. (1963) Physiology of the stomatognathic system. *Journal of the American Dental Association Dental Cosmos*, **46**, 375

Pameijer, J. H., Brion, M. and Glickman, I. (1970) Intra-oral occlusal telemetry, 4. *Journal of Prosthetic Dentistry*, **24**, 396

Pameijer, J. H., Glickman, I. and Roeber, F. W. (1968) Intra-oral occlusal telemetry, 2. *Journal of Prosthetic Dentistry*, **19**, 151

Panmeijer, J. H., Glickman, I. and Roeber, F. W. (1969) Intra-oral occlusal telemetry, 3. *Journal of Periodontology*, **40**, 253

Powell, R. N. and Zander, H. A. (1965) The frequency and distribution of tooth contact during sleep. *Journal of Dental Research*, **44**, 713

Schmidt, J. R. and Harrison, J. D. (1970) A method for simultaneous electromyographic and tooth contact recording. *Journal of Prosthetic Dentistry*, **24**, 387

Chapter 7

Disturbances and disorders

From the time they erupt, the teeth are subject to alteration of their occlusal surfaces and supporting tissues by caries, periodontal disease and wear. The shapes of the teeth, the bone that supports them and the spaces between them are genetically predetermined and these factors do not always provide for optimal function. The phenomenon of adaptation provides for the best function in most circumstances, but this is not always adequate for the health of the masticatory system. It is on this basis of disease, change and adaptation that the various disturbances and disorders will be considered.

A fine distinction may be said to exist between the terms 'disturbance', 'disorder' and 'disease' and it may be pedantic to separate them. But it is necessary, in considering the effects of function in the masticatory system, to be able to distinguish between an alteration or interruption of function and any breakdown which may be the result. It is necessary also to distinguish between these two conditions and disease itself, which is a pathological response to infection or tissue change.

Definitions of the two terms used in this book are therefore given as follows:

A *disturbance* is any interruption or alteration of the established occlusal function of the masticatory system.

A *disorder* is any response to a disturbance which causes a pathological change in the tissues of the masticatory system.

Disturbances in the masticatory system may be developmental or functional.

Developmental disturbances

Malocclusions

These are the result of a malrelationship between both growth and tooth size and position. They are classified according to the first molar relations (I, II and III), or as normal, prenormal and postnormal relations. They are also referred to as primary malocclusions, which arise in the developing dentition, as opposed to secondary malocclusions, which arise in the adult as a result of tooth loss and consequent adjacent tooth movement.

Disturbances resulting from primary malocclusions are as follows:

1. Overcrowding with consequent rotation of individual teeth or development of teeth inside or outside the arch. These disturbances can lead to cusp interferences and displacing activities of the mandible, although in the

developing dentition adaptation by tooth movement generally prevents this disturbance. Other consequential disturbances are unstable occlusal relations (cusp to cusp instead of cusp to fossa) and gingival disorders between the teeth due to insufficient room for the interdental epithelium.

2. Increased or decreased vertical overlap or horizontal overlap which can lead to unstable incisor function or the need for adaptive lip seal.
3. Deviation of upper and lower central midline which can indicate incisor interferences or cusp interferences in the posterior segments.

These disturbances often receive orthodontic treatment during adolescence. Unstable posterior cusp relations are occasionally a sequel of this treatment, however, and an occlusal analysis is recommended to ensure stability of the posterior segments in function.

Lack of development of the dentoalveolar tissues

This is generally seen in the posterior segments, uni- or bilaterally, and results in overclosure of the mandible, if bilateral, and unilateral lack of functional occlusion if restricted to one side (Figure 7.1a,b). These conditions constitute the posterior open bite. This disturbance can also occur in the upper anterior segment due to a lack of growth of the premaxillary bone.

Overdevelopment

Overgrowth of bone in the developmental regions of both condyles results in the anterior open bite (Figure 7.1c) or, if excessive, the acromegalic mandible. Such an overgrowth can also occur in the premaxilla bone.

Cleft palate and associated growth defects

These, and the corrective surgery performed for them, can present the orthodontist and prosthodontist with a well-known range of problems.

The response of the masticatory system to developmental disturbances is generally one of adaptation. As the growth and development of bone and the dentoalveolar tissues proceed, adaptation by tooth movement and muscle activity to these disturbances take place and disorders are uncommon. This is not always so, however, and the adolescent or young adult has to be watched for signs and symptoms of disorders resulting from developmental disturbances.

Functional disturbances

These are numerous but not so varied in origin as their number suggests. The list for consideration is as follows:

• Secondary malocclusions
• Unilateral and reduced function
• Supra- and infracontacts
• Loss of occlusal curve
• Unstable cusp relations
• Cusp interference

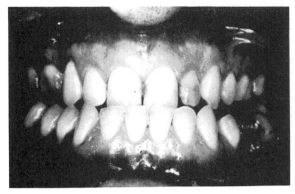

(a)

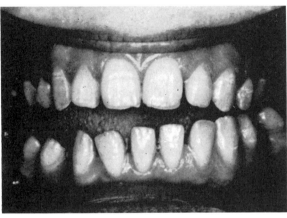

(b)

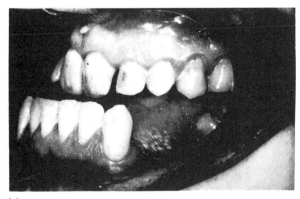

(c)

Figure 7.1 Developmental malocclusion. (a) Lack of development of buccal dentoalveolar tissues. Posterior 'open bite'. (b) Unilateral lack of development of buccal dentoalveolar tissues. (c) Mandibular overgrowth and 'anterior open bite'. Mandible in IP

- Alteration of intercuspal position
- Mandibular overclosure
- Parafunction (bruxism)
- Attrition of the occlusal surfaces
- Food impaction and the plunger cusp
- Denture disturbances.

These disturbances are inter-related and one is often the cause of another. They are conditions for which treatment is not always sought by the patient, and the dentist has to assess the need for treatment as a preventive measure against the development of disorders. They will be considered separately, although more than one is usually present.

Secondary malocclusions

These are altered tooth positions resulting from loss of one or more teeth or from periodontal disease. The loss of a tooth leads to migration of the adjacent tooth or teeth only if the occlusion between them and their opponents is insufficiently stable to prevent it. Some migration usually occurs until a stable occlusion is re-established and this can lead to one or more of the other disturbances. Overeruption of unopposed teeth in this situation is common although it can be prevented by the muscle forces of tongue or cheek (Figure 7.2a). Loss of periodontal support for the unopposed tooth is a common effect and can proceed to a disorder (see Figure 9.1b,c). It is particularly difficult to treat if a replacement for the missing tooth is planned (Figure 7.2b). A disturbance impossible to treat restoratively but not yet causing a disorder is illustrated in Figure 7.2c. An example of the unopposed tooth likely to cause a disorder of muscle or joint activity is that of the last molar tooth (Figure 7.2d,e). This patient had severe pain in the region of the right joint that subsided when the left third molar was extracted. Where periodontal disease is present, with or without loss of teeth, occlusal function can cause migration and further secondary malocclusion.

Unilateral and reduced function

Missing teeth, painful or sharp teeth, gingival or mucosal disorders can lead to mastication being confined to one side or even to the labial segment. Unilateral function in the complete dentition is, however, common enough to be considered normal and the association of being right or left 'handed' in mastication is sometimes claimed. This is not justified as a developmental factor since the two joints are connected to one bone. Adaptation to unilateral function is usually adequate to prevent disorders, but, conversely, the restoration of bilateral function is often a helpful treatment measure when pain in one or other joint region develops. An extension of this disturbance is lack of posterior tooth support which is commonly associated with the mandibular dysfunction syndrome. This can be manifest by the loss of one or more teeth in a buccal segment; and sometimes the loss of an occlusal surface has been sufficient to cause pain in the joint region. Questions to patients about the efficiency of their chewing ability often elicit such responses as: 'I have lost my bite' or 'I have a hole in my bite'. Reduced masticatory function is a widespread disturbance and disorders are uncommon as a direct result of it. On the other hand, its restoration is often beneficial when the musculature has suffered.

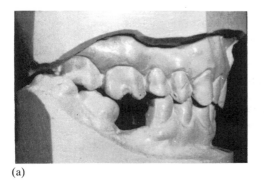

(a)

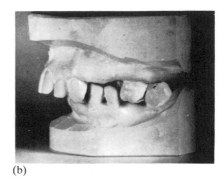

(b)

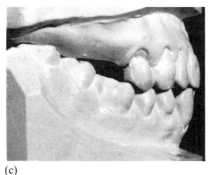

Figure 7.2 Secondary malocclusions. (a) Missing tooth with good adaptation. (b) Over-eruption with mandibular overclosure. (c) Opposing teeth in contact with residual ridge. (d) and (e) Over-erupted third molar causing displacing activity from retruded contact. (d) to IP

(c)

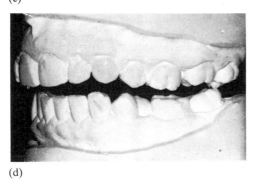

(d)

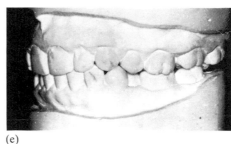

(e)

Supra- and infracontacts

A *supracontact* between opposing teeth occurs when a filling or crown has been overcontoured or when a tooth has become exfoliated by a periodontal abscess. It may constitute the sole contact and usually induces a parafunctional habit. It cannot be left alone. Until corrected it will cause tilting of the mandible on closure or a further pathological response in the periodontal tissues. A supracontact should be differentiated from a deflective contact that causes a deflection in the path of movement to IP which may remain unchanged.

An *infracontact* constitutes a lost of occlusal surface by attritional wear or by an undercontoured crown. It can also be caused by altering the shape of an opposing supporting cusp in order to relieve a 'high' filling or crown. Patients may complain of 'biting into a hole' or 'lost support for my bite'. This has often been associated with the mandibular dysfunction syndrome and represents an unfavourable response by the muscles to an alteration in the pattern of closing or chewing. In other words it can lead to a disorder.

Why it is that a missing tooth may not cause the symptoms mentioned while an infracontact may, is not clear. It may be that the proprioceptors around the tooth in infraocclusion are transmitting stimuli weaker than those which have established the reflex muscle activity in the particular case and that this alters the muscle pattern unfavourably. Where the tooth is missing there are no proprioceptors and a stable new pattern is adopted.

Loss of occlusal curve

This follows the loss of posterior teeth in a bounded saddle situation (see Figure 11.2) and provides another example of secondary malocclusion. It is often followed by extrusion or tilting of teeth opposing the gap and by tilting of the teeth adjacent to the gap. It is a disturbance likely to cause further disturbances and other disorders. Attempts to correct this break in the occlusal curve should be made before replacements are planned, otherwise further disturbances may be promoted by the restoration.

Unstable cusp relations

These are contacts in intercuspal position between cusps and opposing ridges or fossae where there is only one point of contact between the two opposing occlusal surfaces. They are a potential tipping force and cause of cusp interference. As has been previously said, good occlusion requires three sides of a cusp to be in contact with three opposing ridges forming a fossa. This constitutes the stable tripod of contact and is the optimal tooth relation. It represents an objective in treatment.

Cusp interference

This is a contact between a cusp and an opposing tooth which interferes with the established closing or chewing movement.

The *causes* of cusp interference are: teeth in the process of being repositioned (following the loss of an adjacent tooth); teeth which have become loosened by loss of periodontal support; teeth incorrectly restored (supracontact); teeth which have been moved by a parafunctional habit; or teeth incorrectly placed in a bridge or denture.

The *effects* of cusp interference are generally one of the following. First, by a neuromuscular response to avoid the interference in order to maintain comfort and efficiency and this is achieved by a displacing activity whereby the mandible adopts an altered intercuspal position; this constitutes an initial contact followed by mandibular displacement. Secondly, the affected teeth may be displaced on sliding contact and replaced when the contact is past. Thirdly, one or both of the affected teeth may move to new positions, thus constituting a premature contact followed by reposition. Fourthly, a grinding habit may be induced in order to remove the interference and thus perpetuate what may have been the cause of the interference.

The total effect may be a combination of more than one of these responses and the system usually adapts without disorder. Unfavourable responses may, however, take place in the muscles, joints or periodontal tissues.

Cusp interferences may take place during mastication, swallowing or during the parafunctional activities of clenching, grinding or tapping closure.

During mastication cusp interferences may occur:

1. On the working side as the mandible moves into IP. As this interference occurs it is usually avoided and a more direct closure (chopping) to IP is performed.
2. On the non-working side when the mandible may tilt in the coronal plane and cause an unfavourable muscle response.
3. During protrusive closure between opposing incisors. This is generally avoided by direct closure although it is more likely to result in a parafunctional habit.
4. On habitual direct closure to IP, particularly when swallowing, when the mandible will be deflected or the affected teeth will move.
5. On retruded arc closure when the mandible will be deflected either forwards or laterally depending on whether the interference is uni- or bilateral. If the deflexion is laterally, an unfavourable muscle response may result.

During parafunction cusp interferences may occur:

1. On the working or non-working sides as the mandible is forced to glide from one side to the other and the effects are likely to be more harmful to the teeth or muscles because the protective reflex responses tend to be overruled.
2. On the anterior segment as the mandible is forced to glide backwards or forwards.

In most natural dentitions and many artificial ones there is little balanced articulation, thanks to the protection by anterior guidance. Parafunctional gliding usually brings the muscle forces to bear on one tooth. The effects are therefore exaggerated, especially when the gliding becomes grinding. These parafunctional habits are common in children, particularly during sleep, and cusp interferences serve either to bring the teeth into stable occlusion or to be repositioned as they develop. In addition to these habits, space availability for the developing teeth may be a cause of altered tooth relationships. As a tooth is forced out of the arch, cusp interference is a common consequence.

Usually, cusp interference during mastication results in fleeting deflective contacts and adaptation prevails. During parafunction the interference is more persistent and forceful and, as a result, more potentially harmful. Parafunctional grinding may even move teeth and *cause* cusp interference.

Alteration of intercuspal position

This is an IP which has been altered by cusp interference, wear or loss of the teeth. All intercuspal positions are habitual when related to occlusion on the retruded arc and there is a continuing tendency for IP to alter because both the occlusal and interproximal surfaces continue to wear throughout life. In this respect, reconstruction of the natural dentition can be justified since occlusal and interproximal wear will be arrested and the opportunities for a stable IP are increased. In the untreated dentition an alteration of IP implies that some of the teeth may have tilted in order to achieve the new IP caused by the deflected mandible. The deflexion (or displacement) of the mandible varies and sometimes is minute; and adaptation is usually, but not always, adequate to prevent an unfavourable muscle response (Figure 7.3). Nevertheless, this alteration is commonly associated with mandibular joint pain which has its cause in the muscle

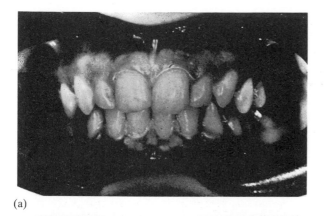

(a)

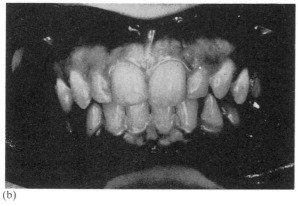

(b)

Figure 7.3 Minor displacing activity to left after initial contact between right canines. (a) Initial contact by IP. (b) IP after displacing activity to left

insertions to the joint tissues. Diagnosis of cusp interference and altered IP can be made by observing the path of closure from rest position to habitual IP and from retruded occlusion to IP.

Mandibular overclosure

This is the IP reached when the path of closure from rest position exceeds the established interocclusal distance (3–4 mm). Expressed mathematically this reads: when RVR + OVR < 4 mm. There is a fine borderline between normal and abnormal and the clinician has to be skilled in assessing what is abnormal in terms of indications for treatment. Many methods for measurement are in use but the important position to recognize is the endogenous (as opposed to the habitual) rest position from which a measurement of the path of closure can be made. A temporary incisal overlay to engage the mandibular incisor teeth at an increased level is often necessary when the patient will respond to a 'better or worse' analysis. Superimposed tracings of condyle radiographs may be helpful in making a diagnosis. In the normal closure there is lineal superimposition; in overclosure the condyle may be distally related at IP (see Figure 4.11b).

Mandibular overclosure may be developmental or acquired.

Developmental overclosure is usually associated with class II jaw relations where the development of the posterior dentoalveolar tissues has been retarded. If the overclosure is developmental, adaptation during growth will almost always prevent unfavourable responses. Loss of teeth may increase the overclosure, however, and disorders result (*see* section on disorders, p. 116). A steep condyle path and increased vertical overlap of the maxillary incisors is often associated with this condition and any restorative procedures should be attempted with caution.

Acquired overclosure follows the loss of posterior teeth and represents a vertical alteration of IP. Disorders which may follow include discomfort at the loss of posterior tooth support, bruising or ulceration of the palatal or lower labial mucosa and mandibular joint pain. These will be discussed in the next section.

Parafunction (bruxism)

This is a disturbance which has to be considered as a separate clinical condition since it can arise irrespective of occlusal disturbances or other oral irritation. Stimuli relayed from the higher centres of the brain lead to hyperactivity of muscles (irrelevant muscle activity, see p. 42). If the muscles affected are in the masticatory system, parafunctional clenching or grinding of the teeth is the result. The impulses resulting in this activity are thought to be some form of emotional upset or anxiety and can be manifest in other groups of muscles. Examples are the clenching of fists, pacing the floor and other activities often more violent. Another acceptable theory is that the irrelevant activity takes place in a region where there is a weakness or defect, as in the mouth where cusp interferences are to be found or in the back where the musculature is perhaps inadequate for the support required for it. This may be speculative reasoning but there is little doubt that muscular action provides an outlet for such emotional states as inadequacy, frustration, anger and anguish. The presence of irritations in the mouth may provide stimuli for these activities or may contribute to them by a feedback system; disturbances of the occlusion can provide such a stimulus. The wearing of unstable dentures provides another such irritation and the effects on the dentures are further instability and discomfort. Parafunctional activities of the masticatory system during sleep were mentioned in Chapter 3 and are not easily explained except through the activities of the reticular and limbic systems of the brain. Dreams may enter the cycle of impulses from these systems and become a cause or an effect of irrelevant muscle activity, resulting in clenching of the teeth. In addition, the posture of the chin on the pillow may, by prolonged stretching of one or more muscles, provide a stimulus for contraction.

Attrition of the occlusal surfaces

This process of wear begins as soon as the teeth erupt and varies according to the quality of the diet, and masticatory and parafunctional habits. Attrition can be localized to one or two opposing teeth or generalized in the dentition (Figure 7.4a–c). Small alterations to the intercuspal position are therefore continuously taking place. Adaptations to this loss of occlusal vertical dimension take the form of further eruption by deposits of cementum over the root surfaces and neuromuscular responses to the altered IP. Also, the pulps of the affected teeth respond by deposits of secondary dentine. Artificial teeth, acrylic and porcelain, are equally subject to this disturbance. This condition is on the border between disturbance and disorder and will be considered again on p. 114.

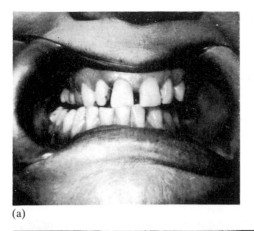

(a)

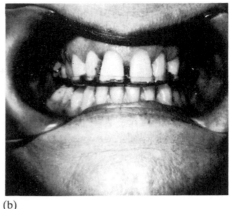

(b)

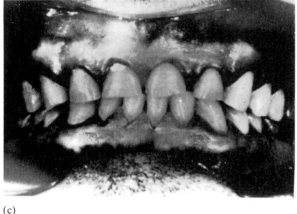

(c)

Figure 7.4 Wear by parafunction. (a) Localized. (b) Treated with bite guard (see also Chapter 14). (c) Generalized; not so easily treated

Food impaction and the plunger cusp

This constitutes a disturbance of function and is generally associated with altered contact points between two teeth and an opposing supporting cusp which occludes in the space between the marginal ridges of the affected teeth. Food particles can then be forced between the teeth by these cusps, which are often called 'plunger cusps'. It will be remembered that four out of the six supporting cusps of the four posterior teeth usually occlude in the opposing marginal ridge areas and are potential plunger cusps. Contact point relations can be altered by tipped teeth, worn marginal ridges, or by incorrectly restored approximal or embrasure surfaces in restorations. A deepening of the interdental col epithelium may also promote this disturbance which occurs when food is forced by the tongue between the teeth during the act of swallowing. Food impaction has a nuisance value and a disorder of the interdental epithelium may result (see p. 115).

Denture disturbances

Partial and complete dentures are subject to most of the foregoing disturbances but their responses are obviously limited by the absence of roots and periodontal receptors. Disorders of the supporting mucosa may result but a denture does have the merit of being removable.

This description and discussion of disturbances emphasizes the need for careful observation by the dentist and for a conservative approach to treatment that will prevent disorders. Disturbances of occlusion are potential disorders and a disturbance is prevented from becoming a disorder by the various processes of adaptation, but this factor can diminish and treatment may be necessary. On the other hand, premature or excessive treatment can itself lead to disorders and the term 'iatrogenic' is not unknown in dentistry (see p. 117).

Disorders

As has been said, a disorder of the occlusion is a response to a disturbance which causes a pathological change in the tissues of the masticatory system. In considering disorders as a group of conditions, a clear idea of the existing disturbances is necessary since one is usually an extension of the other. The following disorders will be described:

- Attrition (or wear) of the occlusal and incisal surfaces
- Ulceration of the interdental epithelium
- Periodontal responses to occlusal forces
- Mobility, jiggling and migration
- Pulp necrosis
- Mucosal ulceration
- Disuse stagnation and atrophy (masticatory insufficiency)
- Iatrogenic disorders
- Denture instability and discomfort
- Occlusal trauma.

These disorders demonstrate a failure to adapt to one or more disturbances, often with an additional precipitating cause. They generally provide a reason for patients to attend the dentist (or doctor) and, as in the disease of caries, when it hurts the damage has often been done. In disorders of the occlusion, pain is not the only symptom; others can be equally damaging and difficult to treat.

Attrition (or wear) of the occlusal and incisal surfaces

This disturbance becomes a disorder when the dentine is exposed and becomes hollowed. It is intermittently sensitive and the occlusal vertical relation gradually closes. The appearance of the teeth deteriorates. The causes are a combination of parafunctional grinding, the quality of the diet and the production of acid by bacterial activity on the carbohydrates ingested. The end-result can sometimes be seen as flattened tooth surfaces with a reverse Monson curve that can be explained by heavier wear of the supporting cusps. The onset is gradual but the disorder can be precipitated by excessive grinding of the teeth.

Another effect of parafunctional forces is the cracked tooth which is a commoner cause of dental pain than is perhaps realized. This disorder can lead to longitudinal fracture of the tooth or to pulp involvement requiring treatment. Preventive warnings should be given as early as possible and overlay appliances provided for night wear.

Ulceration of the interdental epithelium

This disorder results from the disturbance of food impaction and the plunger cusp. The development of an ulcer in the epithelium between the teeth is often predetermined by its col shape but the loss of an effective contact point and a cusp–ridge occlusion is usually the precipitating cause. If untreated, a periodontal disorder will follow and the occlusion (usually by plunger cusp) will continue to act as an aggravating factor. The symptoms are those of discomfort, bleeding, a bad taste in the mouth and bad breath from it. Treatment by restoring the embrasure can be difficult because of the tendency for the more posterior tooth to drift distally. Splinting the involved teeth may be indicated.

Periodontal responses to occlusal forces

This is mentioned if only to exclude it as a disorder of the periodontium and it will be discussed further under occlusal trauma. The claim that a disorder of the periodontal tissues results from sustained adverse occlusal forces in the absence of any other initiating factor has never been proved. However, this does not exclude these forces from being aggravating factors to an already established lesion of the periodontal tissues.

Mobility, jiggling and migration

Mobility or loosening of a tooth can be caused by an opposing occlusal force but, in the absence of a gingival or periodontal lesion, it will recover its stability when the occlusal force is removed. In the presence of a periodontal lesion and some degree of exfoliation occlusal forces will aggravate the mobility. Cusp interferences can therefore be created by periodontal breakdown and provide a cause of premature contact and tooth displacement. A vicious cycle of cause and effect is thus created.

Jiggling is the unscientific but descriptive term given to the movement of a tooth in one direction by a force (tooth, muscle or appliance) and its repositioning by an opposing force (tooth, muscle or removal of the appliance). Thus, a maxillary incisor tooth with loss of periodontal support can be pushed forwards by an opposing mandibular incisor and be repositioned by the activity of the lip muscles. Another example is the retraction of proclined maxillary incisors (usually with inadequate lip support) by a removable appliance worn at night and their repositioning during the day by tongue or opposing tooth when the appliance is withdrawn. In the former example, a periodontal lesion was a predisposing cause; in the latter the treatment was the cause. A disorder may develop in the latter case, if the 'treatment' is sustained, by traumatic necrosis of the periodontal tissues. This activity may also predispose to disturbances in root development of the teeth in the adolescent patient. Intercuspal occlusion and parafunctional habits will aggravate both these examples and, as with mobility, become involved in the cycle of cause and effect.

Migration refers to the movement of a periodontally involved tooth by an opposing tooth or muscle action without the expectation of its reposition. The tooth will move until a stable position between opposing muscles or teeth is reached. This condition usually involves the maxillary incisor teeth which may migrate forwards or laterally. An inadequate lip seal is usually an associated cause. It is not uncommon for these teeth to drift outside the lips, after which the lower lip

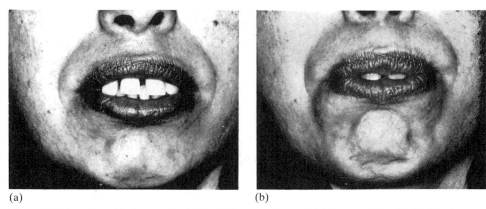

(a)   (b)

Figure 7.5 Migration of incisor teeth with lips failing to make seal. (a) Rest position. (b) Swallowing at IP

becomes an additional displacing force (Figure 7.5). In such a case conservative treatment can become difficult, if not impossible.

There is always a combination of causes in these disorders and, in addition to those of periodontal lesion, occlusal and muscular forces, there is often the loss of posterior teeth and mandibular overclosure. One further pathological response is necrosis of the periodontal tissues following prolonged jiggling, which need not be preceded by a gingival and subsequent periodontal lesion. This is a rare complication.

Pulp necrosis

This disorder can be the result of persistent clenching on an individual tooth when the blood vessels passing through the apex are damaged and eventually destroyed. Death of the pulp follows and the resultant necrosis is sterile. Toxins from the pulp may pass through the apex into the periodontal tissues, causing a pathological response. Circulating bacteria may then initiate a diseased condition which the occlusal forces will further aggravate (Figure 7.6). This condition may be painless throughout and it may take radiography or discoloration of the tooth to reveal it. A vague pain may be noticed from time to time, however, and should be noted in the taking of a history.

Mucosal ulceration

This is the result of injury by mandibular incisors on the mucosa behind the maxillary incisor teeth or by maxillary incisors on the labial epithelium in front of the mandibular incisor teeth. The cause is a progressive overclosure of the mandible and is usually associated with loss of posterior teeth. In addition to the pain on closure and irritation when eating, the mucosa may become detached from the affected tooth surfaces. It is a slowly deteriorating condition and dentists are often reluctant to treat it until it is too late for effective treatment.

Disuse stagnation and atrophy (masticatory insufficiency)

Reduced function promotes stagnation of food on the teeth and surrounding epithelium. The possible consequences of caries and gingival irritation need no

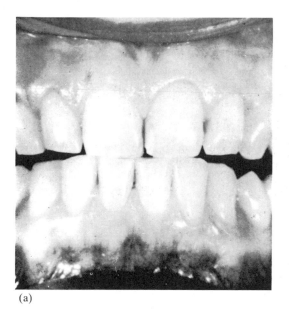
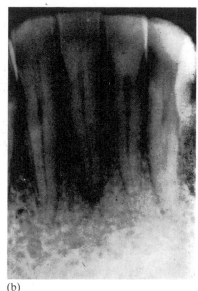

(a)   (b)

Figure 7.6 Localized parafunction and death of pulp. (a) Acknowledged habit. (b) Radiograph of affected tooth

emphasis. Ulceration and bleeding of the affected epithelium may follow when the teeth are brushed or during occasional encounters with tough foods.

Disuse atrophy can develop when a tooth is wholly out of contact with an opposing tooth or residual ridge. The condition most commonly affects the second or third molars. Changes take place in the periodontal membrane: fibroblasts tend to appear and the collagen fibres are replaced by a reticulum of fibrous connective tissue. The alveolar bone tends to have fewer and thinner trabeculae and such teeth do not respond well to restored function if they have been functionless for long periods. The replacement of periodontal fibres by fibrous connective tissue renders the teeth unable to support occlusal or abutment forces and the bone requires more rapid repair than can be provided for the sudden functional requirement. However, if function is restored gradually, as by placing an opposing denture base without a tooth for a time, and then by adding the tooth, restoration of the affected tissues can take place.

Iatrogenic disorders

These are defined as pathological responses to treatment. They were mentioned in the concluding paragraph of the section on disturbances and constitute a group of disorders which may include:

1. *Awareness of the teeth.* This can follow a failure to correct a 'high' filling or crown (supracontact). Reduction of an opposing cusp (usually supporting) instead of the fossa of a filling can lead to changes in the intercuspal position. This may become intolerable to the patient who, until then, has been 'unaware' of his or her teeth.
2. *Insufficient occlusion.* This can be caused by an undercontoured restoration (infracontact) and can lead to food being stacked on the restoration or

channelled to the contact area. Both can become intolerable and lead to interdental food stagnation. Infracontact may also predispose to the mandibular dysfunction syndrome, especially where a bridge or denture has been made with pontic teeth short of occlusion.

3. *Painful teeth.* Pulpal reaction to grinding procedures on natural teeth are not uncommon and when this is accompanied by an unacceptable alteration of the intercuspal position a resentful patient is the result.

4. *Mandibular dysfunction syndrome (MDS).* This may be created by the dentist in restorative and denture procedures where increases or decreases in the OVR have not been tolerated. Horizontal alteration of the intercuspal position may lead to parafunctional habits between the teeth which themselves can cause the syndrome.

5. *Bruised or ulcerated mucosa.* This can be caused under dentures where cusp interferences cause the denture bases to move and bruise the supporting mucosa. Too often, attempts to correct such a disorder are made by removing the border or supporting surface of the denture when the correct treatment is to remove the interference and establish level occlusion.

One of the dangers to be avoided in any restorative treatment involving the occlusal surfaces of one or more teeth is that of failing to correct an existing disturbance before making the restoration and thus promoting further disturbance and possibly disorder.

There may be ethical problems involved in dealing with other dentists' work which require care and courtesy, not forgetting that one's own may be under examination by other eyes. Conversely, the opportunity of praising a colleague's work should never be missed.

Denture instability and discomfort

Denture instability was mentioned as a disturbance and is often tolerated by the patient who has the ability to adapt and control a denture which does not have the properties of retention nor stability. This adaptability is usually associated with the denture teeth being in stable positions relative to the muscles of tongue, lips and cheeks. This should always be an objective in setting denture teeth (Chapter 12). When this is not achieved and when the occlusal and articular relationships on the dentures do not correspond to the jaw positions and movements, tipping forces are exerted on the teeth and the denture bases either move or press on the supporting mucosa. The resulting instability or discomfort constitutes a disorder. Alternatively, if the bases are well fitting, the mandible may be forced into an altered interocclusal position, but the muscles may not tolerate the alteration, as sometimes happens in the natural dentition. This too, may constitute a disorder. Finally, the persistently cracking complete upper denture is almost always due to occlusal imbalance with parafunction added.

Occlusal trauma

This term has dominated studies of occlusion since it was introduced by Stillman and McCall (1927) as 'traumatic occlusion'. The terms are perhaps not interchangeable since the one suggests injury from occlusion and the other occlusion which *causes* injury. Either way, it cannot be left out of any list of disturbances or disorders of occlusion. However, it has engendered much confusion and should be used in a spirit of inquiry rather than dogma, which has often been its role.

The term has been defined as an injury to the periodontal tissues of a tooth as the result of occlusal forces by an opposing tooth or teeth. Occlusal trauma has been classified as primary or secondary: primary occlusal trauma referring to the effect of abnormal forces on healthy periodontal tissues, while secondary occlusal trauma refers to the effect of occlusal forces on an already diseased periodontium. The term has caused disagreement and misunderstanding among clinicians and scientists and the reason is not hard to find: the term begs the question; it presumes a fact not proven, namely, that occlusal forces cause injury to the periodontium. The proposition has been made that it would seem to be so, therefore it is so. This hypothesis has never been adequately tested, let alone proven. It is true that occlusal forces cause teeth to move and become mobile if the force is allowed to persist; but the teeth will recover their stability if the forces are removed. Such forces will aggravate an existing periodontal lesion but they have not been shown to initiate such a lesion unless a gingival lesion already exists. In such a situation the occlusal forces may precipitate the periodontal breakdown. Equally, such a periodontal lesion will recover if the periodontal defect is repaired.

Occlusal forces, especially those directed along the axial plane, can cause strangulation of the vessels entering and leaving the pulp chamber of the tooth through the apex; death of the pulp can result (Figure 7.6). Injury can also be caused by incisors on opposing gingivae, as already mentioned, but neither is this condition the one generally understood as occlusal trauma. Trauma can also be used to describe the wear on the occlusal surfaces caused by parafunctional grinding habits. The term 'traumatogenic occlusion', used by Box (1930) and implying the possibilities of producing trauma, was less presumptuous. None the less, it implied that injury could be caused by lateral occlusal forces on the periodontal membrane, and this has not been shown to occur without other causes.

'Occlusal trauma' is a term which can be applied to wear of the occlusal surfaces of the teeth, necrosis of the pulp vessels or to injury of the gingival or palatal mucosa, but not to a destruction of the periodontal tissues.

Comment

Disturbances of occlusion exist in the majority of mouths and many go unrecognized, causing few complaints. Failure to adapt to a disturbance, however, will result in a disorder, when a pathological response can be demonstrated. There will always be a tendency for occlusal disturbances to deteriorate since tooth surfaces once disturbed do not repair themselves. Also, a repositioned tooth will not recover its original position because opposing adjacent teeth will move in order to attain stability. Probably the most important aspect of recognizing disturbances is to ensure that they are corrected before further replacements of tooth surfaces, or of the teeth themselves, are made. Disorders constitute complaints by the patients and some pathological process is involved. The cause has to be diagnosed, the occlusion analysed and the disturbance treated. These topics will be the subject of the remaining chapters.

References

Box, H. K. (1930) Traumatic occlusion and traumatogenic occlusion. *Oral Health*, **20**, 642
Stillman, P. R. and McCall, J. O. (1927) Significance of traumatic occlusion. *Dental Items of Interest*, **49**, 330

Chapter 8

Articulators

In the previous chapters emphasis has been laid on the need to understand the tissues and functions of the masticatory system and it may seem unphysiological to attempt the transfer of such a system, of any live system, to a mechanical device devoid of muscles, blood supply, or a correlating nervous function. However, the curiosity to see the teeth during function and the difficulty of seeing them (because the lips are usually closed) has prompted dentists to transfer casts of the teeth to hinges representing the mandibular joints. Hinges with teeth on them have been reported from early Egyptian remains, although these were probably the prostheses themselves rather than casts copied from natural teeth. Certainly, hinged dentures date back to antiquity and, as Woodforde (1968) puts it in his story of false teeth, 'for hundreds of years after the collapse of the Roman Empire all kinds of dental skills deteriorated in Europe'. This suggests an inviting field of study for dentists with a training in archaeology. The dark ages of dentistry are reported largely from the fairground and the apothecary's shop and it was not until the nineteenth century, when dentistry began to emerge as a profession with an academic as well as a cultural background, that reports of men like Bonwill (1887), Walker (1896) and Gysi (1910) began to show the possibilities of the jaws being mechanically copied. The story of articulators has yet to be compiled and written and no doubt there will be surprises for contemporary dentists when man's ingenuity in the antique past is revealed. However, a recent survey by Mitchell and Wilkie (1978) of articulators used in the past century will awaken student memories for some older practitioners and reveal the beginnings of a craft that has become a science for the younger students of prosthodontics.

For the purposes of this text an attempt will be made to define and classify articulators, following which four objectives for their use will be outlined. Principles involved in copying jaw movements on these instruments will be discussed and the methods currently used described.

Definition and classification

The articulator is usually a hinged instrument on which casts of the teeth can be mounted in planned relations to each other so that mandibular positions and movements can be copied. Some do not even have a hinge and examples are the Hagman balancer and the Stansbery tripod. The more contemporary Verticulator is a holding instrument which will accept a single record, usually a functionally-generated path, and will disclose premature contacts in the vertical plane.

However, the majority of articulators have a double joint simulating the mandibular condyles. The exception to this principle is the curiously named 'plane-line' single joint instrument which is no more than a plain hinge that bears no measured relation to the retruded axis of the mandible (Figure 8.1); it is widely used with a 'squash bite' record for transferring the relation of the casts. Accuracy of any resultant work cannot be expected.

Horizontal movement was first introduced to articulators with Bonwill's brass wire 'anatomical' articulator (Figure 8.2). The hinge between the upper member and main frame was plain enough and the lateral and protrusive movements allowed by the springs were limited, to say the least, but an instrument which permitted articulation between opposing teeth had been designed and used, and has led to the developments in articulators with which we are familiar today.

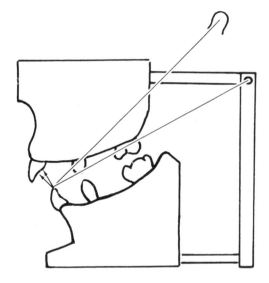

Figure 8.1 Diagram of a plain-hinge articulator. Difference in arcs of closure is shown between the centres of rotation of the articulator and the retruded condyle axis where a facebow transfer has been used

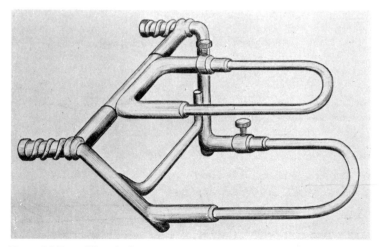

Figure 8.2 Bonwill's articulator

Contemporary articulators are classified into two categories:

1. *Semi-adjustable* articulators are those that receive statically registered positional records and, with a facebow transfer of the retruded axis (either actual or arbitrary), will reproduce an accurate path of closure and reasonably accurate protruded and laterally protruded paths of movement.
2. *Fully adjustable* articulators are those that receive pantographic tracings of the lateral border and protruded movements of the mandible and the actual retruded axis. The articulators will reproduce these movements and the retruded arc of closure with accuracy.

Objectives

Objectives for using articulators are as follows:

1. Functional analyses of occlusion and articulation in the natural dentition.
2. Reconstruction of the natural dentition.
3. Fabrication of fixed bridges and removable partial dentures for bounded saddles.
4. Setting teeth for complete dentures and removable partial dentures with free-end saddles.

For objectives (1) and (2), the fully adjustable articulators are usually required where the accurate reproduction of border movements and rotational Bennett shifts are necessary. A minute error in reproducing the direction of these movements can lead to cusp interferences or to failure in recognizing them.

For restorations where the existing IP (with its incisal and canine guidances on protrusion and lateral protrusion) is to be used, and where pantographic tracings are not possible (as in edentulous mouths), and where occlusal corrections are required for complete and partial dentures, the semi-adjustable instruments are indicated. At all times, however, these articulators are preferable to the plain hinge.

Semi-adjustable articulators

The semi-adjustable articulator has mechanical condylar elements which can be adjusted for lateral and descending movements of the mandible by positional interocclusal records. The condylar elements may have tracks or three-sided boxes to guide the condyles and may be situated on the lower or upper members. The level of closure is established by an adjustable incisal guidance pin (straight or curved) on the upper member engaging a table on the lower member (Figure 8.3). The transfer of the upper cast is made by a facebow record, and of the lower preferably by a precontact record on the retruded axis.

Arcon and condylar mechanisms

These are terms given by [Bergstrom (1950)] to distinguish between those semi-adjustable articulators that have the condyles on the lower member, as in the mandible, and are referred to as *arcon* instruments, and those where the condyles are on the upper member and receive the adjective *condylar*. Examples are shown in Figure 8.3.

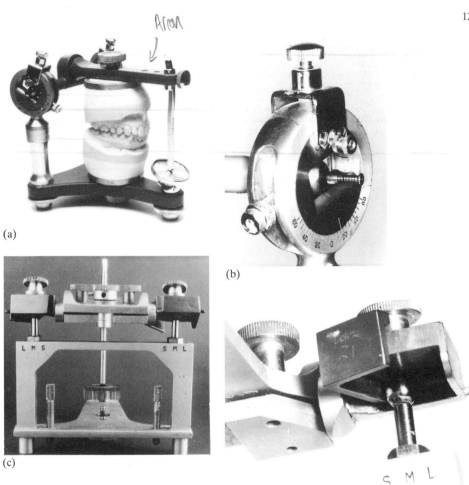

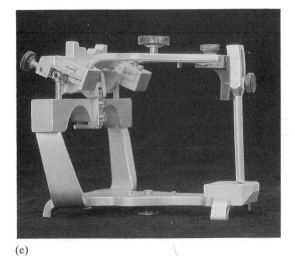

Figure 8.3 Articulators currently in use.
(a) Dentatus. (b) Condyle (condylar)
assembly with extendible rod. (c)
Whipmix rear view. (d) Condyle (arcon)
assembly. (e) Denar Mark II (arcon)

[handwritten at top: ∴ dist bet condyles + mand teeth in protrusion ≈ 6mm.]

The arcon articulator provides greater accuracy in the transfer of the angle of condyle descent by the protrusive positional record. On the arcon instrument the distances between the mandibular teeth and the condyles will be the same in the mouth as on the articulator. On the condylar instrument, where the condyles move distally in protrusion, this distance will be doubled, usually 12 mm instead of 6 mm. As those condyles move upwards as well as backwards the angle made by the line joining mandibular incisors, in protrusion, and the condyle on each side will be steeper in relation to the horizontal plane on the condylar articulator than the angle made by the line joining the same two points on the arcon articulator (Figure 8.4).

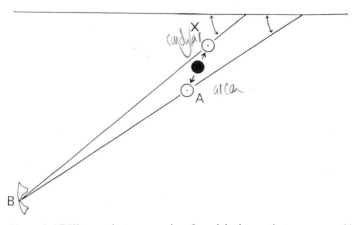

[handwritten labels on figure: condylar (at X); arcon (at A)]

Figure 8.4 Difference between angles of condyle descent between arcon (A–B) and condylar (X–B) mechanisms

This may not be a significant difference but the arcon articulator will produce a more accurate copy of the relation between the opposing teeth in protrusion and lateral protrusion, with all that this implies for the anterior guidance of the mandible.

Incisal guidance pin and table

These features provide a stop for closure of the upper arm of the articulator. The pin should be curved at its upper end so as to form an arc with the axis of rotation of the upper arm as centre, and be fixed by a locking screw. Thus, the upper arm can be raised and lowered without the pin moving on the table. This feature is not present on the Whipmix instrument. The table should be adjustable to follow the paths created by the lingual surfaces of the maxillary incisor and canine teeth. Alternatively, the table can be made of acrylic resin and additions made to it to follow the excursions influenced by the shapes of these surfaces. In reconstruction procedures this feature can be used to follow guidances created in provisional crowns and, subsequently, if correct, in creating the lingual surfaces of the definitive incisor and canine crowns.

The facebow

The transfer of the upper cast to the articulator is made using a facebow. This is an adjustable calliper carrying a 'bite-fork' that records imprints of the maxillary teeth (on wax or compound) in relation to the retruded axis of the mandible. The cast can then be placed on the imprints and the facebow attached to the hinge axis of the articulator. An indicator attached to the horizontal bow can be placed against the infraorbital ridge and this permits the facebow to be oriented to the Frankfort plane of the articulator, to which the upper cast is now secured by plaster (Figure 8.5c). The upper teeth on the cast can then be said to rotate on the same axis of opening and closing as the mandibular teeth rotate in the mouth, provided the mandible remains on its retruded axis. One can hold the upper member and rotate the lower, or seat the lower on the bench and rotate the upper, which is the common practice. The mounting of the lower cast will be described on page 128.

The use of the term 'bite-fork' is perhaps unfortunate because it implies that the facebow has a part to play in the registration of the jaw relation. This mis-conception should be corrected by having the patient hold the bite-fork in place by the thumbs, or the nurse by the fingers, and *not* by the patient closing on the bite-fork with the mandibular teeth, when tilting is likely.

The arbitrary and actual retruded axis

The type of facebow in common use has adjustable rods or ear-pieces which are located, in the case of the rods, over points 12 mm in front of the tragi of the ears on a line between them and the external canthi of the eyes (Figure 8.5a). Those with ear-pieces fit in the ears and the holes for attachment to the articulator (Whipmix) come forward outside the ears and can reach the points 10–12 mm in front of the tragi. These are the *arbitrary* axial points and would not be adequate for diagnostic or reconstruction procedures. The *actual* retruded axis can only be registered by a kinematic facebow (or axis locator) temporarily cemented to the mandibular teeth and having adjustable side-arms that will pinpoint over the actual retruded axis when this has been found by the dentist and is reproducible. There are several methods for ensuring retruded axis rotation and that of Dawson (1979) is the one of choice. Here, the base of the thumb is placed against the chin (Figure 8.6b) rather than the top joint against the centre of the chin, which tends to move the chin to one side or the other (Figure 8.6a). The feeling of 'give and rotation' should be unmistakable. When this axis has been registered and is going to be used for reconstruction procedures (and may have to be reused for remounting) it may be desirable to tattoo the points.

When making the registration of the actual retruded axis it is advisable to apply squares of graph paper against the axis areas; this can be done using topical anaesthetic as an adhesive, especially if the points are to be tattooed. In removing the kinematic facebow, the condyle pointers (which are sharp) should be marked (with a piece of rubber dam or special marker) and withdrawn to prevent scratching the face. The pointers can then be readjusted to the intercondylar distance at which the axis was registered (Figure 8.6c). It is important, where accuracy is required, to have this distance transferred to the articulator, otherwise the cast will not be correctly oriented to the intercondylar distance of the face (Figure 8.6d) and the initial movements from, and final movements to intercuspal position, as determined by the Bennett lateral shift movements, will be different between mouth and articulator, making cusp interferences likely. In order to accommodate this intercondylar distance the condyle mechanisms are adjustable lateromedially in the fully adjustable instruments. In the semi-adjustable versions, some have adjustable condyles and others have extendable rods to meet the condyle pointers

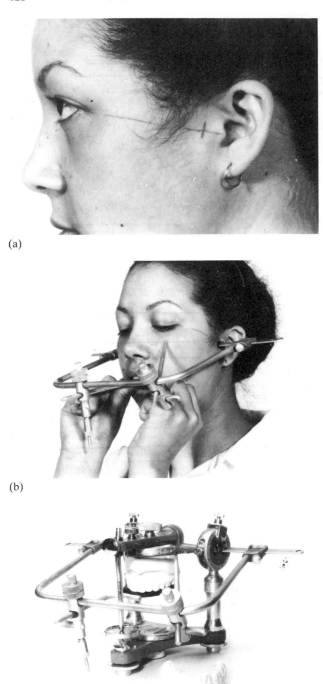

(a)

(b)

(c)

Figure 8.5 Arbitrary retruded axis transfer. (a) Left side marked. (b) Facebow registration. (c) Facebow record transferred to articulator. Upper cast mounted. Lower cast ready to be mounted

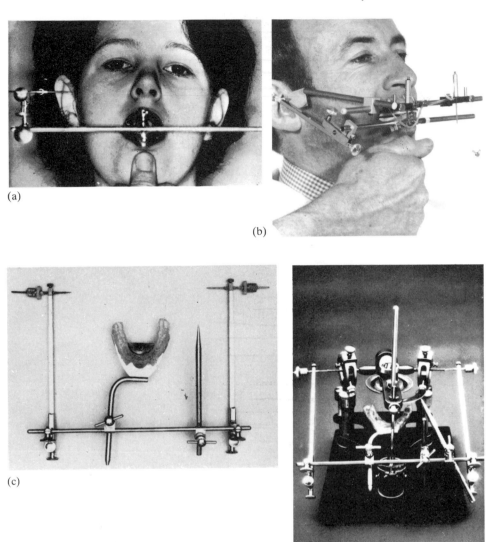

Figure 8.6 Actual retruded (terminal hinge) axis transfer. (a) Almore axis locator. (b) Kinematic axis location. Use of Denar locator and maxillary anterior bow (with styli) to support axis locating flag. (c) Axis locator has been used for facebow record. (d) Facebow record on articulator, ready for mounting upper cast. Orbital indicator touching axis-orbital plane of articulator. Extendable condyle rods meet condyle pointers on facebow (unaltered)

on the kinematic axis locator, thus transferring the actual intercondylar distance (Figure 8.6d). The diagram illustrated in Figure 8.7 indicates the possibilities of inaccuracy in not transferring the actual intercondylar distance.

It is worth repeating that the facebow transfers a reproducible rotary retruded movement of the mandible to the articulator. Without it, only the position is transferred, with an incorrect path of movement to it.

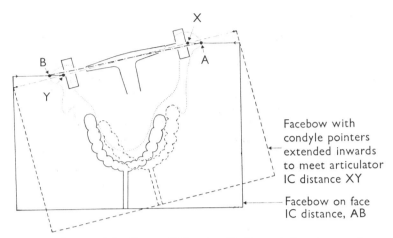

Figure 8.7 Intercondylar distance (IC) on face (A–B, –·–·) altered to meet intercondylar distance on articulator (X–Y, –––). Result is altered orientation of cast to axis on articulator

Transfer of the occlusal position

It has to be stated somewhat dogmatically that there are only two mandibular positions that can be registered with possibilities for checking them. These are the existing intercuspal position and the retruded relation, which has a definite superior component (Dawson, 1979). In the words of Stuart (1979) it is the 'uppermost, midmost and rearmost position'. If the existing IP is selected, as for single-unit or bounded saddle restorations, the lower cast can often be placed against the upper, secured and attached to the lower member of the articulator, usually by plaster. The so-called 'wax squash-bite' is never recommended because the wax will distort on removal and the mandible may displace on closure following contact with the maxillary teeth. For the retruded relation record a precontact registration on the retruded arc is required and methods will be described in more detail in Chapters 11 and 12.

The *Gothic arch tracing* for recording the retruded relation is well known and is attributed to Gysi, who used it in the making of complete dentures, and is still used chiefly in the jaw registration for such dentures. The registration is made at the vertical level selected for the investigation or work required (or as close to it as possible to allow for the appliances carrying the stylus and plate). This, too, will be described in Chapter 11, and later in this chapter when discussing the fully adjustable articulators. Meanwhile, it is important to realize that the apex of the arch must have a sharply defined angle, indicating muscles in good function. If the lines are not sharp and not repeated, the record will not be acceptable. A tiny hole is often drilled at the apex to engage and fix the stylus while the plaster registration is made. Payne (1969) made a study of Gothic arch tracings on five edentulous patients and found this record to be 'a reliable guide to the position of habitual closure' but that it is not the most retruded position. This is an ingeniously devised study and is worth repeating. Nevertheless, the Gothic arch is the key point indicating the retruded relation in fully adjustable articulators.

Checking the jaw relation

There are several methods for ensuring a reproducible retruded relation and two will be described in Chapter 11 and again in Chapter 12. The use of a pictorial method for making this check was developed by Buhner and reported by Lundeen (1974) in a study to compare condylar positions obtained by different methods. A Whipmix articulator is used with graph paper attached to the sides of the upper condylar housing. The condyle balls on the lower arm are removed and replaced by a bar carrying vertical blocks at each end in which horizontal holes are drilled to allow pointed rods to slide laterally in and out, and to touch the dimples on the side of the condylar housing. This makes the rods act as centres of rotation on the same line as the opening and closing axis of rotation of the articulator. The graph paper is now placed over the side walls of this housing. The upper cast is mounted using a facebow transfer, and the lower cast against the upper using a record registered on the retruded arc and plastered to the lower member of the articulator. The condyle balls are now replaced with the bar carrying the pointed condyle rods and marks are made by the rods on the graph paper. A new record is made and placed on the lower teeth. The upper arm carrying the upper cast is placed against this record and the pointed rods moved to touch the graph paper. A comparison as to which is the more retruded can now be made and this procedure should be repeated until two retruded records are achieved.

This Buhnergraph was used by Lundeen to compare three types of records (heavy, light, and with the myomonitor) and proved excellent for making comparisons. Illustrations are provided in Lundeen's article.

Materials used for making registrations include stone plaster, Kerr's bite registration paste, hard wax supported by metal across the palatal area, double thickness strips of wax separated by tin-foil, compound, acrylic resin and various forms of synthetic rubbers, provided they are not subject to recoil. An anterior stop using fast setting acrylic resin is often advisable in order to stabilize the mandible while the materials used for registering the buccal segments are setting.

Condyle angle adjustments

While the mandible is moving, the condyles are said to be rotating and/or orbiting. While opening on the retruded axis, both condyles rotate on a horizontal axis. When moving to the right, that side is the working side and the right condyle rotates on a vertical axis. The left is the orbiting condyle and the left posterior teeth are non-working.

The adjustable mechanism in the condyle assembly is used to transfer the angle of condyle descent, as recorded on the precontact protruded registration. Its use for this purpose is usually confined to complete denture construction and is adjusted by moving the angle until the artificial teeth or occlusal rims fit into the imprints on the record made in the mouth. If the orbital indicator on the facebow has been used to relate the bow to the Frankfort plane on the face, the adjusted angles on the condyle mechanism should be the same as those transferred from the patient's condyles. If this indicator has not beeen used, the angle will be the same but the figure on the mechanism will be different because all condyle angles on the articulator are relative to its horizontal plane.

When lateral records are used, the angle made by the orbiting (non-working) condyle is usually steeper than the straight protrusive descent. The angle between the protrusive path and the path of the orbiting condyle in lateral movement is known as the Fischer angle and varies between 3° and 10°. If lateral records have not been made, it is advisable to increase the condyle guidance by 5° over the protrusive guidance when making adjustments to the lateral articulation for complete dentures. This angle can be seen on pantographic tracings of the lateral border movements (see Figures 8.12a and 11.1).

When casts of the natural dentition are being assessed for condyle guidance, the contacts on incisor protrusion and canine lateral protrusion will determine the incisal and canine guidances. The condyle guidances can then be adjusted to follow these tooth-determined movements which are protective of posterior articulation. *The anterior component of articulation thus takes precedence over the posterior determinant.*

Bennett angle

In order that the inward component of the orbiting condyle path can be transferred, the condyle pillars on the condylar articulators (Hanau and Dentatus) should be rotated inwards. The angle which the path of the orbiting condyle makes with the median plane is called the Bennett angle (B) and varies between 5° and 30°. As this inward (and downward) movement has an outward component (on the working side), it is an angle difficult to calculate. Nevertheless, Hanau had a formula for it and it reads $B = \frac{1}{8}H + 12$ where H is the protrusive angle. Students may be forgiven for forgetting about this calculation, especially as Gysi adjudged it basically wrong and set up geometrical constructions to prove his point. In the semi-adjustable articulator this angle is usually set at 15°; if greater accuracy is required a pantographic tracing transferred to a fully adjustable instrument will provide it.

Paths of movement on the articulator

It is assumed that the paths of movement of the condyles on the articulator between the protruded and intercuspal positions are the same as those in the patient. This accuracy cannot be assumed since the articulator condyle paths are straight lines, whereas in the joints they tend to be curved. Some adjustable articulators have curved condyle paths but these too can be inaccurate assumptions. Where lateral

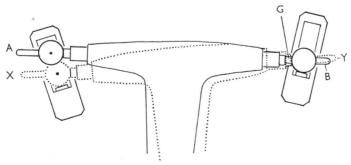

Figure 8.8 Lateral shift permitted on Hanau (Dentatus) type articulator, see gap G. If shoulder of axle is kept in contact with condyle sphere on orbiting side the condyle axis will shift laterally on orbiting movement. AB to XY. It is an arbitrary movement and no accurate lateral shift is possible at IP

paths are concerned, the semi-adjustable articulator has no accurate copy of the lateral (Bennett) shift movements. In the Hanau and Dentatus instruments a straight lateral shift is possible after the condyle axis has moved forwards (Figure 8.8). In the mouth this begins immediately the movement from intercuspal position begins and, conversely, as the mandible moves into intercuspal position from a lateral incoming movement. This component of lateral movement may be critical in avoiding deflective cusp contacts, and where the quality of the work demands such accuracy a fully adjustable articulator is recommended.

Advantages and disadvantages

Semi-adjustable facebow articulators, therefore, provide four aids to copying mandibular movements on the laboratory bench:

1. Transfer of retruded path of closure.
2. Transfer of angles of condyle descent in protruded and lateral precontact relations of mandible to maxilla.
3. Approximate lateral shifts.
4. Incisal guidance table which will adjust to incisal and canine articular movements.

In addition, greater accuracy can be achieved by those instruments having an arcon condyle mechanism and adjustable intercondylar distance. There are three shortcomings of these articulators:

1. The arbitrary facebow is an approximation of the actual retruded axis.
2. The precontact records are made within the borders of the parcel of motion and are not reproducible.
3. The paths between the positional records are straight-line approximations of the actual condyle movements.

These shortcomings are not intended to detract from the considerable advantages of adjustable articulators over plain hinges which cannot, by definition, be called articulators.

Semi-adjustable articulators in current use

Some features of the Dentatus ARH, Denar Mark II, Whipmix, and SAM will be briefly described.

The Dentatus ARH (see Figure 8.3a,b) is a condylar instrument but has anterior condylar stops which are helpful in comparing jaw relation records. It possesses extendable condyle rods for adjusting to the actual intercondylar distance of axis locators. The metal incisal guidance table is adjustable anteroposteriorly and laterally but will not accept a patient-determined self-curing resin record. Lateral (Bennett) shifts cannot be accurately copied (see Figure 8.3) but the Bennett angle can be adjusted with a lateral positional record.

The Denar Mark II (see Figure 8.3e) has the arcon condylar mechanism and will adjust to the axis locator intercondylar distance. It can be used with the Slidematic facebow (Figure 8.9) which comprises a jig assembly, carrying the tooth imprints, which is detachable from the bow and can be transferred to the articulator in place of the incisal guide table and allows the upper cast to be mounted. This reduces the need for the whole facebow to be transferred from surgery to laboratory. The

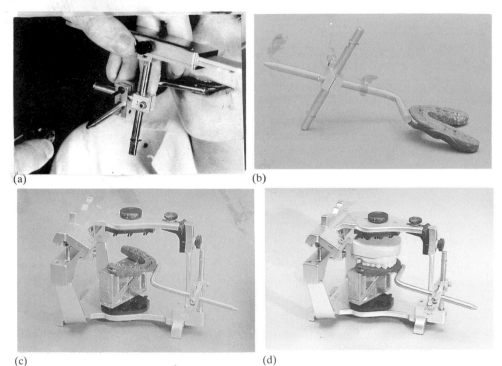

(a)   (b)

(c)   (d)

Figure 8.9 (a) Securing bite fork assembly relating maxillary teeth to retruded axis; (b) Bite fork assembly removed from bow ready to be sent to technician; (c) Mark II Denar articulator with incisal table removed, mounting block attached at 0° and vertical arm of bite fork assembly seated into mounting block; (d) Upper cast seated on bite fork ready for mounting to upper arm of articulator. (Courtesy of R. J. Ibbetson, Eastman Dental Hospital)

condyle mechanism is made of nylon and a set of curved paths are available with variable immediate and progressive side shifts, if required.

The Whipmix (see Figure 8.3c,d) has the arcon condyle mechanism and adjustable medial and upper walls. The Bennett angle can be adjusted with a positional record. The plastic incisal guidance table can be used to define incisal and canine paths with self-curing resin from the mounted casts when planning treatment. The instrument will receive the Buhnergraph mechanism for comparing retruded axes of rotation before and after splint therapy.

The SAM articulator has arcon condyles. Any discrepancy between IP and retruded axis can be measured on graph paper in both sagittal and horizontal planes using an indicator in the lower member. The plastic incisal table can accept an incisal guidance record made in self-curing resin. Adjustment of intercondylar distance is not possible but Bennett shift guides can be inserted and ground if necessary.

Pameijer (1985), in his excellent and beautifully illustrated text, deals more fully with these and other articulators.

Fully adjustable articulators

The objective with these instruments is to provide a copy of the reproducible border movements of the condyles and mandible, namely the arc of opening and closure on the retruded axis and the horizontal envelope at one level. These border movements are not always producible, let alone reproducible, because of muscle disability (pain or stiffness) on one or both sides. Assuming border movements unrestricted by disability, however, it is possible to make an accurate retruded axis registration and tracings of the horizontal envelope of motion in three planes, on each side of the face, by styli on prepared writing tables. These are transferred to the articulator which can be adjusted to follow the tracings.

It may be said that to reduce human neuromuscular movements to a series of curves and rotations is asking too much of man's ingenuity, that jaw movements are too refined and delicate to be copied, and that copying nature is a presumption too bold to attempt. But it is justifiable to assume that the movements, however delicate, have rotational and translatory components, and that if they are reproducible an attempt can be made to copy them.

Transfer of border movements

In order to be able to transfer border movements to an instrument which will copy them, several fully adjustable articulators have been devised. Essentially they consist of four adjustable parts:

1. A condylar axis with an adjustable intercondylar distance. This is not an axle but two independent hinges with the condyles attached to the lower member (an arcon instrument).
2. Left and right condyle assemblies consisting of upper and rear walls which can be adjusted to follow the paths of movement of the rotating and orbiting condyles (Figure 8.10).
3. Guide mechanisms, usually on the upper member, which will permit the lateral shift (Bennett) movements to be copied (Figure 8.10).
4. An incisal guidance pin and table. These permit the height of the upper member to be altered and the horizontal inclination of the table to be adjusted laterally and anteroposteriorly, which will allow the OVR to be altered and the incisal and canine guidances to be copied or created. If the articulator can be adjusted to copy these movements, tracings may not be necessary.

The advantages of transferring the border movements to the articulator are twofold: first, accurately copied mandibular movements can be seen by both dentist and technician, and treatment planned accordingly; secondly, restorations can be created to conform to, and not interfere with articular mandibular movements.

Retruded axis transfer

The correct performance of this operation is essential to the accuracy required for transfers. If the axis transfer is not retruded, not only will the axis of closure on the instrument be incorrect but the pantographic tracings which follow will be incorrectly transferred. Instruction and practice in the feel of the mandible when it is fully retruded are therefore essential. Only when the condyle axis is retruded will the condyle pointers rotate, and this provides the confirmation of retruded axis rotation. By keeping the mandible in this position and extending the pointers to touch the sides of the face the retruded axis centre of rotation can be marked and subsequently tattooed on both sides of the face.

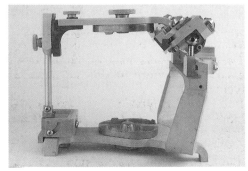

(a)

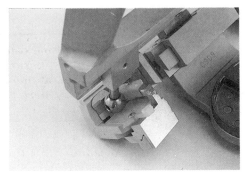

(b)

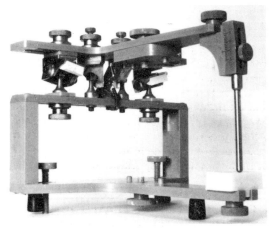

(c)

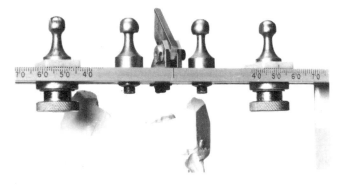

(d)

Figure 8.10 Fully adjustable articulators. (a) Denar. (b) Denar: fully adjustable condyle (arcon) assembly. (c) Stuart, with fully adjustable condyle (arcon) assemblies. (d) Condyles and medial (Bennett) condyles

Tattooing

It may be desirable to mark the axis points permanently on the face since the axis transfer is often not made until the pantographic tracings have been completed. Also, if restorations are being planned, facebow transfers may be required at various stages and it would be an unnecessary expenditure of time to make a retruded axis registration each time a transfer was required. The permanent marking is made with a skin-coloured tattoo, using a hypodermic needle or a special form of applicator consisting of three tiny needles welded together which carry the tattoo powder between the three points. The tattooed marks are visible only to the dentist and can remain for a number of years.

The transfer of the retruded axis to the articulator is made prior to the pantograph of the horizontal border movements.

Registration of the border movements

This is carried out by the pantograph which is a device for registering the left and right border movements of the mandible. Registrations are performed on three planes on each side of the midline while the teeth are separated by a central bearing screw. The pantograph also registers the protrusive movement which is not a border movement but begins and ends at a border position. It comprises an upper and lower frame, each consisting of three bars bolted together. The side-arms of the lower frame can be adjusted so that the condyle pointers touch the tattooed axis marks. The lower frame is in fact the axis locator, to which are added six writing tables, three on each side, in different planes. The upper frame carries six styli, each at right angles to each opposing table. The frames are attached to the maxillary and mandibular teeth respectively by means of clutches, either seated securely or temporarily cemented. They are separated by a central bearing screw adjusted to the closest distance between the teeth but permitting unrestricted lateral movements between the clutches (Figure 8.11). In some pantographs the vertical and horizontal side tables are on the upper frame with the styli on the lower. The differences lie in having to read the tracings made on them in reverse of those made on anterior horizontal tables.

The attachment of the frames to the teeth and the assembly of the styli at right angles to the tables (to provide unrestricted movement of the styli) require careful instruction and practice. The instruction of the patient to provide the border movements also requires practice but, when correctly performed, the tracings made by the movements will be reproducible. Guichet (1979) makes these instructions to the patient a strict ritual which can produce a pantographic tracing in 11 minutes. It should be repeated that these movements will be reproducible only if the muscles are free from inhibitory spasm, stiffness or pain (see Figure 11.1).

The tracings

The protrusive and lateral movements are recorded individually and each must begin at the retruded position. Assisted practice is necessary and the patient must get the feel of the retruded position. Consequently, this is practised before each tracing movement by a forceful forward and back movement by the mandible. As taught by Guichet, using the Denar pantograph which employs compressed air to

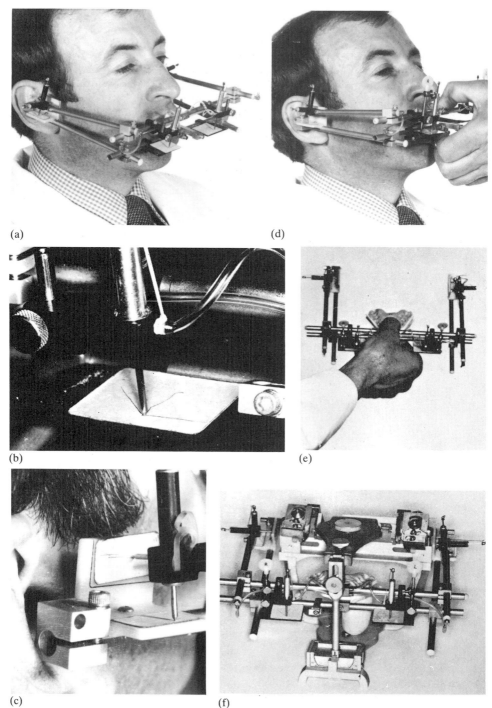

Figure 8.11 Mandibular recording assembly (Denar). (a) Mandible retruded and ready to make first movement. (b) Tracings on anterior tables. (c) Tracings on posterior tables. (d) Assembly about to be removed. (e) Pantograph removed. (f) Pantograph transferred

keep the styli raised against the gentler downward force of six elastic bands, the following procedure is used:

1. An air cut-off is held by the operator who gives the command 'forward and back' several times until operator and patient are certain that the retruded position has been reached, each time pressing the air cut-off on retrusion until the styli hit the same spot each time. The 'forward' movement is then commanded with the styli down from the retruded position and released at full protrusion. The procedure, therefore, is: 'forward and back'; press, release; repeat; then, press; 'forward'; release; 'back'.
2. For left lateral: 'forward and back'; press, release, and repeat; press, 'move slowly to the left'; release; 'back'. It may be necessary for the operator to press gently backwards with the hand on the contralateral side of patient's chin to assist this movement.
3. For right lateral: repeat as for left movement.

Tracings will vary from a sharp Gothic to a rounded arch with wavering lines anterior to the arch, indicating joint disturbances, uncertain movements and clicks.

The six tracings are then protected with transparent adhesive covers. They represent the Gothic arches on the two anterior tables, and the working and non-working (orbiting) condyle movements on the four posterior tables (Figures 8.11b, c and 8.12a). The two bows are then joined together, with each stylus in the retruded position. Condyle pointers are secured through the vertical condyle tracing tables and placed against the retruded axis marks on the face. These should be secured with a collar device which can be withdrawn before the assembly is removed in order to prevent scratching the face. A light rigid bow with adjustable pointer is then laid on or attached to the upper bow and the pointer is adjusted to touch the third reference point. This will transfer the level at which the tracings were made. Any subsequent transfers of the maxillary teeth should be made at this level and using this device.

The tracing assembly is then removed from the clutches and the condyle pointers restored to the intercondylar distance. The clutches are removed from the teeth and reattached to the maxillary and mandibular bows respectively. The whole assembly is then transferred to the condyles of the articulator which are adjusted to fit the intercondylar distance between the two condyle pointers. Each instrument has a mounting frame assembly which holds the recording bows. The articulator is then positioned so that the condyle pointers accurately touch the rotation axis of the upper arm which then becomes the retruded axis. The clutches are attached (by plaster or other device) to the maxillary and mandibular arms of the articulator. They are subsequently separated from each other so that the maxillary clutch can move more freely over the mandibular clutch on the central bearing screw and open and close on the retruded axis.

Adjustment of the articulator

Each fully adjustable instrument has its manual. This should be studied in detail and the order of adjustments to the joint assembly followed precisely. The adjustments to the intercondylar distance, the superior and posterior walls and the medial walls for the Bennett shift movements can only be understood and carried out if the recordings have been carried out by the operator. Experience is invaluable and no instruction by words will take the place of sitting down with the

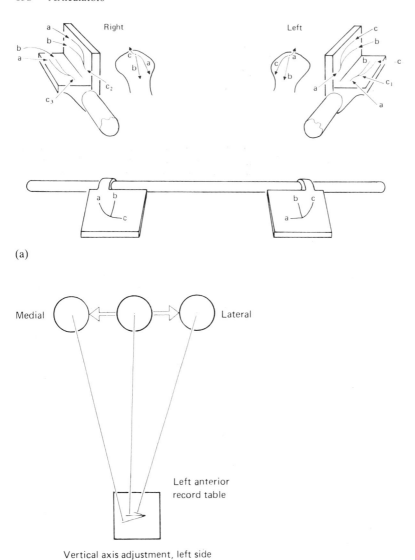

(a)

(b)

Figure 8.12 (a) Tracings of mandibular border movements. All tables attached to mandible. a, mandible moves to left; b, mandible protrudes; c, mandible moves to right; c_1, immediate side shift right (adjust medial wall); c_2, surtrusion or detrusion right (adjust top wall); c_3, rotation to right (adjust rear wall). (b). Adjustment to vertical axes

instrument, its pantograph and with an experienced operator to provide guidance. Some observations from diagrams, however, may be helpful.

Figure 8.12a shows the paths followed by the condyles in protrusive and both lateral retrusive movements. These markings correspond to the tracings made during the border movements of the mandible. It should be borne in mind that, in this diagram, all the tables are attached to the mandibular bow and these are the

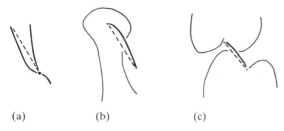

(a)   (b)   (c)

Figure 8.13 (a) Tracing from right posterior table (see Figure 8.12a). (b) and (c) Tracing related to right condyle and right opposing molar teeth. **Note**. Tracing table moves back and out while condyle and mandibular tooth move down and in. Dotted lines indicate paths of movement on semi-adjustable articulator

moving elements. The styli remain stationary. The following observations are made:

1. The angle of descent of the orbiting condyle is usually steeper than that made by the protruding condyle as seen on the posterior vertical table. Adjustment to these tracings is made by altering the angle of the superior wall of the condyle assembly (see Figure 8.10b).
2. The immediate and progressive side shifts are seen on the horizontal posterior tables as the non-working condyles move to the sides away from the tables. Adjustment is by alterations to the medial wall of the condyle assembly.
3. The lateral thrust of the rotating (working) condyle can be seen on the shorter tracing on both the horizontal and vertical tables as the mandible moves to that side. The condyle in rotation may move upwards or downwards as it thrusts laterally. The terms *surtrusion* and *detrusion* have been given by Stuart to describe these upwards or downwards thrusts respectively. Adjustment is made on the rear wall.
4. The anterior tables show the relative backward movement of the styli as the protruding condyles cause the tables to move forwards. The arcs made by condyles in rotation are shown as the Gothic arches on each table. The outer arc on each side is made by the opposite condyle and the inner arc by the condyle on the same side in rotation. Adjustment is made by alterations to the vertical axis (the intercondylar distance) (Figure 8.12b). This, however, will not alter the orientation of the cast which was mounted at the intercondylar distance marked on the face.
5. The difference between the condyle paths on the fully adjustable and positional record articulators is seen in Figure 8.13. The dotted straight line represents the movement obtainable with positional records. The curved line of actual condyle movement can only be achieved by the mandibular recording.

Transfer of casts and three assumptions

The upper arm of the articulator will now copy the border movements of the mandible at the level transferred. A further facebow transfer of the maxillary teeth in relation to the retruded axis and to the anterior point of reference will allow the upper cast to be mounted on the articulator. A precontact interocclusal record on the retruded axis is then made when the lower cast can be mounted on the articulator in relation to the upper cast. The closure to retruded contact on the articulator can then be *assumed* to be the same as in the mouth. The *assumption* is also made that the lateral border movements transferred at one level of jaw separation will be copied at other levels of jaw separation provided the transfer has been made on the retruded axis and using the anterior point of reference.

A *third assumption* is that as all border movements can be copied on the articulator, as can all movements within the borders of the vertical and horizontal paths of motion. This assumption can be accepted provided there is no hindrance by the condyle assembly to freedom of movement of the upper arm. Thus all movements which the mandible can make in relation to the maxilla through tooth contact can be seen on this type of articulator. This means that each mandibular cusp, ridge and fissure will move in the same arc of opening, working or non-working movements as in the mouth. The importance of this transfer in diagnosis, treatment planning and in restorative treatment is considerable. It is possible to see inhibited jaw movements interrupted by clicks, pain or muscle stiffness. In diagnosis any transfer of casts less accurate cannot provide useful information on the behaviour of teeth in contact with each other.

Together with the information from the consultation and the examination, both clinical, radiological and gnathosonic, these mounted casts can provide a view of the *empty* movements of the mouth from buccal and lingual aspects which can give a good indication of their behaviour in function. The genuine need for restorative treatment can then be more realistically assessed.

Recent developments

Recent developments in fully adjustable articulators began with a series of experiments by Lee (1969), who devised apparatus to engrave jaw movements in three solid plastic blocks (attached to a lower clutch) by burs on an air turbine (attached to an upper clutch). The clutches were separated by a central bearing screw and the upper supported the lower. A set of recordings (engravings) related to the retruded axis were achieved by the patient moving to the right and left borders and to protrusive directions. Patients who were premedicated with sodium nembutal were examined and a consistency of patterns was established.

In making graphic recordings of mandibular movements, Clayton, Kotowicz and Myers (1971) had laid down criteria for establishing research data: the styli on the pantograph should be at right angles (zeroed) to the tables; tracings will differ if angled forward or back; tracings should be guided; and the OVR should be standardized for each series of tracings.

Lundeen, Shryock and Gibbs (1978), using Lee's instrumentation, evaluated the character of mandibular border movements in 163 subjects aged between 20 and 65. They gave the figures of 2.5 to 3.5 mm to Bennett movement that would cause flattening of lateral movement pathways and have little anterior guidance. This would make the mandibular cusp pathways shallow and render reconstruction procedures difficult. A lower Bennett shift (0.75 mm) with steep anterior guidance would reduce the tendency to molar cusp interference. The influence of the non-working condylar path was most evident in the frontal plane. In 163 subjects the average Bennett shift was 0.73, with 80% of 150 or less.

Guichet (1979), writing about the Denar system and its application to 'everyday dentistry', refers to 'occlusal diseases' and how the 'tops of the teeth', acting as occlusal irritants, can programme muscle groups to cause muscle tension, premature wear of the occlusal surfaces, pulpitis, tooth fractures, periodontal disturbances, and joint and muscle disturbances, with the consequent need for modifications of the occlusal surfaces. Guichet claims, with some justification, that the Denar system is educational as well as diagnostic and curative.

Celenza (1979) made an analysis of articulators and pointed out that absolute precision was not required for all restorative procedures, such as for complete dentures where precise movements by the teeth and bases could neither be recorded nor reproduced. The use of positional records and their mechanical equivalents on semi-adjustable articulators are adequate for procedures such as removable partial and complete dentures, single-unit and three-unit crown and bridgework.

Lundeen (1979), from these and further studies, concluded that most patterns of condylar movements resemble each other and has developed a 'movement analyser' to identify characteristic patterns relative to known parameters. From several hundred recordings he established a set of five patterns from which the majority of patients' movement patterns could be selected.

Clayton et al. (1976) established a pantographic reproducibility index (PRI) for detection of temporomandibular joint dysfunction. Two clinical studies substantiated its effectiveness in identifying muscular and occlusal problems and monitoring treatment.

Clayton and Beard (1986) have developed a computerized pantographic reproducibility index which prints out the settings for the articulator at the end of each movement sequence and makes it unnecessary to transfer the pantograph to the articulator. This is the Pantronic (Denar Corporation) and it will indicate the degree of muscle dysfunction present. It can also be used to assess the success of splint therapy, occlusal and restorative treatment, and changes in levels of dysfunction for research data.

In the same publication, Beard and Clayton (1986) compared electronic and mechanical pantographs and concluded that the electronic version (Pantronic) produced more consistent results than the mechanical in assessing dysfunction-free patients. In addition they were able to establish that operators with varying experience need not cause fluctuations in making these assessments.

Anderson, Schulte and Arnold (1987) made an *in vitro* study of an electronic pantograph and compared it with the mechanical version. They concluded that the electronic version proved the more consistently accurate in assessing the immediate and progressive side shifts and the protrusive angle of descent.

Thus, ingenuity and the adaptation of current electronic advances to neuromuscular investigations seem to be sifting out possibilities for treating facial pain associated with mandibular dysfunction. To date, occlusal therapy, though often successful, has not had the surety of a pathological diagnosis, but the day when it will is coming closer.

Recording movements during function

Reference has already been made to Lewin's *Electrognathographics* (p. 96) and this followed the use of a small bar magnet cemented to the mandibular incisor teeth during mastication (Lewin, Lemmer and Van Rensburg, 1976; Lewin and Nickel, 1978). The jaw movements were then tracked by a set of linearizing antennae attached to the head. By this method the rotations and translations of the mandible can be recorded and measured. Thus the effect of chewing various items of food can be measured and correlated. The magnet has been designed by Siemens GK, and serves as a source of energy. The magnetic field emanating from it is defined but asymmetrical and this makes possible the measurements through the geometric axes of the magnet. Siemens GK have also designed the detector systems with Hall-effect transducers which will detect the asymmetrical magnetic field. Six of these detectors are arranged, two to a plane, in three planes. The signals emanating from the transducers during displacement of the magnet are fed into the electronic circuits of the device that has an oscilloscope screen. This will display the graphic representation of the various activities performed. The overall error is in the region of 5%, which includes the noise of the transducers, the electronic circuits and the inaccuracy of the geometric alignment of the detectors. The most recent design of headgear supporting antennae is light and the patient being examined can be unaware of it after a few minutes wear.

Characteristic patterns of movement have been established, intraindividually, in frontal and sagittal planes, and comparisons between the effects of function and dysfunction are becoming available (van Rensburg, 1980).

The mouth as an articulator

It is often claimed that the mouth is the best articulator since it is the movements which the mandible makes which determine the shape of the restorations being made or the occlusal adjustments necessary. The reasons why the mouth does *not* make a satisfactory articulator are as follows:

1. Adaptive movements are readily made if any interferences are encountered and the end-result of closure may not be the one desired. The difficulty of making a reproducible interocclusal wax record on any path of closure, except on the retruded axis, is proof of this. Direct wax patterns suffer for the same reason.
2. It is difficult to see tooth contacts, particularly lingual cusps, and the use of cheek retractors does not promote natural movements.
3. It is difficult to add to wax patterns or alter tooth positions in wax in the mouth.
4. The tongue, cheeks and lips are liable to dislodge wax patterns, teeth and articulating paper.

However, many restorations are created and adjustments made with the mouth as articulator. Provided the closing and any articular movements made are reproducible, this can be an acceptable practice. Experience and results will tell their story.

Comment

The question 'Which articulator to use?' is often asked and can best be answered, albeit vaguely, by the reply 'How much do you want to know?' The amount of information required from a patient and from the state and usage of his or her dentition will vary with the patient's initial requests and with what the dentist regards as necessary for the long-term health and function of the mouth in question. Only a minority will justify the painstaking procedures outlined in this chapter. If occlusal disturbances are to be prevented from becoming disorders, the time taken to make a thorough analysis will be justified. Consultations with colleagues will always be valuable and the use of fully adjustable articulators indicated. Time spent at the stage of analysis will usually be rewarded and the next chapter will extend this concept.

References

Anderson, G. C., Schulte, J. K. and Arnold, T. G. (1987) An in-vitro study of an electronic pantograph. *Journal of Prosthetic Dentistry*, **5**, 577

Beard, C. C. and Clayton, J. A. (1986) Electronic PRI consistency in diagnosing TMJ dysfunction. *Journal of Prosthetic Dentistry*, **55**, 255

Bergstrom, G. (1950) On the reproduction of dental articulation by means of articulators. *Acta Odontologica Scandinavica*, **9** (supplement 4), 7

Bonwill, W. G. A. (1887) The geometrical and mechanical laws of the articulation of the human teeth – the anatomical articulator. *American System of Dentistry*, **2**, 486

Celenza, F. V. (1979) An analysis of articulators. *Dental Clinics of North America*, **23**, 305

Clayton, J. A. and Beard, C. C. (1986) An electronic computerised pantographic reproducibility index for diagnosing temporomandibular joint dysfunction. *Journal of Prosthetic Dentistry*, **55**, 500

Clayton, J. A., Crispin, B. J., Shields, J. M. and Myers, G. E. (1976) Pantographic reproducibility index (PRI) for detection of TMJ dysfunction. *Journal of Dental Research*, **55**, 161

Clayton, J. A., Kotowicz, W. E. and Myers, G. E. (1971) Graphic recordings of mandibular movements: research criteria. *Journal of Prosthetic Dentistry*, **25**, 287

Dawson, P. E. (1979) Centric relation: its effect on occluso-muscle harmony. *Dental Clinics of North America*, **23**, 169

Guichet, N. F. (1979) The Denar system and its application in everyday dentistry. *Dental Clinics of North America*, **23**, 243

Gysi, A. (1910) The problem of articulation. *Dental Cosmos*, **52**, 1

Lee, R. L. (1969) Jaw movements engraved in solid plastic for articulator controls. *Journal of Prosthetic Dentistry*, **22**, 209

Lewin, A., Lemmer, J. and van Rensberg, L. B. (1976) The measurement of jaw movement. Part II. *Journal of Prosthetic Dentistry*, **38**, 312

Lewin, A. and Nickel, B. (1978) The full description of jaw movement. *Journal of the Dental Association of South Africa*, **33**, 261

Lundeen, H. C. (1974) Centric relation records: the effect of muscle action. *Journal of Prosthetic Dentistry*, **31**, 244

Lundeen, H. C. (1979) Mandibular movement recordings and articulator adjustments simplified. *Dental Clinics of North America*, **23**, 231

Lundeen, H. C., Shryock, E. F. and Gibbs, C. H. (1978) An evaluation of mandibular border movements: their character and significance. *Journal of Prosthetic Dentistry*, **40**, 442

Mitchell, D. L. and Wilkie, N. D. (1978) Articulators through the years: Part I: up to 1940; Part II: from 1940. *Journal of Prosthetic Dentistry*, **39**, 330; 451

Pameijer, J. H. N. (1985) In *Periodontal and Occlusal Factors in Crown and Bridge Procedures*, Dental Centre for Postgraduate Courses, Amsterdam

Payne, A. G. L. (1969) Gothic arch tracing in the edentulous. Some properties of the apex point. *British Dental Journal*, **126**, 220

Stuart, C. E. (1979) Use of the Stuart articulator in obtaining optimal occlusion. *Dental Clinics of North America*, **23**, 259

van Rensburg, L. B. (1980) Recording jaw movements during function. Presented at Annual Congress FDI, Hamburg

Walker, W. E. (1896) Articulator and a new method of articulation. *Atlanta Dental Journal*, **2**, 295

Woodforde, J. (1968) *False Teeth*, Routledge and Kegan Paul, London

Chapter 9

Analysis and diagnosis

Disturbances in occlusal relations are often overlooked in the routine examination of a patient's mouth. Caries and bleeding gums require immediate attention; replacement of missing teeth and appearance problems are often equally pressing; instructions on hygiene and prevention occupy as much consultation time as can be spared in the busy practice. Occlusal disturbances are so common as to be assumed within the normal limits of the average mouth and they seldom cause the patient to complain. It is, therefore, understandable that the philosophy of let well alone is justified. It can be argued that a disorder can be caused by attempts to improve what is an acceptable disturbance. 'Striving to better oft we mar what's well.' So said William Shakespeare early in the seventeenth century, and this ambivalence may persist until a disorder occurs. The practitioner must then be ready to make a careful examination and diagnosis and, if necessary, a thorough analysis of the occlusion. Whether this step is taken before or after the disorder appears is a matter for individual judgement. The replacement of missing teeth presents an example of the need for analysis where occlusal disturbances can all too easily be incorporated into restorations. Certainly the practice of dentistry becomes more interesting if the functional status of each mouth is assessed according to its potential comfort and efficiency, to say nothing of its potential harm.

The diagnosis of a patient's occlusal disturbances is based on consultation and examination followed by analysis of occlusal function. This analysis is carried out by clinical, gnathosonic and articular examinations.

The consultation

The objective in a consultation is to establish a preliminary diagnosis, which can be defined as the identification of a disease or disorder by means of the symptoms described. It is always helpful in a consultation to establish an understanding by the patient of what the practitioner is trying to find out. This is best done comfortably in chairs, away from the operating area, and preferably in a room other than the surgery. The customary welcome and details of name and referral should be directed at developing a good rapport with the patient. It may be helpful for the practitioner to make a general statement of purpose before proceeding to the questionnaire. For example: 'Before asking about your dental problem may I say that my concern is with the health of your mouth, with its efficiency and comfort and, if necessary, with its appearance'. The consultation should begin by having the patient describe any symptoms rather than answering a check list. The open is preferred to the closed question. For example: 'Tell me if anything is wrong in your mouth' is more helpful in diagnosis than 'Which tooth hurts?' And, if pain is mentioned: 'Describe the pain' is preferred to 'Is it a sharp or dull pain?' The more leading, closed question can follow if there is difficulty in establishing a diagnosis.

Eight questions concerning function are suggested:

1. Do you have any difficulty in eating? Are you able to chew tough foods?
2. Do you prefer one side or do you use both in eating?
3. Do you feel any discomfort during or after eating? In the mouth or side of the face?
4. Do you hear or feel any noises in your jaw when eating?
5. Do you have difficulty or discomfort in opening wide?
6. Do you clench your teeth in moments of tension or concentration? Tap, slide or grind your teeth together? On waking?
7. Do you use your teeth for any other function: holding, opening, tearing, biting on pen, pencil or pipe? Bite your nails or lips?
8. Does food become lodged between any of your teeth? Do the gums bleed?

These questions are a requirement if there is any suspicion of facial pain or joint dysfunction but are helpful in a routine consultation, when considering the status of a patient's occlusal function (see Appendix for MDS questionnaire).

Past dental and medical histories can now be investigated. Caries incidence, extraction dates and difficulties, orthodontic treatment and denture history may prove helpful, as may information on any jaw injury, either by extrinsic force or from the stretching involved in prolonged or difficult dental treatment, yawning or hard chewing. Medical history should include information on any joint or muscle disorders, blood dyscrasias, skin complaints and any condition currently being treated, including drug therapy.

Such a consultation can be extended or shortened depending on the patient's requirements in seeking dental care and on the interest of the dentist in oral health generally and occlusal function in particular.

The consultation generally closes with a general question on: 'Have you any other comments about the health and efficiency of your mouth?' and the suggestion that 'I should like to examine your mouth and teeth and perhaps take some radiographs'.

The examination

In addition to routine charting of decayed, missing and filled teeth and noting the condition of the gingival and oral epithelium, information is required on several features of the teeth and gingivae with a view to establishing a diagnosis of any disturbance or disorder of occlusal function. This examination should include:

1. The state of cusp wear both on individual teeth and on the teeth in general. This can generally be related to patterns of grinding the teeth either currently or in the past. Loss of enamel and dentine is not naturally restored and could have occcurred in the past. The possibility of its having been caused by the dental stone should be excluded, as should the less likely occurrence of a fibrous or sandy diet.

2. The inclination and stability of repositioned teeth. Mobility and antagonistic movements of any teeth. Central incisor midline.
3. Cusp–fossa and cusp–ridge relations. This will indicate the possibilities of further repositioning of the teeth or of premature contacts.
4. Contact area relations. Open contacts and plunger cusps indicate the possibilities of food lodgement.
5. The state of overeruption of unopposed teeth.
6. Bleeding of the interdental epithelium. This may indicate disease but more commonly a failure to maintain interdental hygiene.
7. The incidence of gingival and intrabony pockets. These may be associated with unstable occlusal forces which may be acting as aggravating factors.
8. Bruised or ulcerated mucosa behind maxillary incisors or in front of mandibular incisors indicating trauma of the mucosa by opposing incisors.

Radiographic examination

Intraoral and interocclusal radiographs will confirm the existence of unfavourable inclinations and overeruption of the teeth, intrabony pockets, and open contacts between the teeth. Interocclusal radiographs may also help to confirm static occlusal relations but the angle of incidence of the X-ray beam has to be taken into account, as has the position used for holding the film (Figure 9.1).

This constitutes an examination of the dentition and epithelium with the mouth open; the possibilities of disturbances or disorders of occlusal function can only be deduced. In order to make a diagnosis based on function in the mouth a more comprehensive analysis of the occlusion becomes necessary.

Analysis of occlusal function

What happens in the mouth during the three meals of each day and during the remaining hours of day and night when it is not occupied with eating is not easy to assess. It may even be wrong to assume that the evidence from a chairside analysis bears any relation to what happens when the patient is behaving naturally and away from the eyes or apparatus of the dentist. But an attempt must be made if improvements in occlusal function are to be made, if disturbances are to be prevented from becoming disorders, or if disorders are to be cured. No attempt to improve or change occlusal relations should be made without making such an analysis. In the first place the treatment might not be necessary, and, secondly, if it is, and is performed incorrectly, the fire may be worse than the frying pan.

At the outset of the analysis, it is necessary to have a clear objective of what information is required and how this information may affect the optimal function of each masticatory system examined. This objective may be summarized as four requirements:

1. Information from the patient on all aspects of function, including parafunction.
2. Information from the examination of the mouth which leads to a comparison between the function as it seems to exist and the optimal function possible for that mouth.
3. The incidence of adaptive function and its potential harm.
4. The incidence of disturbances and disorders.

There are three methods of making an analysis of occlusal function: the clinical, the gnathosonic and by the articulator.

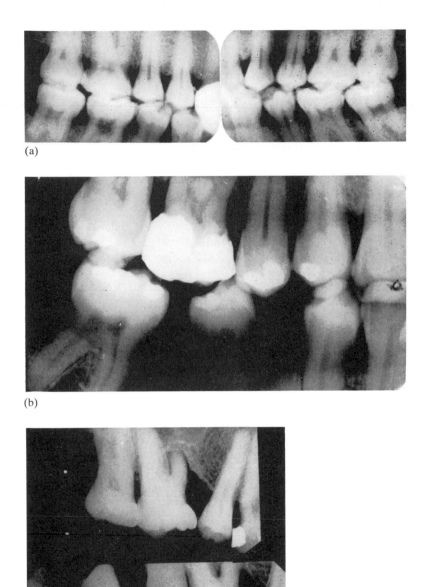

(a)

(b)

(c)

Figure 9.1 Interproximal radiographs. (a) Cusp–ridge occlusion. (b) Antagonistic occlusal forces with potential extrusion of maxillary second premolar and incipient intra-bony pocket of distal maxillary first premolar. (c) Antagonistic occlusal forces with advanced periodontal disease, with buccal segment view

Clinical analysis

The information from the questionnaire and the examination of the open mouth should given an indication of what to expect from the examination of the mouth in its various movements. It should provide a basis for comparison between the mouth examined and the best possible function for that mouth. What is now envisaged is an examination of the mouth with a view to assessing adaptive and parafunctional movements. In the case of the latter, some questions on the possibilities of emotional stress causing irrelevant muscle activity will be helpful in making a diagnosis.

The following aspects of function should then be observed.

Eating

The patient is given a piece of hard biscuit and asked to eat it. Following this function, he is asked to confirm which side he prefers, if anything hurts, if any teeth get in the way, and if food lodges anywhere. If this does not provide positive answers a second mouthful is tried. Observations of this function should include how the chin moves and whether there are any forcible contractions of the circumoral muscles (suggesting adaptive movements), both during eating and swallowing. If teeth are 'getting in the way' an attempt should be made to determine whether this is a working or a non-working side premature contact. This function may be an embarrassment to some patients and can be delayed till the end of the analysis or exluded if it is not considered necessary. It is, however, particularly helpful in patients with denture problems.

Speech

Observations of the circumoral muscles in speech will indicate difficulties in making a lip seal and if the teeth are subject to unopposed forces. The incisor relations should also be noted and, in the case of denture patients, the existence of any tooth contact noises. Difficulties with 'm', 'f' and 'v' sounds requiring excessive movements of the lips or chin may suggest overactivity of the lateral pterygoid muscles and a cause of muscle fatigue and pain. The 's' and 'ch' sounds, particularly in denture patients, should be noted with a view to assessing wrong tooth positions or shape of the muscle (polished) surfaces of the dentures. The closest speaking space will indicate faults in incisor positions and the OVR (see Chapter 6).

Rest position, lip competence and habitual closure

The *rest position* represents the rest vertical relation (RVR) of the face and is a vertical plane of reference for the mandible in relation to the maxilla. The distance between it and intercuspal position (RP to IP) via habitual closure should be 2–4 mm (Figure 9.2). The distance between RP and RO (occlusion on the retruded axis) will be slightly less than RP to IP. Rest position is not on the retruded axis but its vertical level is still a reference plane when dentures or reconstruction are being planned on this axis. Lip competence at rest position is a requirement for stable incisor relations.

The objective in observing these features is to assess if rest position is endogenous and not habitual and if there are any cusp interferences on habitual closure. The observations are carried out with the patient seated, relaxed and the head unsupported. Instructions such as 'Make the mouth comfortable, teeth

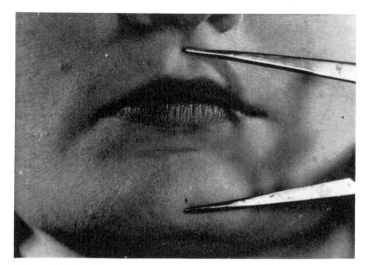

Figure 9.2 RP to IP = 3 mm. Measure with dividers, this picture shows normal closure from rest position. See distance of spot on chin from lower arm of dividers

parted, lips relaxed' or 'Close and swallow and say the letter M', help the patient to adopt RP. Any movement around the lips or chin will suggest effort being made by the lips and the adoption of a habitual posture. Closure to IP may then be uncertain and cusp interference may be encountered. In such an instance the instruction to part the lips may be followed by a gradual relaxation of the mandible to RP. This movement between RP and habitual posture is productive of fatigue.

Lip competence at RP can be difficult to assess for reasons suggested in Chapter 4. A test to determine the borderline lip incompetence consists of asking the patient to close the teeth and lips. Then: 'Part the teeth'. If the lips are incompetent they will tend to remain together as a result of habit, especially if a closed-mouth appearance has been the objective of the habit. It is a significant piece of information since the stability of the maxillary incisor teeth and the activity of the postural muscles may be affected if the lips are incompetent.

The patient is then asked to close lightly on the back teeth and to report if one or all the teeth are touching. Then: 'Close lightly and close tightly', and report any movement between the two positions. Once these closures have been practised the lips are parted by the operator and the movement is observed. Care should be taken to avoid incisor tooth contact and the word 'bite' should never be used since it implies incision.

Cusp interferences seen from RP are usually those associated with overclosure, since the horizontal deflexions of the mandible have become adaptive movements. It is then difficult to assess the original path of closure. Premature contacts with tooth displacement may be seen (or felt) as mandibular displacements since the relaxed closure from RP is not forceful enough to displace the tooth. These can be confirmed by firm closure.

Firm closure

The patient is asked to close firmly on the back teeth from an open-mouth position and asked if this is comfortable and if it is a secure position. Any discomfort is noted with a view to this being a cause of interference or the site of a periodontal disorder. Pain may indicate a cracked tooth or one demonstrating premature contact. This closure is repeated while the operator's forefinger is lightly placed on each upper tooth in turn. Premature contacts and mobile teeth can be diagnosed by a feeling of femitus. The midline between the mandibular and maxillary central incisors can again be checked and any deviation of the mandibular in relation to the maxillary indicates that a movement of teeth has taken place and that an adaptive change in the intercuspal position has occurred.

The sounds of occlusion on firm closure as a method of diagnosis will be described in the section on gnathosonic analysis.

Parafunctional closure and movements

A further examination of facets of wear is made and these are pointed out to the patient who is then asked to press the teeth together and make the facets fit. This mandibular position may not coincide with the intercuspal position and may exist in one or more lateral or protruded positions. This evidence is also shown to the patient, in a mirror, and he is questioned if this represents a current habit. The wear may have taken place some time in the past: canine wear is common in the adolescent, often during sleep. If the habit is current, the patient is advised of its possible harm both to the teeth and as a cause of fatigue in the muscles. The patient will often deny being aware of such a habit but may acknowledge it at a subsequent visit (see Figure 7.4).

Articulation movements

The patient is asked to open and to close 'coming in from one side and then from the other'. This may or may not represent the incoming movement in mastication but it should give an indication of cusp interferences on working and non-working sides. After making several such movements, the patient is asked to stop at first contact on one side and then the other and the articulation pattern can be assessed. This examination is then repeated for the incoming protrusive movement. The whole procedure is repeated for the outgoing movements, beginning at intercuspal position and moving laterally on each side and then protrusively. Difficulties experienced by the patient in making the movements will indicate that they are probably not used and that a simple (or chopping) closure in mastication is used instead.

The articulation can then be classified as *mutually protected* (canine or incisor guided), or *unilaterally* or *bilaterally balanced* (see Chapter 5). Short or missing canines or incisors are often associated with uni- or bilateral balanced articulation. Alternatively, there may be interferences in such lateral excursions that can be harmful in parafunctional movements. These contacts can be observed more easily on casts mounted on an articulator with a pantographic transfer of border movements. The value of being able to see these articular movements on a fully adjustable articulator will be mentioned in the section on articulator analysis. For the purpose of the clinical examination it may be helpful to look upon uninterrupted articular movements as *isotonic* and parafunctional articulation as *isometric* contraction of muscles.

Retruded axis contact

This is probably the most significant movement and position to be assessed. It is sometimes the most difficult to examine and often the most puzzling to interpret and explain.

As was explained in Chapter 4, the retruded axis (or terminal hinge axis) is an imaginary line running between both condyles when they are fully retruded in their respective fossae. In this position the mandible can rotate about this axis for a distance of up to 20 mm on an arc described by the midpoint of the two mandibular central incisors. This is a reproducible arc for each patient and the occlusion which takes place on it (retruded occlusion or contact) is reproducible. Following retruded occlusion (RO) the mandible glides to IP. It has been suggested that intercuspal occlusion takes place on this arc (retruded intercuspal occlusion) in childhood but in early adolescence all teeth tend to move forwards and intercuspal occlusion becomes habitually anterior to the retruded arc.

The significance of the retruded axis closure is the direction in which the mandible travels following RO. If the occlusion is bilateral and the resultant movement to intercuspal occlusion is forwards and slightly upwards (see Posselt's vertical envelope of motion, p. 57), this is recognized as habitual but normal. If RO is on one side only and the resultant movement to intercuspal occlusion is to one side or the other, this indicates a potentially harmful adaptive movement. It means that each time the mandible closes to IP the muscles may not be contracting according to their stable patterns and the condyles are adopting a more rotated position in their respective fossae. This can result in muscle fatigue or joint click.

In examining this movement it is helpful to have the patient perform it but this is not usually possible without some assistance from the operator and practice by the patient. In the first place, the movement may not be possible because of stiffness or discomfort in the muscles. Secondly, the adaptive movement to IP has become habitual and considerable effort is required to resume the movement of retruded closure.

One procedure is to sit the patient upright with the head supported. The operator rests his thumb-nail on the lower incisor teeth (Figure 9.3a) and assists an opening and closing movement on the retruded axis. The thumb-nail arrests the movement and removes the proprioceptive stimulus caused by occlusion. This prevents the adaptive movement to IP. When the mandible seems to be swinging on this axis, closure is allowed, whereupon the patient is asked to stop as the teeth touch on the retruded arc. The completion of the movement to IP can then be observed. This requires practice and the operator requires the experience to know when the mandible is on the retruded axis and to differentiate this from a resisted retrusion.

There are other methods of chin holding and the amount of force used can only be learned by practice and results. The method most favoured currently is to have the middle of the thumb above the point of the chin and the chin cupped in the hand, thus preventing the chin being pushed to one side or the other (see Figure 8.6b). The patient is then asked to try to repeat this movement unassisted, and occlusion is prevented by holding a tongue or cement spatula against the maxillary teeth (Figure 9.3c). The most consistently helpful instruction is 'Push your upper teeth forwards'. The patient is then asked to 'Push forward and back, keeping your teeth in contact with the blade'. Then: 'Pull right back'. At this stage the patient may push the chin forwards but this can be corrected with a mirror. When the fully retruded relation is achieved, say: 'Open and close with the chin back . . . get the

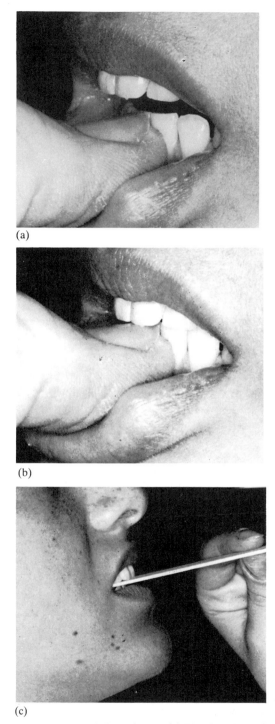

(a)

(b)

(c)

Figure 9.3 Retruded arc closure. (a) Thumb nail on mandibular incisors guiding mandible. (b) Thumb nail used as stop. (c) Patient self-assisted with wooden spatula for pulling back mandible

feel of it'. Then pull the blade away and advise: 'Repeat that open and close movement and stop when your teeth touch'. Then: 'Slide till all your teeth touch'. This should provide the evidence of the slide from RC to IP and should not exceed 1 mm and be straight upwards and forwards.

Penetration of a soft wax wafer on the retruded axis may indicate sites of retruded occlusion (Figure 9.4). The analysis of this movement can also be observed on casts mounted on an articulator with a retruded axis transfer and this will be described in the section on articulator analysis. It is emphasized that this is only an analysis and whether steps are taken to alter or correct any deflective contacts depends on the diagnosis.

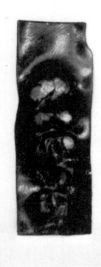

Figure 9.4 Wax penetration on retruded arc

Where a denture is worn the operator must ensure its retention; two methods are illustrated in Figure 9.5. Method (a) is preferred since the right hand is free to guide the closure. It is rarely possible to allow the patient to perform this movement without the assistance of a clamp to stabilize the lower denture. Even with such a device and a fixative it can never be certain that the denture has not moved.

Maximal active opening of the mandible

The patient is asked to open as widely as possible and to close the teeth comfortably. The observations should include: extent of opening, which should be more than 40 mm measured between the maxillary and mandibular incisors; any deviation of the mandible indicating resistance to free movement of the condyle or meniscus on the side to which the mandible deviates; any noise (click or crepitus) in one or other joint, which is usually accompanied by an uneven opening or closing movement. Auscultation, using a stethoscope, can be helpful in confirming the presence of joint noises and on which side they occur.

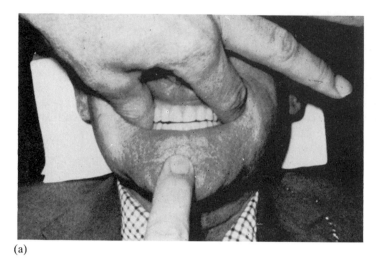

(a)

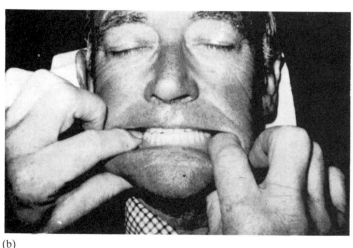

(b)

Figure 9.5 Retruded arc closure with complete dentures in place. (a) Preferred method. (b) Lower denture only held

Palpation of the condyles and muscles

This is most effectively performed while standing behind the patient with first or middle fingers lightly held over both condyles. Palpation of the condyles for tenderness is made at rest position, firm closure, and on opening widely and closing. The fingers are then moved slightly forwards into the depression in front of the condyles where the inner fibres of the masseters and possibly the lateral pterygoids can be palpated. The positions and movements are repeated. Palpation inside the ears may help in eliciting click and help the patient to tell which side the click occurs. Palpation of the masseter muscles over the mandibular rami may also elicit tenderness as may the temporalis muscles on both sides of the head. Finally, the origins of the lateral pterygoids may be palpated by inserting the forefingers behind and slightly lateral to the superior tuberosities inside the mouth where tenderness on one side may be experienced (the pterygoid sign). Tenderness from any of these regions will usually indicate injured muscles. Over the condyle itself tenderness may suggest a synovial disturbance, although the diagnosis of muscle injury is often the correct one.

During this analysis of occlusal function the operator should be able to diagnose the existence of any disturbance or disorder and to assess the tolerance and adaptability of the patient to them. He should be deciding if the patient requires treatment, as distinct from the patient's request for it.

Mandibular dysfunction syndrome

For patients who present with facial or joint pain or dysfunction suggestive of this syndrome, a form of examination can be found in the Glossary, and Chapter 13 is devoted to this topic.

Gnathosonic analysis

The impact sounds made by the teeth meeting in intercuspal occlusion have been analysed and classified by Watt (1970). His methods are directed at estimating the sounds made by stable and deflective contacts and constitute a gnathosonic analysis of occlusion.

Watt stressed 'the need for a classification that relates broad variables of function to morphological variables'. More specifically, he has been able to discover the discrepancies which exist between the muscle position (the position to which the muscles, acting harmoniously, bring the mandible in order to produce intercuspal occlusion) and the tooth position (the intercuspal position altered by tooth movement or change of occlusal surface). The premature or deflective contacts which cause these 'discrepancies' may be minute in nature but are sufficient to be recordable by the method devised by Watt. By synchronizing the sounds emitted from tooth contacts (suitably amplified and recorded) with ultra-high-speed cinematography, Watt concluded that these sounds provide 'useful analogues of occlusion'. This is known as the gnathosonic method of analysing articulation.

Three classes of impact sounds can be distinguished:

Class A. All sounds are of short duration (less than 30 ms) indicating that all tooth contacts are stable.

Class B. Some sounds are short and some prolonged, indicating that some are stable and some unstable contacts.

Class C. All sounds are prolonged (over 30 ms) indicating that all the tooth contacts are unstable.

Clinical method

The equipment required to produce traced gnathosonic records is obviously not available to the practitioner but a stethoscope or, preferably, a stereostethoscope placed on the infraorbital regions can be used to identify the three cases (Watt and Hedegard, 1967). Practice and comparison with the other methods mentioned in the previous section will bring a skill that can be most helpful in reaching a diagnosis of unstable contacts.

The patient is seated in the chair with the head supported while the operator stands behind the patient so that he can place the two ends of the stereostethoscope with equal pressure. Alternatively, the patient can be seated in a chair with the head against a wooden door, when the operator can stand in front of the patient. The door will amplify the sounds slightly, especially if it is hollow. The patient is then asked to tap the teeth together eight to ten times into the most comfortable closure of his back teeth. In addition to listening to the impact sounds, the opening and closing movements are observed for any deviation or curving of the movements which would indicate imbalance or stiffness of the muscle activity. The quality of the sounds is noted and the patient is asked if any pain or discomfort (which may be felt in a tooth or muscles) was felt.

Conclusions

In class A cases, where there is neither pain, discomfort nor deviation from the open and close movements, the classification A1 is given. Where the sounds are short but the mandible opens and closes on a curved or uneven arc indicating unbalanced muscle activity, the classification A2 is given. In class A2 cases it is often possible to detect a slight blurring of the sound on separating the teeth. This separation noise is detectable on the gnathosonic records and suggests that one or more of the teeth have moved on occlusion and are heard to slide back on the slower opening movement. An alternative explanation is that the muscle activity on closure has proved uncomfortable and the separation movement is uncertain.

Watt emphasizes that a stable occlusal sound in the presence of pain may prove to be a class C occlusion after muscle relaxation has been accomplished. Also, an unstable occlusal sound in the presence of muscle hypertonicity may prove to be stable when the hypertonicity is relieved. Pain limits movement. Stiff muscles produce uncertain movements. It is therefore important to emphasize that the occlusion should not be classified when pain symptoms are present.

In class B cases where the sounds are mixed the conclusion is that the degree of unbalanced muscle activity required to bring the teeth into stable contact is greater than in class A2 cases. These sounds may also suggest that a loose tooth or teeth have become temporarily repositioned on closure and that the contact is therefore a sliding one.

Class C occlusions exist in those cases where the patient is unable to find a stable position of closure. All the sounds are prolonged and separation noises exist in the majority.

Discussion

The conclusions which Watt draws from his observations are that the adaptive closures in the majority of mouths do not necessarily result in a precise intercuspal occlusion. It would seem that there is imbalance in much mandibular activity and that this causes, or is caused by, minor occlusal interferences. There is therefore a close relationship between these two disturbances of occlusal function, namely, unbalanced muscle activity and minor occlusal interferences. The conclusions from gnathosonic studies emphasize the fine degree of tooth movement or adaptive jaw movement which may alter the existing intercuspal position. These alterations may require corrections of a relatively minute nature in order to restore comfort and efficiency to occlusal function. This assumes that there are symptoms or signs to justify treatment.

It should be emphasized that these observations are made in the empty mouth. Therefore, it would be fair to conclude that the disturbances are caused in the empty mouth, namely, by grinding habits which can cause tooth movement or muscle fatigue with consequent unbalanced muscle activity. However, persistent chewing of resistant foods is a likely cause, as would be chewing on pipes or pens.

Clinical applications

In addition to the value of gnathosonic analysis in making a diagnosis there are two further clinical applications which should be mentioned.

First, prior to making fixed or removable prostheses it provides a simple and quick method (for the trained ear) of assessing the intercuspal position and, after the appliances have been placed, of checking it. The sound of a 'high' filling, crown or pontic (supracontacts) is unmistakable. A class A intercuspal occlusion should therefore be established before any prosthesis is made.

Secondly, it provides a continuing check on the intercuspal occlusion, in view of its tendency to change.

The ten-point test for occlusal function

The following points should provide a revision of what has been described and a reference list for assessing occlusal problems.

 1. Patient's assessment of function and parafunction.
 2. Stability of rest position and lip competence.
 3. The interocclusal distance and any cusp interference from rest position.
 4. The incisor midlines and any altered tooth inclinations.
 5. Palpation and sounds of intercuspal occlusion on firm closure.
 6. Length and direction of slide from retruded to intercuspal occlusion.
 7. Wear facets as indicators of parafunction.
 8. Articulation movements to and from IP.
 9. Maximum active opening of mandible: deviation and noises.
10. Palpation of joints and muscles.

The compilation of this list is the result of a generous series of letters from Professor Krogh Poulson (1971).

Hand-held study casts

Before proceeding to the topic of articulator analysis, the useful practice of looking at occlusal positions on hand-held study casts will be briefly discussed.

The casts should be made from fully extended alginate or reversible hydrocolloid impressions. The plaster bases should be trimmed so that the teeth fit into intercuspal occlusion when placed on the bench on their back or side surfaces (Figure 9.6). When picked up from these positions they will be in intercuspal occlusion. They should be freed from plaster bubbles and impression faults so that the eye is not distracted by imperfections. They should be pleasing to look at. The following disturbances can be noted.

1. Facets of wear and otherwise altered occlusal surfaces: indications of parafunction and improperly contoured restorations.

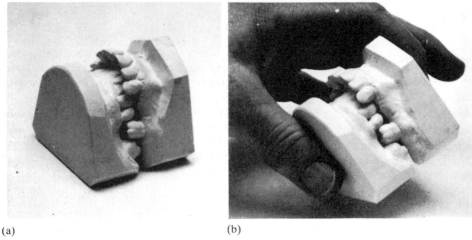

(a)   (b)

Figure 9.6 Hand-held study casts. Note occlusal curve disturbance

2. Tipped teeth and potential causes of cusp interference.
3. Migration of teeth and the need to check tongue–lip muscle activity and to examine for periodontal lesions.
4. Overerupted teeth and closs of occlusal curve.
5. The possibilities of altered intercuspal position.
6. Open contact points and possible plunger cusps.
7. Certain developmental anomalies.

Other aids to diagnosis from these casts include the classification of buccal segment relationships, central incisor midline deviations, horizontal and vertical incisor overlap rotations, overcrowding and views of the teeth from the lingual side.

When seen in conjunction with a set of radiographs, provisional conclusions can be made on the effects of occlusal forces on already disordered periodontal tissues and indications for treatment can be decided. However, *hand-held study casts can only provide guesses at occlusal positions and articulations*. Where radical treatment measures are being planned they should serve as indicators for articulator analysis. At all stages in analysis and diagnosis it is important to consider the potentially harmful effects of gap-filling restorative measures before any occlusal disturbances have been diagnosed and treated.

Articulator analysis

Occlusal function is performed, for the most part, behind closed lips, and attempts to study it are much hindered by its being out of sight. The parting of the lips reveals only buccal and labial contacts and even those are partly obscured by the vertical overlap. In addition, parting of the lips by the operator usually results in adaptive movements which are not those of the natural function being analysed. Consequently, the ability to see casts of the teeth on an articulator moving on the same paths which they follow in the mouth provides a substantial aid in diagnosis and treatment planning. The requirement of accuracy has not yet been fully met but it can be provided in direct proportion to the quality of the instrument selected and the expertise of the operator using it.

Descriptions and usage of articulators were the subject of Chapter 8 and it remains now to apply the instrument to the need and to emphasize certain principles. For purposes of diagnosis where cusp interferences are seen or suspected, it is desirable, even necessary, to have the advantages of the fully adjustable articulator, but not every practice has one. Lundeen's (1979) observations from 'several hundred recordings' allowed him to advise that a choice could be made from five patterns for the majority of patients' border movements. This will make the use of border movements more available for diagnosis. The accurate transfer of the retruded axis is essential and if a semi-adjustable instrument is the one of choice it must have either extendible condyle rods or horizontally adjustable condyles in order to provide the correct orientation of axis to articulator. Thus, the transfer of the upper cast by facebow from the retruded axis marks and mounting of the lower cast by precontact retruded record will allow closure of upper to lower cast to be an accurate copy of mandibular to maxillary teeth. Any cusp interferences seen on this path of closure should correspond to those seen in the mouth. It has to be said that the mounting of study casts on a plain hinge has little value in analysing the movement of closure, and certainly no more than hand-held casts. The mounting of casts with an arbitrary facebow transfer and precontact retruded record on a semi-adjustable articulator is a big step in the right direction but its limitations should be understood. The fine adjustments made by the neuromuscular responses in the mouth cannot be accurately copied by these latter transfers.

Choice of articulator

The four semi-adjustable and two fully adjustable instruments mentioned in Chapter 8 are six out of many.

Rigidity and flexibility would seem to be opposite qualities but both are required: the former for accurate movement and the latter for adaptability. The arcon instrument is always preferred to the condylar for accuracy of protrusive and lateral movements but the difference is small. Plastic condylar housings and incisal guidance tables make it easier to copy incisor and canine guidances by additions of acrylic resin, and a curved incisal guidance pin allows the point of the pin to remain stationary on the table when the upper member is moved up or down. There are, therefore, pros and cons to all instruments and one has to take advice from users and teachers as well as to use one's own judgement.

Procedures

Location and transfer of the retruded axis

This has been described in Chapter 8, except for the method of moving the patient's mandible and ensuring a secure fit of the clutch to which is attached ths axis locator.

Practice is necessary to achieve the relaxed retruded open and closed movement. Whether the patient is supine or upright the head should be supported and the operator behind the patient. The patient's chin should be cupped in the operator's most used hand which should feel for the 'give and let go' by the patient. The patient should be encouraged to recognize this feeling during the practice session. The clutch should have a piece of soft wax over the incisors to help prevent vibration; the cementing material should have that combination of rigidity and ease of removal which is not always easy to achieve. An acrylic special tray ending at the greatest convexity of the mandibular teeth with a metal bite-fork (for attachment to the locator) processed to it will usually serve well. It should be as thin as possible occlusally to allow maximal closure. The teeth are coated with a thin layer of Vaseline and the clutch cemented with zinc-oxide–eugenol impression paste. One side-arm with condyle pointer is then attached and the retruded axis performed. The side-arm is adjusted until the pointer is rotating (hence the graph paper). The paper is removed and the point on the cheek marked. This is repeated on the other side, after which the clutch and locator are removed. The facebow side-arms are now added and the facebow transfer made. Care is taken to have slide markers on both pointers so that they can be withdrawn (to prevent scratching the face) and replaced, thus preserving the intercondylar distance.

The retruded precontact record

This is registered using two thicknesses of hard wax, softened in a water bath and strengthened by a palatal metal sheet. The wax should not be penetrated (indicating tooth contact and probable deflexion). Alternatively (Figure 9.7c,d), two double layers of hard wax (separated by tin foil) softened in warm water can be used. The anterior stop method incorporating a frame for holding the registration medium is another alternative (Figure 9.8a,b,c,d). The record is then used for mounting the lower cast to the upper on the articulator. Closure of the upper

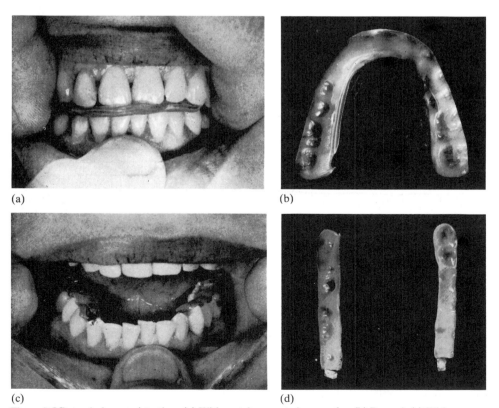

(a)

(b)

(c)

(d)

Figure 9.7 Retruded arc registration. (a) With metal supported wax wafer. (b) Record. (c) With wax-strips. (d) Records

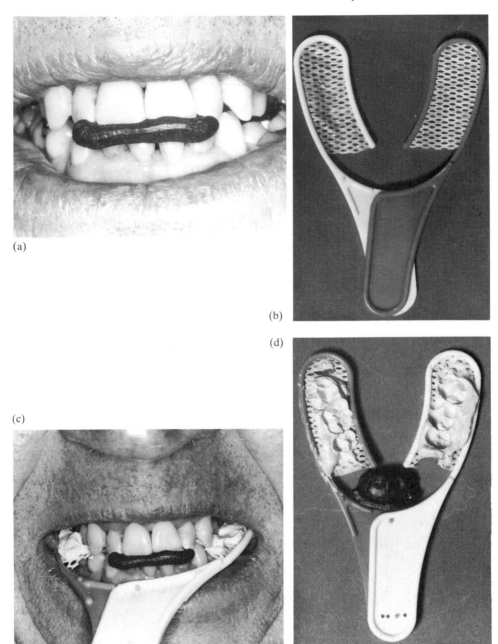

Figure 9.8 Jaw registration. (a) Anterior stop. (b) Paste holding device (Coe). (c) Registration. (d) Record

member will demonstrate the first contact on the retruded arc, after which the upper member will displace backwards until the teeth slide into intercuspal occlusion. This represents the lower teeth sliding forwards from retruded occlusion to the intercuspal position.

In making this registration it is important to ensure that the mandibular muscles are relaxed. Any resistance to the retruded arc movements by stiffness, pain or voluntary effort by the patient should first be resolved. If any uncertainty exists the record should be confirmed by repeated records checked by the split cast (p. 189) or other method.

The value of being able to see the retruded arc of closure and subsequent movement to IP lies in the direction which the mandible moves following RC. If this movement has a lateral component it means that the muscles have adapted to a lateral habitual IP and that unbalanced muscle activity can be expected. A forward movement to IP is the normal expectation. This will prove a valuable guide if occlusal adjustment procedures are being planned (Chapters 10 and 11).

Incisal and canine guidance

The incisal guidance table is adjusted so that the incisal pin will remain on the table as the upper incisor teeth are made to glide backwards on the tips of the mandibular incisors. This is repeated for the lateral movements guided by the canines (and perhaps the incisors). The condyle guidance mechanisms are freed and can be fixed at the angles determined by the incisal and canine guidances.

The lateral (Bennett) shift

Only the fully adjustable articulators can accurately copy this movement since it begins immediately the rotations of both condyles begin. Many of the adjustable articulators allow a lateral component of movement but it is either determined by the horizontal inclination of the guide paths (see Figure 8.10) or guessed by a hand-directed movement. The value of being able to see the immediate side shift in the Bennett movement is again emphasized and for this aid in diagnosis the fully adjustable instrument is required.

The fully adjustable articulator

If this type of articulator is selected for treatment it is imperative that it is used for analysis and diagnosis. The location of the retruded condyle axis is registered and marked on the face. The frames are then used for the pantographic tracings which must repeat themselves after the covers have been placed over them. The frames are then locked together in the retruded position of the mandible and a pointer is attached so as to relate the level at which the tracings were made to a fixed point on the face. The condyle pointers are adjusted to touch the retruded axis marks and their positions relative to the frame noted so that they can be withdrawn to prevent scratching the face on removal and be replaced accurately for mounting. The clutches and frames are then removed from the mouth and reassembled on the articulator. The intercondylar distance of the articulator is adjusted to fit the patient's intercondylar distance and the upper and lower clutches are plastered to the upper and lower members of the articulator respectively. The clutches are then adjusted to follow the tracings, after which the casts of the upper and lower teeth can be mounted using the adjustable facebow and a retruded axis precontact interocclusal record.

Pantographic diagnosis

If the tracings show irregular movements within the borders, especially those on the anterior tables, muscle dysfunction is indicated. The mandible is finding difficulty in reaching the borders and there is likely to be injury, areas of scar tissue or spasm within the muscles. Also, if the tracings do not repeat themselves after the covers have been placed, there are likely to be problems which should be resolved before proceeding with any diagnosis or treatment. The wearing of an incisal overlay will usually resolve such inhibited movements.

Provisional wax-up

After mounting the study casts it is always advisable to show them to the technician and patient and also to a colleague if there are doubts cast or choices to be made. The plaster teeth should then be prepared and a wax-up of the proposed restorations made. This will give indications of tooth preparations and any coverage necessary, space required and shapes for pontics and the occlusal forms relative to opposing and adjacent teeth.

Comment

Obviously, routine dental care does not require these painstaking examinations and analyses. What is advised, however, is a few questions and observations concerning the comfort and efficiency of the mouth, emphasizing to the patient that these qualities contribute to good function and health which, in turn, help to prevent disturbances and disorders. The ten-point test will provide an adequate examination which is not time-consuming and will indicate if further investigations are required. If disturbances are present and disorders suspected the more comprehensive functional, gnathosonic and articulator investigations are advised.

References

Lundeen, H. C. (1979) Mandibular movement recordings and articulator adjustments simplified. *Dental Clinics of North America*, **23**, 231

Watt, D. M. (1970) Classification of occlusion. *Dental Practitioner and Dental Record*, **20**, 305

Watt, D. M. and Hedegard, B. (1967) The stereostethoscope. An instrument for clinical gnathosonics. *Journal of Prosthetic Dentistry*, **18**, 458

Chapter 10

Occlusal adjustment of the natural teeth

The objectives in restorative or corrective measures concerned with the occlusion of the teeth are to provide even contact in IP, equal bilateral contact on retruded closure (usually on one molar tooth on each side), and to prevent cusp interferences during mastication and empty-mouth articular movements. These objectives will help to provide efficient and comfortable occlusal function and to make patients unaware of their teeth.

Cusp interferences in the natural dentition are defined as contacts between opposing teeth which interfere with the established closing or chewing movements of the mandible and with bilateral contact on the retruded axis. They can cause disturbances to occlusal function. Cusp interferences can take place during mastication, swallowing and empty-mouth parafunction. They can be corrected by occlusal adjustment. This is a procedure which occupies a controversial place in the treatment of occlusal dysfunction because it is irreversible. It often forms part of the treatment plan prior to making partial dentures or bridgework and is a recognized procedure in the treatment of the mandibular dysfunction syndrome where displacing activities of the mandible have been diagnosed. Much occlusal adjustment of the natural dentition is carried out empirically and this can be helpful in reducing supracontacts on fillings and forces on mobile or periodontally infected teeth, provided certain principles are observed. On the other hand, disorders of the masticatory system can be caused by the indiscriminate removal or reduction of cusps in the emergency treatment of some of these conditions.

Occlusal adjustment is defined as a planned removal of selected occlusal areas of the teeth in order to restore stability to the mandible on closure and to remove interferences to and from IP in functional and parafunctional movements. The older term, 'selective grinding', is perhaps more realistic but this is the age of the euphemism. It cannot be too strongly emphasized that these procedures are irreversible and no amount of secondary dentine will restore a lost occlusal shape.

The term occlusal adjustment can, of course, be used in a wider sense to describe procedures on the teeth that restore lost occlusal height or prevent harmful parafunctional habits, but in this chapter the term refers to reshaping of the tooth surfaces by selective removal.

Indications

1. The mandibular dysfunction syndrome where there is a lateral deflexion to IP from retruded occlusion.

2. Preparatory treatment for fixed and removable prostheses where displacing activities on closure have been diagnosed.
3. Postorthodontic treatment in adults, with limited application for adolescents.
4. Postperiodontal treatment.
5. Improvement of appearance of incisor and canine teeth.
6. As part of a plan in the treatment of mobility and migration.
7. As emergency treatment of tooth extrusion following periodontal abscess or of injury to opposing mucosa in cases of overclosure.

It will be noted that the first four require a plan for the development of stable IP and free articulation and that the remainder are localized measures.

Contraindications

1. Severe overclosure and displacement, except as part of the prosthetic plan.
2. On sensitive, worn and adolescent teeth, with some exceptions for the last.
3. Patients who are preoccupied with their teeth and for whom the mouth and teeth have become an outlet for irrelevant muscle activity.

Plan and mounting

A plan for adjustment is essential and should be based on an analysis of habitual occlusal function and of the movement between retruded and intercuspal occlusion. This should be carried out first on mounted casts using a retruded axis transfer and retruded arc record. This record should be checked against two or more similar records using a split cast mounting (see p. 189). Records for transferring protrusive and lateral movements should be made according to the accuracy required (see p. 158). The retruded contact, habitual intercuspal position and canine and incisor guidance can then be assessed and decisions made to remove cusp interferences to and from intercuspal position and during working and non-working side movements. A record of interferences to be corrected is illustrated in Figure 10.1.

Ret   Pro

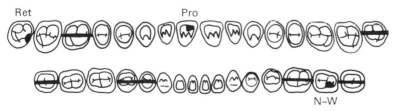

N–W

Figure 10.1 Retruded (Ret), protruded (Pro) and non-working (N-W) interferences

Adjustments on casts

This is now carried out using a sharp knife or dental excavator and noting each cut as it is made. This will help the beginner to see the effect of adjustment at close viewing and at each stage, and will ensure that the more experienced practitioner maintains objectives.

There are nine principles involved in providing good occlusion and articulation by occlusal adjustment:

1. Provide bilateral contact on retruded occlusion with a forward glide to intercuspal occlusion free from interferences.
2. Provide intercuspal occlusion on retruded axis if this is required by diagnosis.
3. Remove cusp interferences (both working and non-working) on protrusive and lateral articulation.
4. Remove posterior tooth contacts on protrusive and lateral articulation if this is required by diagnosis.
5. Provide group contact between opposing incisors on protrusion.
6. provide tripod contact between cusp ridges and opposing fossae wherever possible.
7. Avoid loss of OVR.
8. Reduce effect of plunger cusp without disturbing cusp–ridge occlusion.
9. Retain the shapes of cusps and fossae.

Procedures

For interferences to retruded occlusion

The following are advised for the situations indicated.

Cusp or fossa

Note. It will have been noted that the terms 'mandibular' and 'maxillary' have been used to describe teeth or tooth surfaces in the mandible and maxilla. In this chapter, 'lower' and 'upper' will be used to denote tooth surfaces so that the various acronyms in general use can be employed as an aid to memorizing the adjustment procedures.

Schuyler's (1935) rule provides the first guidance for trimming: if a cusp does not make premature contact in lateral and protrusive articulation, trim the fossa. If it does make contact in these movements, trim the cusp. It is rare that a cusp has to be reshaped in the natural dentition but if it does, retain the shape by trimming around the cusp, reducing it gradually.

Fossa

To produce a more retruded contact, trim the mesial facing inner inclines of the upper fossae or the distal facing inner inclines of the lower, thus MU or DL (Figure 10.2). This will permit a more distal seating of the lower cusp into an upper fossa or

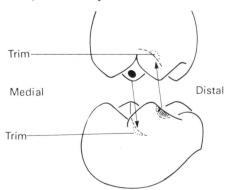

Trim

Medial   Distal

Trim

Figure 10.2 Fossa adjustment to provide more retruded intercuspal position. Mesial upper or distal lower. MU DL

a more distal seating of a lower fossa around an upper cusp. This may apply to any part of the occlusal surface between the mesial and distal marginal ridges.

Marginal ridges

Rather than cut into the ridges themselves and so initiate or aggravate a plunger cusp action, the mesial facing cusp ridges of the lower buccal (supporting) cusps or the distal facing cusp ridges of the upper lingual (supporting) cusps may be trimmed; thus, MIBL or DILU (Figure 10.3). This may tend to cause a slide forward into a habitual occlusion but, if limited to one or at the most two teeth, the remaining teeth in intercuspal occlusion should prevent this slide.

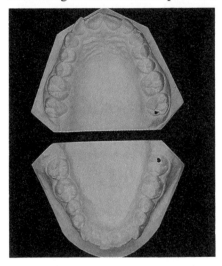

Figure 10.3 For interferences to retruded occlusion on marginal ridges, trim opposing cusp ridges: mesial inner of buccal lower or distal inner of lingual upper. Thus MIBL or DILU

For interferences which produce a lateral glide into habitual intercuspal position

This can prove helpful in the treatment of the mandibular dysfunction syndrome.

1. The teeth on the side *to* which the mandible is deflected are trimmed on the *non-working inclines*, namely, the *mesial inner inclines of the buccal lower cusps* or the *distal inner inclines of the lingual upper cusps* (Figure 10.4); thus, MI of BL or DI of LU. Trimming should be carried out diagonally on these non-working inclines so that there will be no interferences when lateral movements are performed.
2. Teeth on the side *from* which the mandible is deflected are trimmed on the *inner inclines of the buccal upper* or *lingual lower cusps* (Figure 10.5); thus, inner of BU or LL. In this situation, however, it would be allowable to trim the functional outer aspects of the buccal lower or lingual upper cusps since it is for intercuspal occlusion that this adjustment is being performed.

For interferences in working and protrusive articulation

1. On the working side in lateral articulation: trim the *buccal upper* or *lingual lower cusp ridges on their inner facing surfaces* (Figure 10.6); thus, BU or LL. On the buccal upper trim *distally*; on the lingual lower trim *mesially*, thus avoiding reduction of buccal lower and lingual upper supporting cusps which might alter the intercuspal position.

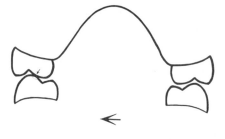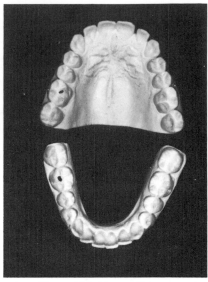

Figure 10.4 For interferences which cause lateral displacement on side to which the mandible moves or for non-working interferences on that side, trim mesial facing inner aspect of buccal lower or distal facing inner aspect of lingual upper. Thus MIBL or DILU

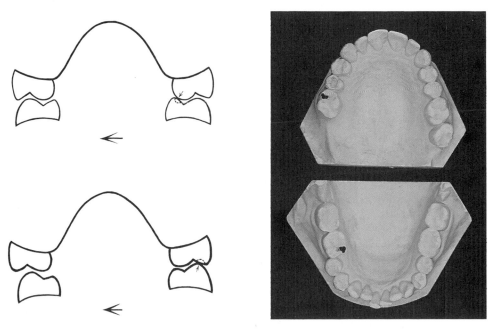

Figure 10.5 For interference which causes lateral displacement to the opposite from which initial contact occurs, trim buccal upper or lingual lower. Thus BU or LL

2. In protrusive articulation: trim as for working side lateral articulation.
3. On incisors and canines in lateral and protrusive articulation: trim the lingual surfaces of the uppers in order to avoid loss of intercuspal occlusion. The incisal edges may be trimmed to provide group contact in protrusion if appearance permits. Care must be taken to avoid removing canine or incisor guidance surfaces.

For interferences in non-working articulation

These interferences take place between opposing supporting cusps on the side opposite to that being used for chewing and care should be taken to avoid loss of occlusion in intercuspal position. The rule, therefore, is to trim the *mesial inner inclines* of the *buccal lower cusps* (i.e. the triangular ridges running inwards towards the fossa from the cusp tips). Alternatively, trim the *distal inner inclines* of the *lingual upper cusps* (i.e. the triangular ridge running inwards towards the fossa from the cusp tip) (Figure 10.4b).

In these procedures each cut made on the casts should be noted in order to prepare a trimming list for the adjustment of the teeth in the mouth. Short cuts should be avoided since they often lead to shortening of supporting cusps and to complaints of 'lost support for my teeth', 'clashing' and awareness of the teeth which was not previously present. Non-working interferences can be prevented by simultaneous bilateral chewing on the posterior teeth.

Procedures on the teeth

The exercise of performing the adjustment on mounted casts not only helps the beginner to see the results and prepare a trimming list but to make mistakes on plaster and not on enamel and dentine. The trimming list should be prepared with reference to specific areas on the teeth.

Before trimming the teeth, the patient should be trained in performing the retruded arc of closure and in ensuring that the same arc is performed each time. The 'cement spatula' movement (p. 151): 'forward and back, forward and back, *right* back' is practised before the opening and closing movement 'with the chin back' is tried. The dentist should feel the retrusion with the base of his thumb on the patient's chin and the patient should then be able to open and close in retrusion without assistance. Protruded and lateral retruded movements should also be practised.

Articulating papers

The ultrathin plastic 'paper' (GMH) with a marking stain on one side only is recommended. Spring-loaded pliers for holding the paper reduces the attention required to keep tweezer beaks held together, but two pairs are required, one for marking the upper and one for the lower. The marks on the opposing teeth can then be checked in succession. If the double-sided paper is used there will be marks on opposing teeth where firm contact has been made and the paper will be punctured. A well-defined spot will be seen on the tooth where sharp ridge or cusp has made contact and a ring on the flatter opposing tooth. Where a sliding contact has been made a line puncture mark will be seen.

The practice of occlusal adjustment will be improved by the following suggestions:

1. The paper should be cut to the length and width of the quadrant being examined with an overlap for the pliers.
2. The teeth should be dry, otherwise a sliding contact may simulate interference.
3. Cheek retraction by an assistant aids visibility.
4. The patient should practise the required movement with the cheeks retracted.
5. There should only be one mark if there is one interference.
6. The use of different colours for occlusion, working and non-working articulation prevents confusion.
7. The teeth should be cleaned and dried between registrations.
8. The patient should be allowed to rest between registrations and to test the effects of each adjustment.

Instruments (Figure 10.6)

Stones and rubber polishing discs are advised and water cooling is essential. The tapered fissure stone (diamond or carborundum) in a slow-running handpiece is the tool of choice for reshaping ridges while the knife-edge stone is preferred for deepening fossae and fissures. All cut tooth surfaces should be polished but the practice of chew-in carborundum paste is discouraged in view of the possibilities of reducing the OVR.

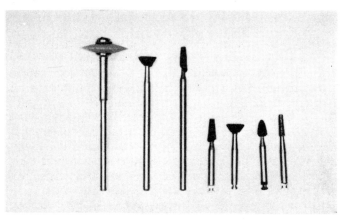

Figure 10.6 Instruments

The foregoing principles and objectives derive from the original teaching of Schuyler (1935), later developed by Lauritzen (1951), Beyron (1954), Jankelson (1960), Ramfjord and Ash (1974) and many other proponents of adjustment. In the hands of painstaking dentists these procedures represent a method of providing improved function. But mistakes have been made and excesses of treatment have led to dental distress ranging from mandibular dysfunction and awareness of teeth to mental depression requiring psychiatric care. It is seldom that, in a mouth with class I occlusion with normal vertical and horizontal overlap and with ridges and fissures intact, such treatment will be required. But where missing and tilted teeth exist with reverse overlaps and large flat fillings, occlusal analysis will often reveal the need for improved function by adjustment. Guiding cusps may have become supporting cusps due to reverse overlaps; fossae and fissures may have disappeared; mobility and migration may not be correctible; periodontal breakdown may have to be treated before any occlusal corrections can be undertaken. But when such problems have been solved and occlusal surfaces have been restored, occlusal adjustment will provide a necessary stage in treatment and the prevention of further breakdown.

Alternative methods

The plea for simplicity should always be heard but occlusal dysfunction cannot be cured by reducing a few cusps and without resort to the principles outlined. Nevertheless, more simple procedures have been outlined and both Silverman (1962) and Ross (1970) are recommended reading for practical methods of adjustment carried out in the mouth. Shore (1976), in a comprehensive text, describes an autorepositioning appliance made of acrylic resin and fitted to the maxillary arch. Rapid set resin is added until retruded occlusion is achieved between the mandibular teeth and the appliance at a minimally increased OVR. This level is gradually reduced until there is contact with the maxillary teeth on the retruded arc of closure. Adjustment is then carried out in stages on the teeth as the OVR is gradually closed by reducing the acrylic bite plane.

Jankelson (1960) identifies cusp interference to intercuspal position by a tap-tap technique or a stretch and relax method of adopting retruded closure. More recently Jankelson (1979) reports on his myomonitor which produces relaxation of the mandibular muscles and then initiates controlled isotonic muscle contraction. This propels the mandible from rest position to a 'neuromuscularly orientated occlusal position in space'. This is referred to as 'myocentric occlusion' and in no measured instance was it found to coincide with the retruded arc of closure. Occlusal ajustment carried out at myocentric occlusion by 'transcutaneous electrical neural stimulation' provides optimal occlusal function, according to Jankelson. Cusp interferences are recognized by penetration of soft occlusal wax and marked by a wax pencil. Singer (1966) uses a 'chewing detector' for covering the teeth. The teeth are specially treated and covered with a varnish. The patient is limited to a liquid diet until the next visit, when the parafunctional contacts are revealed. It is used, therefore, for examining tooth contacts between meals and overnight. Adjustment is carried out at the chairside as thought best.

Glickman (1979) describes occlusal adjustment as being necessary to relieve microtrauma associated with periodontal injury, muscular dysfunction and mandibular joint disorders. The objective is to correct cusp interferences and so achieve mandibular stability in IP. Interferences are recognized during three movements: functional, from one border position to another and by using Jankelson's myomonitor into an optimal IP, as outlined in the previous paragraph. The methods are, therefore, both static and excursive. The areas trimmed are: (1) buccal inclines of the mandibular buccal cusps against the lingual inclines of the maxillary buccal cusps; and (2) labial surfaces of the mandibular incisors against the lingual surfaces of the maxillary incisors. Glickman describes the correction of these surfaces as grooving, spheroiding and pointing. The mounting of casts on an adjustable articulator for study and practice is recommended and ten steps in procedure are described.

Riise (1982) describes a rational performance of occlusal adjustment in two steps. In step I the adjustment is performed in the closing movements and in step II during contact excursions. In step I, adjustment starts with the patient in the supine position and providing guided closing movements into the retruded contact position. The patient should feel completely relaxed (as should the operator) and should exert light and hard pressure in succession on closure. Adjustment is made on the mesial facing aspects of the maxillary teeth. Only occasionally should the adjustment be made on the mandibular teeth. The patient then sits upright, looking ahead and ensures that the occlusion is even.

In step II, with the patient again supine, the operator guides the mandible in free contact excursions (right, left and forward) and these contacts are marked. The patient again performs the movements with light and hard pressure. Adjustments should not start until all contacts have been indicated and diagrams of areas to be adjusted are noted. The adjustments should be performed only on the maxillary teeth except where a cross-bite exists. Then, the maxillary teeth are considered mandibular and are adjusted. Tests for free movements are carried out in both supine and upright seated positions.

Kleinrok (1984) has developed an intraoral tracing device (Functionograph) that enables recordings of both free and tooth-guided mandibular movements to be made intraorally on the same tracing plate. Ninety-six patients with 'articulatory disturbances' were examined and the records showed that the tooth-guided movements were asymmetrical and related to the location of the disturbances. A simple objective diagnosis could be made of intercuspal and gliding contacts. Improvements in the symmetry of the tracings followed the correction of the cusp interferences. Details of three cases are given.

Localized occlusal adjustment

There are several disturbances and disorders which can be adjusted directly in the mouth without recourse to mounted casts, although a clear objective and awareness of potential harm are always necessary. These conditions are: mobility and migration, extrusion following periodontal abscess, extrusion of incisors in mandibular overclosure causing ulceration of opposing mucosa, extrusion of the unopposed last molar tooth, appearance defects on anterior teeth and supracontacts on recent restorations.

Mobility and *migration* are treated (see Chapter 14) according to a plan. Careful but minimal reduction of the occlusal surface causing the movement is usually necessary to relieve the aggravating factor in these conditions.

Periodontal abscess can be relieved of its pain by removing the occlusal force. On the assumption that the tooth is going to be successfully treated, adjustment should be performed with a view to future cusp–fossa relations. Where possible the fossa should be reduced.

Overclosed incisors should be minimally reduced in order to relieve the injury being caused. This can only be a temporary measure since the affected teeth will continue to erupt and be repositioned. A treatment plan should be made to stabilize such teeth and correct the OVR if necessary (see Figure 14.3 and p. 262).

The *unopposed last molar* is a common cause of displacing activity and the mandibular dysfunction syndrome, and its extraction is usually advised. Immediate treatment is to remove the deflecting surface of the extruded tooth (see Figure 7.2d,e).

Appearance defects of incisor and canine teeth can often be improved by small adjustments to their incisal edges. Caution is advised to prevent overshortening which may disturb lip posture and cause speech defects. The patient should be warned of the dangers which also include reducing removal of unsupported enamel in large class III fillings and penetration of the dentine. Better to accept a small improvement than to regret an irreplaceable loss.

Supracontacts on crowns and fillings should be reduced with a view to maintaining cusp–fossa relations. The temptation to reduce a supporting cusp should be resisted. Loss of support following such 'treatment' can be a cause of reduced function and muscle pain.

Occlusal adjustment of amalgam fillings can include the development of triangular and marginal ridges which will help to develop tripod contact, relieve interferences and improve function.

Occlusal additions

The advent of composite resins has made it possible for additions to be made to the enamel surfaces of teeth and the glass ionomer cements for additions to dentine. The latter material can then be etched and a layer of composite resin added. Boksman (1983) has demonstrated reconstruction of a complete natural dentition, severely abraded, by using composite resins. He recommends the heavily filled variety that has more durability than the microfilled resins. Rubber dam is necessary and the enamel edges should be chamfered for etching and attaching the resin. The occlusal level should not be increased more than 2 mm. Van der Knij, van Velzen and Wabeke (1986) have used the acid etch technique on the lingual surfaces of canines to restore the rise required for canine guidance. The author has restored worn and excessively adjusted cusps using this method, with some success and probably with some luck. The occlusal position has to be predetermined and practised and the amount of composite resin must be neither too much nor too little.

Occlusal adjustment and counselling

A comparison between occlusal adjustment and counselling was conducted by Kopp (1979). Thirty patients with mandibular dysfunction involving the joints were examined at three visits six weeks apart. At the first visit all received counselling. At the second they were divided into two groups: one received occlusal adjustment and the other no treatment. The degree of dysfunction was assessed by the patients according to Helkimo's (1976) five grade scale. Subjective dysfunction after counselling was reduced by 60% but there was no effect on clinical dysfunction. Clinical dysfunction was reduced by 67% following occlusal adjustment but there was no further effect on the subjective dysfunction score. It was concluded that counselling may reduce the subjective symptoms, and occlusal adjustment the clinical signs, of dysfunction but individual variation in response was substantial. A helpful list of references is appended.

Mock equilibration (Goodman, Greene and Laskin, 1976)

Because none of the acceptable occlusal treatments for MDS have been evaluated under controlled conditions, 25 patients suffering the syndrome were analysed and treated with mock equilibration (adjustment limited to non-occluding surfaces) together with 'strong positive suggestions'. The occlusal analyses had revealed a variety of 'so-called occlusal disharmonies'. Nevertheless, of the 25 patients, 16

(64%) reported 'a total or nearly total remission' of their symptoms. These patients have remained symptom free for periods ranging from 6 to 29 months. The remaining 9 patients were classified as 'unsuccessfully treated'. Thus, the placebo effect is claimed and the assumption that occlusal disharmonies are causative of facial pain is undermined. One would like to have had a critical look at the occlusions but the implied warning against indiscriminate adjustment should be heeded.

Comment

It has to be repeated and emphasized that this form of treatment is almost always irreversible and the effects of it, incorrectly applied, can lead to disorders of muscle activity and facial pain, undue awareness of teeth or lack of them ('I cannot find my bite' or 'There is a hole in my tooth'), hypersensitivity in the teeth adjusted, and even to depressive illness because of alteration to the tooth surfaces. Short cuts and indiscriminate or inspirational removal of occlusal surfaces can cause distress and are to be avoided at all costs. Instead, the objective of instantaneous intercuspal occlusion round the arch must be achieved, with each supporting cusp occluding in an opposing fossa or between two marginal ridges. One clear snapping sound should be heard. From IP to protrusion there should be gliding contact between opposing incisors without interferences; to lateral protrusions, a rise between opposing canines on the side to which the mandible is moving.

Occlusal adjustment following orthodontic treatment for teeth which have been moved should be prescribed cautiously and not until retainers have been worn for a predetermined length of time. Following periodontal surgery and the healing of tissues, analysis of closure and of articular movements will usually reveal interferences which should be corrected in order to achieve that same snapping closure and free gliding movement. Thus, occlusal adjustment requires cooperation between specialities in both hospital and general practice.

References

Beyron, H. L. (1954) Characteristics of functionally optimal occlusion and principles of occlusal rehabilitation. *Journal of the American Dental Association,* **48**, 648

Boksman, L. (1983) Use of composites in the treatment of lost vertical dimension. *Journal of the Ontario Dental Association,* **60**, 24

Glickman, I. (1979) *Clinical Periodontology,* 5th edn, Saunders, Philadelphia, p. 947

Goodman, P., Greene, C. S. and Laskin, D. M. (1976) Response of patients with myofacial pain–dysfunction syndrome to mock equilibration. *Journal of the American Dental Association,* **92**, 755

Helkimo, M. (1976) Epidemiological surveys of dysfunction of the masticatory system. *Oral Sciences Review,* **1**, 54

Jankelson, B. (1960) A technique for obtaining optimum functional relationship in the natural dentition. *Dental Clinics of North America,* **March**, 131

Jankelson, B. (1979) Neuromuscular aspects of occlusion. *Dental Clinics of North America,* **23**, 157

Kleinrok, M. (1984) Occlusal adjustment under the control of intraoral recording with the aid of the functiograph. *Journal of Oral Rehabilitation,* **11**, 181

Kopp, S. (1979) Short term evaluation of counselling and occlusal adjustment in patients with mandibular dysfunction involving the TMJ. *Journal of Oral Rehabilitation,* **6**, 101

Lauritzen, A. G. (1951) Function, prime objective of restorative dentistry. A definitive procedure to obtain it. *Journal of the American Dental Association,* **42**, 523

Ramfjord, S. P. and Ash, M. (1974) *Occlusion*, Saunders, Philadelphia, p. 255

Riise, C. (1982) Rational performance of occlusal adjustment. *Journal of Prosthetic Dentistry,* **48**, 319

Ross, I. F. (1970) *Occlusion: a Concept for the Clinician*, Mosby, St Louis

Schuyler, C. H. (1935) Fundamental principles in the correction of occlusal disharmony, natural and artificial. *Journal of the American Dental Association,* **22**, 1193

Shore, N. A. (1976) *Temporomandibular Joint Dysfunction and Occlusal Equilibration*, Lippincott, Philadelphia

Silverman, M. M. (1962) *Occlusion*, Mutual Publishing, Washington DC

Singer, F. (1966) Occlusions, functions and parafunctions. *International Dental Journal,* **16**, 385

van der Knij, P., van Velzen, F. J. and Wabeke, K. B. (1986) Cuspid guidance and acid etch techniques in the restoration of cuspid protected occlusion. *Nederlands Tijdschrift voor Tandheelkunde,* **93**, 172 (English abstract)

Chapter 11

Occlusion in fixed prosthodontics

Most procedures on the teeth involve considerations of occlusion. Failure to restore occlusal contacts which blend with adjacent and opposing teeth can lead to disturbances in muscle activity and possibly to injury, spasm and fatigue. On the other hand, life can be sustained without teeth, or with small numbers of them, unencumbered with dentures, partial or complete. The good fortune of such people, however, does not constitute a case for less dental care. Practices everywhere are attended by middle-aged patients with deteriorating dentitions containing heavily restored teeth requiring patchwork repairs to broken enamel walls or recurrent caries. For them a plan can be justified for radical treatment in order to provide healthy pulps or well-filled root canals as bases for secure restorations that will not require emergency appointments for yet another repair. The question has then to be posed: at what stage is full reconstruction the genuine need? Tolerance to dysfunction can be preferable to regret following too ambitious a treatment plan or one carried out with too little training or experience. Nevertheless, the need and the decision remain to be faced and, whether it be for one occlusal surface or many, attention to the occlusal surfaces is of prime concern and will provide the topics of this chapter.

Application of principles

There are six principles of muscle activity and occlusal function which apply to all restorative procedures and are worth restating.

1. There is an innate pattern of jaw movements which governs the function of mastication. Reflex adaptation to interferences of this pattern by alterations of tooth shapes and relationships will take place usually without disturbance, but the tolerance of the teeth, muscles and joints is not unlimited.
2. The teeth respond to occlusal forces by omnidirectional movements within their supporting tissues. The teeth will return to their original positions on removal of the forces provided the forces do not cause reposition of the teeth.
3. The most stable occlusion between opposing teeth is that of a tripod contact between supporting cusp ridges and opposing fossa ridges. This principle includes the provision of adequate horizontal and vertical overlap by the guiding cusps and anterior teeth.
4. The majority of dentitions are habitual and stable. If diagnosed as being unfavourably altered by cusp interferences or loss of teeth, the dentitions should

be restored on the retruded arc at a vertical level 2–3 mm above that of rest position.

5. A stable pattern of tooth contacts which occur in excursive movements of the mandible is evident in the majority of mouths. Such contacts can be seen between opposing incisors and canines as part of the anterior guidance in class I and II, division 2 jaw relations. In class III, some class II, division 1 relations and those with edge-to-edge incisor contacts there is no anterior guidance.
6. Two phases or levels of occlusion exist: the first, light contact, and the second, full contact when the teeth of both arches are firmly in occlusion. At the second phase the teeth have all moved slightly and it is not possible to duplicate these tooth positions and their occlusion on plaster casts. The cast teeth are related to each other at the first phase of contact.

Rehabilitation and reconstruction

These terms are introduced to differentiate between restoration of mandibular function and reconstruction of tooth surfaces. *Rehabilitation* is defined as procedures directed at restoring optimal muscle and joint function. When applied to the masticatory system, these include bilateral back teeth chewing movements which will encourage this function and the avoidance of parafunctional activities. *Reconstruction* is defined as procedures directed at restoring or replacing the occlusal surfaces of the teeth in order to promote optimal occlusal function.

Pretreatment analyses

This topic has been discussed in Chapter 9 but some aspects require emphasis and specific attention.

1. Firm closure into IP should be rendered comfortable and stable before beginning any major restorations. The occlusion should make a clear sound.
2. The contacts in mandibular excursions should be limited to the opposing incisors and canines except in the case of class III jaw relations or edge-to-edge intercuspal occlusion, in which case cusp interferences should be noted and perhaps removed.
3. Hand-held study casts can be helpful for assessing tooth loss and breakage, plunger cusps, open contacts, facets of wear, overerupted teeth and possibilities for disturbances leading to disorders.
4. A maxillary study cast mounted with facebow on a semi-adjustable articulator with the mandibular cast placed in IP and mounted to the lower arm of the articulator will allow comparison between contacts in the mouth and on the articulator. Shimstock is recommended for these tests. If there is an obvious discrepancy between these mounted casts and the occlusion in the mouth, a retruded precontact registration should be made and the record used to remount the lower cast.
5. The mounting of casts on a fully adjustable articulator is recommended if problems of group function and/or class III relation are to be solved. Here, the operator can assess the areas of contact which may have to be adjusted to prevent protrusive, working and non-working interferences. For students in crown and bridgework, the confident and accurate use of the pantograph and consequent mounting of casts is a compulsory training.

Pretreatment requirements and determinants

Such analyses should lead to the establishment of intercuspal occlusion, of which the patient can be unaware before treatment is begun, and to anterior guidances in all protrusive directions that will protect the posterior teeth from interferences while chewing. For this to occur, incisors and canines must be sound in tissue structure and in their periodontia. Any suspect conditions should be treated and rendered supportive of their responsibilities in mandibular contact (articular) excursions. The descending angles of condyle guidance (the posterior determinant) should be assessed, either from the natural lingual contours of the anterior crowns or from crowns with created contours to provide this protection (the anterior determinant). This may require provisional crowns which can be adjusted until the desired angles of descent are achieved. The anterior always takes precedence over the posterior determinant.

The following criteria are therefore suggested.

1. Adequate posterior teeth disclusion in protrusive and lateral excursions.
2. Patient is comfortable while eating.
3. Speech is unimpaired.
4. No increased mobility of the anterior teeth.
5. No sensitivity of the anterior teeth.
6. No loss of crowns (provisional or definitive) because of habit grinding and/or failed cementation.
7. The anterior guidance, as determined by the lingual surfaces of the maxillary incisors and canines and angles of descent of the condyles freed from tooth contacts or central bearing screws, should be governed by harmonious muscle activity.

Modifications in treatment procedures

As a result of achieving these criteria, the operator will be in a better position to adjust restorations in the mouth and this will reduce the need for complex procedures to mount casts for single restorations. In many cases, two hand-held casts with a clear idea of where intercuspal occlusion is and the mandibular excursions are should obviate the need for mounted casts. It has also to be said that, if a stable IP exists, closure into any of the registration materials can, and often does, produce inaccurate relations of opposing casts when mounted. When it comes to more complex reconstruction procedures, the use of a fully adjustable articulator may only be necessary if there is absence of anterior guidance or if group function is to be established and controlled for potential cusp interferences.

On the other hand, the use of pantographic tracings before and after treatment will indicate improvements (or otherwise) in the flow of border movements (Figure 11.1). A knowledge and experience of all aspects of observed and recorded jaws relations is desirable when restoring teeth to optimal function.

The single restoration

This includes all restorations from the class I alloy to the bonded crown.

The class II alloy

The class II alloy is probably the one restoration on which most demands have been made in the past century of restorative dentistry and the one where marginal ridge insecurity has often led to the action of the plunger cusp and to failure of the restoration. Careful observation of the opposing supporting cusp in all relative excursions should lead to careful placement of the matrix and allow excursions to take place while the alloy is setting, and preliminary carving to be carried out. This is more easily done in the maxillary tooth where the overlap allows the matrix

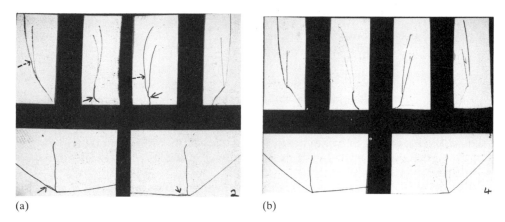

(a)   (b)

Figure 11.1 (a) Pantographic tracings showing clicks (arrows) and deviations due to muscle avoidance (broken arrows). (b) Tracings following treatment. (From Greenberg, 1986)

holder to be avoided. However, the Automatrix on a mandibular posterior tooth will often allow free excursions to be made. The objective is to allow tripod contact with the opposing tooth to be carved, and this can be achieved by carving until the alloy is freed from shiny contacts. However, care should be taken to avoid infraocclusion. The paths marked by the opposing cusp can be deepened at their base to form the grooves between the triangular ridges using a sharp-pointed carving instrument.

Removal of the matrix should be delayed until there is no chance of fracturing the marginal ridge. The matrix should be cut vertically and the edge most available held firmly by pliers and removed buccally. If a copper band is used it should be cut by a slowly rotating size 1 fissure bur before removing buccally by pliers. There should still be time to carve the marginal ridge, and supplemental grooves can be added later with a slowly rotating bur. Timing and experience with the material being used are of the essence. It should also be remembered that the shredding efficiency of the occlusal surface is improved by well-formed ridges and supplemental grooves.

The resin and glass ionomer cement restorations

It cannot be said that these are permanent restorations for the occlusal surfaces of posterior teeth. They have, of course, been popularized by tooth colour appeal and the case against amalgam alloy as a health hazard that has not been proved. They do wear proximally and occlusally and occlusal form is not maintained. However, their use will doubtless continue and, if advice on bilateral chewing and 'No grinding of the teeth, please' can accompany their insertion, some of the restorations may survive, though not with their occlusal contours. A layer of thin tin foil placed over the surface of the inserted filling material (of the correct amount), and the patient instructed to close while the material sets, may give a shine to the restoration which may reduce wear. However, this does not permit a properly contoured occlusal surface. This is not to discredit the many advantages of these materials as restorations and as build-up materials prior to crown coverage of broken down ('bombed-out') posterior teeth, to say nothing of their adhesive properties. They can be particularly useful in restoring the teeth of elderly patients and as preventive restorations in young teeth as fissure sealants.

The cast metal inlay and crown

If direct wax is used, the method is similar to that employed for the alloy. It should be emphasized that the force used in closing on wax may cause the occlusal level to be depressed (see (6) in the foregoing principles). This will result in an inlay with an occlusal level raised at first light contact. Care should therefore be taken to ensure that the occlusion and articulation should be clear on the wax with the teeth *lightly* in contact.

With the indirect method, where an impression and subsequent cast is made of the prepared tooth and the adjacent teeth, a record of the opposing teeth is required. The 'wax squash' method, where two thicknesses of softened wax separated by a layer of foil are used, is discounted because of the occlusal force necessary to make the registration. This causes depression of the teeth and a record with the opposing teeth further apart than they are at rest. The consequent 'high bite' on the completed restoration is inevitable. Further, the strain induced in the wax by this force leads to distortion of the wax on removal from the mouth, thus providing a further cause of inaccuracy. Any material used to register the relationship between opposing teeth in intercuspal occlusion will be either too thin to be usable (plaster, silicone or thiakol rubbers) or too thick for accuracy (see above).

Two alternative methods are suggested: two complete mounted casts and hand-held opposing casts.

Two complete mounted casts

For reasons already explained it can be dificult to place two plaster casts in the same intercuspal occlusion as in the mouth. The chief reason is that plaster teeth are not provided with periodontal membranes and will not ease into precise intercuspal occlusion. However, a reasonably accurate intercuspal position for the lower cast in relation to the upper cast can be achieved by adopting the following procedure.

1. Facebow transfer of maxillary cast to a semi-adjustable articulator.
2. Both casts are freed from plaster bubbles and any other hindrances to intercuspal occlusion.
3. The lower cast is placed by hand against the upper cast at intercuspal occlusion

and secured with an adhesive wax. It is then attached to the lower arm of the articulator using minimal expansion plaster.

The articulator occlusion should then be checked for all contacts and adjustments made to the plaster occlusal surfaces until there seems to be accurate occlusion. Even this care will not guarantee the same precise closure as in the mouth and it is permissible, even advisable, to place a layer of tin foil on the tooth opposing the tooth for crowning. If this layer is burnished firmly on to the plaster tooth and secured it will provide a suitable surface against which to wax the proposed crown. Alternatively, a small amount of closure can be achieved by adjusting the plaster occlusal surfaces. The amount (say, 0.5 mm) should be checked on the incisal guide pin.

Waxing is carried out by cones for the supporting cusps into the opposing fossae and then for the guiding cusps. If the articulator movements are considered accurate the upper arm can be moved laterally and protrusively in order to ensure that the wax cones are not interfering. The cusp ridges, marginal ridges and, finally, the triangular ridges are then waxed, each time checking occlusion and articulation (see pp. 192–3 for waxing technique).

When the unpolished casting has been made and returned to the articulator, the occlusion and articulation can be checked and adjusted using ultrathin articulating paper. Another method is to dust the casting with a zinc stearate powder (used in the wax technique, p. 193), which will shine with interfering contacts. Finally, the opposing tooth contacts are checked with shimstock foil and the casting is ready for seating on the tooth. If there are errors in occlusion the fault lies in the method and not with the technician.

The same additive principles apply to the application of porcelain though more difficult to execute.

Hand-held casts for single posterior crowns

With the training gained by using semi- and fully adjustable articulators, and by having observed the intercuspal position and tooth contacts during excursive (articular) movements in the mouth, it should be possible to relate the hand-held casts accurately in IP and movements while carrying out the drop-wax procedure (see p. 193). This requires practice by dentist and technician, who should *both* be trained in this method.

Anterior crowns

Where a single crown is being made and the all important incisal guidance is obvious, hand-held complete casts can be used in the hands of a well-instructed technician. Where four or six crowns are to be made and the incisal guidance is obvious, it is advisable to leave one central unprepared in order to retain the guidance for the others being made. The remaining central can then be made using the retained guidance. If all six anteriors must be crowned at the same time, it is advisable to make six provisional resin crowns and adjust the anterior guidance on them until they are comfortable and secure. The definitive crowns can then be made using one provisional central for guidance, as previously described. However, it should be pointed out that both lateral and protrusive guidances have to be provided and it is wise to retain two teeth (central and canine) for this purpose. This procedure should also be followed when full reconstruction is to be carried out (see later).

Errors and excuses

There are possibilities for errors in all methods of relating plaster casts of teeth to one another:

1. Any displacement of the teeth is not copied in the related cast.
2. Plaster expands on setting.
3. The interocclusal registrations are inaccurate unless made on the retruded axis.
4. Registration materials are seldom soft enough to avoid displacing the teeth and are not dimensionally stable after removal from the mouth.

The use of silicone or thiokol rubber materials has been recommended for making these registrations but they have the disadvantage of a prolonged setting time, during which jaw movement and separation can take place. Also, the record is often too thin to be reliable, and can be subject to recoil.

There are many excuses for failure to reproduce accurate occlusion but a clear idea of the limitations will help in overcoming them. The technician should not be blamed, provided his restoration fits the die and the occlusion is seen to be correctly developed on it. One improvement that would help to solve the problems of occlusal transfers would be a registration material of minimal viscosity (the consistency of whipped cream) that would set instantaneously, on demand. It should also be tough and dimensionally stable after removal from the mouth. Chemists, please note!

Quadrant restorations and the unilateral bridge

Where all the teeth in one quadrant are being restored or a bridge is being made, a treatment plan based on an occlusal analysis is desirable. Missing and unopposed teeth lead to migration, overeruption and adaptive function, respectively. Occlusal adjustment and shortening may be necessary before the teeth are prepared (Figure 11.2), otherwise the disturbance will be built into the restoration. A warning is also

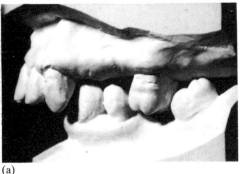 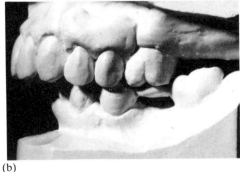

(a)   (b)

Figure 11.2 (a) Bounded saddle occlusal curve disturbed by tilted lower molar, over-erupted upper molar, and overclosed OVR. (b) Upper molar (26) reduced and crowned as bridge abutment; pontics 24 and 25 covered by acrylic insert. OVR restored by lower bridge (with sanitary pontic) as part of reconstruction

given against the use of textbook anatomy in a mouth where cusps have been worn or where the teeth no longer display their original contours or relations. Here, form is in danger of becoming uniform and of cusps causing interference in function. Quadrant dentistry may be part of a plan for the reconstruction of both arches but it is assumed that the existing intercuspal position will be used. Following the preparation of the teeth, three methods of transfer to the articulator are suggested. In each a facebow transfer of the upper cast is made, thus allowing the maxillary teeth to move on the arbitrary retruded arc of opening and closing.

1. Place the lower against the upper cast, provided the position is obvious and there is an unprepared molar cusp on the quadrant being restored. This will prevent rocking of the cast with the unprepared side acting as a fulcrum. Plaster bubbles must be removed and care taken to avoid moving the mandibular cast when plastering it to the articulator.
2. Fast-setting resin (Duralay is preferred) is added to the prepared teeth and built up so that an occlusal registration can be made against the unprepared teeth. The prepared teeth should be treated with a detergent (Microfilm) to ease removal of the record. This is then placed on the prepared teeth of the cast and the fit assured. The mandibular cast is then mounted using this unilateral record.
3. A precontact interocclusal record. A wafer of two thickness hard, dimensionally stable wax is softened in a water bath. A compound or resin stop is fashioned over the maxillary incisor teeth and the precontact level determined. This should be just prior to the existing IP. A notch is cut out of the wax in this region and the softened wax held against the maxillary teeth with the left forefinger and thumb. The right hand is then free to ensure that the mandibular incisor teeth touch the anterior stop while the wax hardens, preferably by the nurse applying cold water. The record is removed, examined for no penetration, and replaced while the occlusal relation is checked. The tooth marks can be clarified for mounting by placing a fast-setting zinc-oxide–eugenol cement while the second seating is checked.

    Waxing should be carried out with cones in the wax additive method (p. 193). This should ensure cusp–fossa occlusion and freedom from interference in articulation.

Complete reconstruction

The decision to restore all teeth in the mouth must be made on a basis of prevention; namely, to prevent the premature loss of existing teeth and the need for any further treatment over an indefinite period. Most mouths can be kept in a reasonable state of health and function by regular repair and hygiene; by the time middle age is reached, the prognosis for the future should be relatively easy to assess. The objectives for reconstruction should therefore be preventive as well as curative, the need genuine, and the work performed with the closest attention to good occlusal function.

Indications

1. Loss of occlusal surfaces by wear or flat fillings and the inability to find a 'comfortable bite'.
2. Missing teeth and subsequent drift of adjacent teeth resulting in disorders that cannot be successfully treated by simple removable prostheses.

3. Incipient periodontal breakdown aggravated by adverse occlusal forces causing or having caused repositioning of teeth.
4. Multiple restorative failures that have to be treated in any event.
5. Restoration of balanced activity to the muscles of the masticatory system.

Contraindications

These include advanced periodontal disease, high caries susceptibility, patients with poor self-care and those who are obviously heading for complete dentures in the foreseeable future. In addition, there are those patients who do not require reconstruction.

Requirements

These include the exclusion of contraindications, an optimistic and cooperative attitude on the part of the patient and his or her partner, the ability of the dentist and the technician to do the work, the funds required to pay for it and, of first importance, the genuine need in the dentition of the patient.

Preconstruction treatment

Before making and deciding the final plan for reconstructing a dentition there are several treatment measures which should be considered.

Caries control in middleage may be akin to closing the stable door after the horse has bolted, but in susceptible mouths all caries and suspect restorations should be treated as if they were going to give trouble at a later date. Provisional crowns may be necessary. During this period hygiene and its effects can be assessed, pulps tested and root canal therapy performed if necessary. The obvious moral is better now than later.

Periodontal therapy for the reduction of pockets and the assessment of future periodontal hygiene and health is always better done before rather than after reconstruction. It will provide a better basis for diagnosis, treatment plan and prognosis.

Orthodontic repositioning of the teeth is possible at any age, although the later the slower. Its success depends on maintaining the restored positions and treating the causes which moved them which, in middle age, are generally a combination of periodontal breakdown and muscle and occlusal forces. The objective for the orthodontist is to achieve an approximate cusp–fossa occlusal relation which can be refined by the reconstruction.

Extractions or *root canal therapy* must be considered before the final plan is made and the patient advised. All the dentist's experience with failed bridgework and loss of pulp vitality should be brought to bear on deciding the future health of the teeth to be reprepared, crowned and used anew. Better a tooth or a pulp to be lost now than to lose a bridge abutment or incisor crown later.

Diagnosis and decision

This begins with the consultation (see Chapter 9). If, at the outset, it is apparent that the patient is bent on reconstruction, this should be discouraged. If it becomes obvious that it is required, the patient should be seen to want it and be discouraged.

The point being made is that the patient should persuade the dentist to carry out the work in spite of warnings about time, inconvenience, discomfort and cost. A second consultation should be conducted with radiographs and hand-held study casts available, and preferably in the presence of a third party (partner, relative or physician). A plan and an alternative plan should be presented and this will often mean a decision between supervised neglect, dentures and reconstruction. If the patient and adviser wish to persist with reconstruction, the dentist must be satisfied that there is a genuine need and that the work will succeed for a stipulated period. Letters should now be exchanged to establish the plan, an understanding of the difficulties, and a realistic approach to the problem of cost and payment. A clear understanding on these aspects of treatment will help to assuage recrimination and disappointment, should these arise.

The plan

Emphasis on the need for a plan cannot be too strong, if for no other reason than to be able to change it. Circumstances alter cases and both dentist and patient should be aware of dangers ahead, with the consequent need to adapt. Success may depend on correctly assessing the adaptability of the dentist's plan and the patient's tissues.

In addition to orthodontic, endodontic and periodontal treatment and the build-up of individual teeth for crowns and for bridge abutments, there are four stages in reconstruction therapy which should be followed and explained to the patient.

1. The establishment of a stable posterior occlusion with comfortable chewing ability, firm, even contacts between opposing teeth on provisional restorations at an acceptable vertical relation.
2. The establishment of a correct and comfortable anterior guidance which will disclude posterior occlusion on all protrusive and lateral protrusive movements. As has been previously advised, this may require provisional crowns being made and leaving some to establish the acceptable guidance.
3. Make and complete the anterior restorations at the correct vertical and horizontal jaw relations.
4. Make and complete the definitive posterior restorations.

Articulator analysis

This topic has been discussed in Chapters 8 and 9 but it should be re-emphasized that mounted casts on a semi-adjustable articulator transferred by an actual retruded axis and with a precontact retruded record are a necessity. Hand-held casts will be available, in any event, for mounting. They will help technician, operator and patient to see the problems and the need to treat. In addition, the extent of treatment as demonstrated by a diagnostic wax-up will aid clarification. If a fully adjustable articulator is to be used, a pretreatment pantograph and mounting will be necessary.

Order of tooth preparation and removable partial dentures

It has been decided that the occlusion of the posterior teeth should first be established and this must be carried out by provisional crowns, using materials that will retain their occlusal level while the anterior teeth are being prepared and crowned. There may be existing opposing posterior teeth that will establish this occlusion and a decision may have to be made from several alternative situations. Removable partial dentures may be involved and metal occlusal surfaces considered. However, the principle of making the definitive anterior crowns at the planned OVR, with protrusive and lateral protrusive guidances incorporated, should be sustained.

Material for the occlusal surfaces

The patient will want to have a say in the choice of materials: this will be between porcelain and gold. Porcelain will be the obvious choice for anterior and possibly for the mandibular posterior teeth, but gold for use with the wax additive technique makes for greater accuracy. Advances in porcelain techniques have made cusp–fossa relations achievable but there are important considerations for both materials (McLean, 1980).

Anaesthesia

Although not the concern of this text, the topic must be discussed with the patient. General anaesthesia in hospital is always tempting for the patient but the number of restorations involved, the impressions to be made and the jaw relations to be registered will require more visits to the hospital than could be justified. The compromise of local anaesthesia and intravenous temazepam is worth consideration. This medication has also proved helpful in registering jaw positions on the retruded arc. When it comes to impressions, the introduction of 0.6% probanthine submucosally can be invaluable in obtaining a dry field, although the dry field is unnecessary if hydrocolloid impression material is used. It is recommended that an anaesthetist performs these services.

Provisional restorations

The patient should be assured that comfortable provisional crowns will be supplied at all stages and this often poses unwelcome problems. The most comfortable provisional crowns are those made using an impression (or vacuum formed mould) of the teeth before preparations are begun. A fast-setting acrylic is placed in the impression and applied to the prepared teeth, taking care to protect sensitive dentine against the heat of polymerization. This will solve the temporary problems of occlusion and the fitting of teeth to partial denture retainers. Time and the cooperation of the technician have to be planned, and the situation to be avoided is the announcement of the next patient before the provisionals are made, let alone cemented, let alone adjusted for intercuspal occlusion. A state of haste and a full waiting room are to be avoided. In reconstruction work it is often advisable to make provisional restorations for the whole mouth to include the new occlusal scheme and so assess the responses of the patient as to comfort and efficiency before proceeding with the permanent work. This will involve more time and expense and these factors have to be weighed against the long-term expectations of the treatment. There are many pathways up the mountain and, in this type of work, the summit is high. Base camps are required on the way to restore the stamina of both patient and dentist. No specific advice can be offered on this decision except to consider fully all possibilities.

Comment

There are many aspects of planning to be considered and their importance cannot be overestimated if pulps, periodontia, muscles, joints and occlusal schemes are to survive the test of preparation and prolonged function in the future. Four visits will have elapsed by now and nothing that has been done is irreversible. A registration of the patient's retruded axis may have been tattooed on the patient's face but this is not noticeable. A pantographic tracing of the patient's healthy border movements may have been registered and transferred to a fully adjustable articulator which will have been adjusted to copy it. This can now be used for the work planned or at a future date, provided the muscles remain healthy. It is not too late to back out, and the question should be seriously asked either by the patient or by the dentist of himself: 'What is the prognosis?' Despite the optimism of the dentist and the trust of the patient, reputations and purses are soon lost if the soil be sour. But if this section is to proceed, let Shakespeare (1602) have the last word:

Our doubts are traitors,
And make us lose the good we oft might win
By fearing to attempt.

Procedures

Tooth preparation

Although this is not a text on restorative procedures, some features of preparations and transfer are suggested.

1. The shape and extension of the preparations should be considered with a view to future periodontal health and caries recurrence. A crown margin extended below the gingival margin is a potential source of irritation to the crevicular epithelium and a site for plaque lodgement. Where possible crown margins should be sited above the gingival margin. This principle applies equally to the buccal and lingual as to the approximal surfaces where, from the aspect of hygiene, it is just as easy to maintain an enamel surface as a gold one with an interdental woodstick or dental tape. Subgingival extensions will depend on caries, the extent of previous operations and crown height for retention. The last factor is an important consideration when allowing sufficient room for the new occlusal surfaces. The preparations should allow adequate space in all dimensions for optimal thickness of the restorative materials being used. It is also necessary to extend maxillary anterior crowns into the gingival crevice for reasons of appearance. On the other hand, a further advantage of limiting gingival extension is the damaging effect of tissue-retracting devices and chemicals on the crevicular epithelium. Electrosurgical removal of the gingival epithelium has proved a satisfactory alternative to these measures in some circumstances, and decisions on all of these factors require consideration.

   The buccal and lingual shapes of crowns should copy the original tooth shapes. Wide crowns lead to wide separation of cusps and this will disturb the direction of occlusal forces and the effects of function will become potentially harmful. A close look at these surfaces in relation to supporting and guiding cusps, as mentioned in Chapter 2, may be helpful. Finally, the approximal surfaces in the natural dentition should be viewed again. Below the contact areas, posterior teeth surfaces are more concave than convex and this makes for easy woodstick or tape hygiene and the promotion of good gingival health. This feature should be emphasized in the completed restorations.

2. Each die must be rigid when seated in the cast and bear an accurate relation to each other die. To assure this requirement, a duplicate cast is often advised. The margins can then be waxed on the removable dies from the working cast and the patterns transferred to the complete cast for occlusal and contact point waxing.

3. The prepared margins of each die must be clearly seen by dentist and technician.

Transfer of the retruded condyle axis

This is made using a facebow with adjustable side-arms. The prepared teeth must be seated accurately on the bite-fork where hard compound refined by zinc-oxide–eugenol (Temp-Bond) is recommended (Figure 11.3). There must be

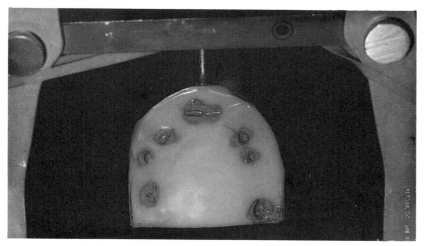

Figure 11.3 Bite-fork corrected by Kerr's registration paste

no movement of the bite-fork on the prepared teeth while the condyle pointers are adjusted to touch lightly on the tattooed axis marks. The holding should be done by the patient or assistant and no attempt should be made by the patient to close on to the bite-fork. The orbital pointer is then adjusted to touch the mark (preferably tattooed) on the face so that this transfer corresponds to the same level at which the pantographic tracing was made. The dentist should then hold the bite-fork and check that there has been no movement. The *upper* master cast can then be secured to the *upper* member of the articulator, making sure that the orbital pointer touches the same plane of reference on the articulator as was used when the pantograph was originally transferred. If the split-cast method for checking the interocclusal record (described below) is to be used, the master cast should be notched before attaching it to the *upper* member.

The interocclusal jaw registration

There are two components to this registration, the vertical and the horizontal, and they are estimated in that order. The occlusal analysis will have revealed if any alteration is required in the vertical relation and no change should be attempted without a trial period while the patient wears an acrylic resin appliance at the altered OVR. Both patient and dentist must then be assured that this alteration is both necessary and comfortable. The horizontal component of the registration must then be practised at the retruded relation and at the acceptable vertical relation. The muscles must be responsive to the need for retrusion and both dentist and patient should be assured that the patient can perform the opening and closing movements of retruded closure, and these should be practised. The spaces between the opposing posterior teeth should be observed to ensure that no interferences exist and that there is adequate room for coverage by crowns on the prepared teeth. It is not too late to make corrections at this stage and start again with new impressions, rather than having to do so after crowns are made.

The following steps are then carried out.

1. An anterior stop of fast setting acrylic resin (Duralay) is placed against two maxillary central incisor crowns and the retruded relation registered at the predetermined vertical level. After the resin has set, the opening and closing movements on the retruded arc are repeated several times to ensure that the retruded path has been followed.
2. The anterior stop is removed and trimmed for easy replacement. It is secured (with fixative if necessary) and the retruded closure practised once more. The registration proper is then made, preferably using two thicknesses of hard wax (Moyco Beautypink) held against the maxillary teeth by the left forefinger and thumb and with sufficient wax removed to accommodate the anterior stop (Figure 11.4; see also Wise, 1982). The record is then refined by adding zinc-oxide–eugenol paste (Kerr's Temp-Bond) or bite registration paste to the tooth imprints and re-registered, making sure that no penetration of the wax by the teeth has taken place which would indicate displacement of the mandible.
3. The lower cast is then attached to the lower member of the articulator against the upper cast using this record.

Checking the record

The precontact interocclusal record made on the RCA is the weakest link in the chain of procedures. If the record has not been registered on this arc, it will not be reproducible in the mouth and the costly occlusal surfaces will not meet accurately when returned to the mouth. It should therefore be checked for reproducibility, which means that it must have been registered on the retruded arc. Two methods are suggested below.

The split cast

This method consists of comparing three or more retruded records and of assuming that if two coincide they will both be on the retruded arc because only on this arc is there reproducibility of closure. Three deep notches are cut in the base of the upper (master) cast which is then coated with a separating medium. Alternatively, a notch former made of acrylic resin can be used (see Figure 11.5). The cast is seated on the bite-fork of the facebow and is plastered to the upper member of the articulator. The mounting cast is thus separable from the master cast. Three or more retruded records (preferably in stone plaster) are now made and the one thought to be the

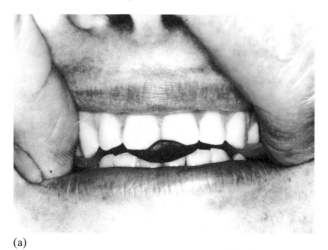

(a)

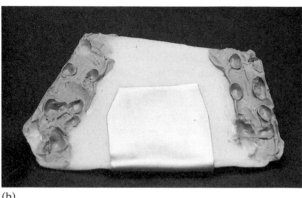

(b)

Figure 11.4 (a) Jaw registration. (b) Record corrected with Kerr's bite registration paste

most retruded is used to attach the lower master cast (against the upper) to the lower member of the articulator. This record is removed and a second one is seated on the lower cast. The upper cast, separated from its mounting cast, is seated on this record and the upper member with its mounting cast is lowered on to the base of the upper cast until the notches engage, or do not. If the notch former now engages the notches more anteriorly (Figure 11.5c), the original mounting was the more retruded. Further records should be seated until two retruded ones coincide, indicating a reproducible retruded relation. This may seem a rigorous discipline but time is better spent at this procedure than in remaking crowns.

Plastic caps and pins

This method consists of making fast-setting plastic caps for three prepared teeth in both arches, each incorporating a pointed pin. Each pair is set to be touching when the first mounting is made (Figure 11.6). The three pairs of pins are then transferred to the relevant teeth and retruded closure made. If there is no coincidence of contact, fast-setting resin, plaster or compound is added to the lower

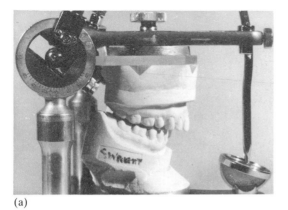

(a)

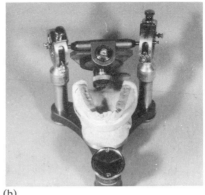

(b)

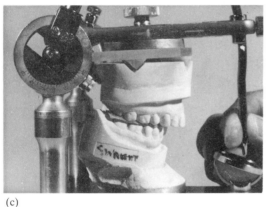

(c)

Figure 11.5 Split cast mounting to check record. (a) Lower cast mounted with record thought to be most retruded. (b) Second record on lower cast. (c) Upper arm wants to seat more anteriorly. Therefore, previous mounting was the more retruded

or upper caps, the retruded closure practised and then, when moving freely, closure is completed. The lower cast is remounted, the pins reset and returned to the mouth. Again, this procedure is repeated until two mountings coincide. This is a modification of Brewer's method of checking such a record and will be described for complete dentures in Chapter 12. When the operator is satisfied that the mounting on the laboratory bench coincides with the retruded arc of contact in the mouth, the waxing can proceed. The method has been used for complete reconstruction with success, but is more suited to complete dentures.

Development of the occlusal surfaces

The removable dies should be lubricated and the occlusal surfaces covered with fast-setting resin or specially prepared adaptable plastic discs (Adaptafoil, Bego, Bremen). These will act as copings on which waxing can be carried out (Figure 11.7a). These copings should leave no residue after burning out and are used because dropping wax on to a lubricated die can render removal without breakage difficult.

There are many combinations of opposing prepared teeth to be waxed and the diagrammatic example is only one (Figure 11.7). The incisors and canine crowns have been completed and impressions of them have been made with those of the

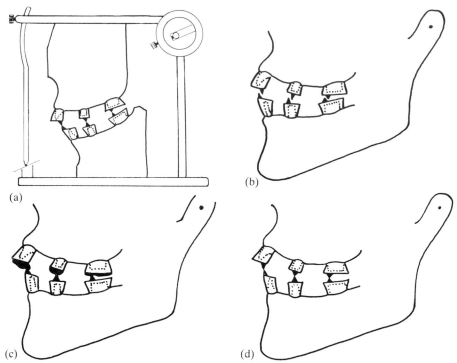

Figure 11.6 Pin method to check record. (a) Pins mounted on acrylic caps to touch. (b) Pins do not oppose in mouth. (c) Re-registration. Upper pins removed and compound used. (d) Pins touch (after being adjusted to touch on articulator, as in (a))

prepared posterior teeth. The objective is to provide cusp–fossa occlusion at the retruded intercuspal position for the posterior teeth and disclusion from it during all articular movements of the mandible. The articulation is thus taken over by the incisors and canines.

Waxing stages

1. Method

A blunt curved probe (or the specially designed Thomas instruments in a set of five) is heated and touched on the wax which clings to the metal. By heating the shaft the wax runs to the end of the probe which can then be touched on to the die in the correct site. By slowly lifting the instrument the wax is left in the form of a cone.

2. Supporting and guiding cusps

The areas of the central fossae should be lightly touched with wax to provide a target for the supporting cusps. Where possible, the preparations should show enough of the original buccal and lingual walls to allow vertical pencilled lines to indicate the sites of the proposed cusps as viewed from the sides. The upper lingual and then the lower buccal cusps are then built in the form of cones and the articulator closed and moved horizontally after each addition to ensure freedom from collision. Once these, the supporting cusps, have been established the guiding cusps (upper buccal and lower lingual) are added.

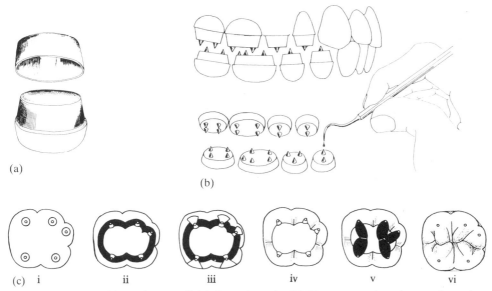

Figure 11.7 Waxing. (a) Plastic cap to finish short of margin. (b) Wax cones on sites of supporting and guiding cusps. (c) Stages in completion of wax additive technique: i, cones; ii, buccal and marginal ridges ('fish mouth'); iii, buccal and lingual cusp walls; iv, complete buccal and lingual contours; v, triangular ridges; vi, supplemental ridges and grooves and developmental grooves; completion

3. Cusp and marginal ridges

These are formed to connect the cusps by flowing wax around the ridge circumference of each tooth and tested for avoidance of contact (Figure 11.7). The extensions to the functional outer aspects of each tooth are flowed on at this stage to provide stability for the wax cones.

4. Triangular and oblique ridges

These are now dropped on in convex patterns. At this stage a dusting of zinc stearate powder is applied by a camel hair brush on to the opposing wax surfaces to prevent adhesion. It will also show a shiny surface where contacts exist. The direction of the ridges is altered at this time if indicated by the shiny marks.

5. Developmental grooves

Fossae are now filled in with molten wax, dusted with the zinc stearate powder and the articulator arm closed into retruded intercuspal position. Areas of contact will be seen and the tripod cusp–fossa occlusion is now refined. The developmental grooves separating the triangular ridges are deepened and this will remove contact between the cusp tips and the opposing fossae. The grooves are then burnished and for this there is a special instrument in the Thomas set.

6. Supplemental grooves

These grooves are added as illustrated in a series of Us or Vs in order to provide a shredding surface. The ridges are then accentuated by flowing on further wax but tested to ensure that there are no contacts during articular movement.

7. Check tripod contacts

It is unlikely that the tripod contacts will be precise as such when the castings are returned to the articulator or to the mouth. However, as the security of retruded IO depends on the perfection of this feature the following adjustments may be helpful. If the Stuart articulator is being used, the ground-in side shift (Bennett) metal guides should be replaced with straight guides so as to encourage a precise retruded closure *with no wavering into lateral movements*. In the Denar articulator the immediate side shift guides can be returned to zero. Each opposing tooth closure should maintain contact with an ultra thin (0005) strip of shimstock placed between them.

8. Check release of shimstock

The ground-in Bennett guides are reinserted (the immediate side shift guide returned to border movement reading) and the articulator upper arm moved into its border movements. The shimstock strips should be released immediately the mandible leaves its retruded intercuspal position. On the other hand, shimstock strips held between the incisors and canines during the protrusive and lateral movements should be firmly held.

Skill and perfection in these waxing procedures are not achieved without instruction and practice. Practice casts can easily be prepared and mounted. Instruments can be fashioned from probes and plastic hand instruments but the Thomas set of five is recommended. Instruction is more difficult to find and study groups around individual operators who have learned the techniques are invaluable.

Castings

Castings should fit the dies without force. Any resistance or scratching when seating will indicate too firm a fit on the prepared teeth. In order to provide a tight marginal fit without force it can be helpful, before waxing, to apply a layer of thin varnish over the dies, short of the margins. Commercial preparations are available. The addition of small 'blisters' to the castings, just above the margins, will prove helpful in removing the castings from the teeth, especially if they are to be temporarily cemented. Castings should be polished and sandblasted before testing occlusion and articulation on the mounted casts. This will be helpful in seeing premature contacts on closure. Contact testing with shimstock strips is repeated as with the waxed version. When satisfied that the castings are in good occlusion and articulation on the articulator the patient is recalled for trial seating of the work.

Trial seating and remount procedures

At this stage a well-known quotation from the poet Burns suggests itself as a daunting prospect: 'The best laid plans o' mice an' men gang aft a-gley', and it is seldom that a complete reconstruction has proved to be in correct occlusion at the first seating, in spite of the pains taken. Inaccuracies creep in at every stage of preparation, impression, registration, record and transfer. In addition, teeth move and castings do not always seat on the prepared teeth as they do on the dies. If things can go wrong they often do (ancient law).

And so further time-consuming effort is required as follows:

1. Prepare a rigid bar or wire to seat over the castings prior to the remount appointment.

2. Provisional crowns are removed and the prepared teeth cleaned.
3. The castings are seated and their fit assured. This may take hours, not minutes, and it may be desirable for the patient to wear them uncemented for 24 hours.
4. Retruded occlusal position checked. If increased, even in the most minor degree, the corrections are better made on the remounted casts than in the mouth, where one inaccuracy leads to another.
5. With the castings seated, a facebow transfer is made and two, preferably three, precontact retruded registrations are made.
6. Fast-setting acrylic resin is placed on the castings in the mouth and the prepared bar seated over the resin. An alginate or plaster impression is then made over the bar and withdrawn from the crowns. The crowns are then removed from the teeth and seated on the acrylic resin in the impression. A new mounting cast is made taking care not to unseat the castings. To prevent this happening a mix of near liquid alginate can be poured around the castings and allowed to set before making the cast. This applies to both arches.
7. The upper cast is mounted using a new facebow transfer and the lower cast to it using the record estimated to be the most retruded. This mounting can then be checked against the other two using the split cast. It is essential that this mounting be made on the retruded axis.
8. Occlusal adjustment is carried out following the principles outlined in Chapter 10.

Permanent seating

The temptation to cement permanently should be weighed against the need for accuracy of fit and of occlusal relations. The following questions should be posed.

Will the patient be unaware of his teeth and not be tempted to perform parafunctional contact movements?
Have all the margins been finished and passed the sharp probe test?
Are the prepared teeth free from pathological response?
Would you have the work cemented in your own mouth?

The cement and methods used are for individual choice but care should be taken to avoid sensitive dentine and failure to seat each restoration. Escapeways for cement and firm force in the seating should be in mind while remembering that dentine can be sensitized or fractured in these operations.

Pre- and post-treatment stages of a treated mouth are illustrated in Figure 11.8a,b.

Additional problems and questions

Pontics for fixed bridgework

Wax occlusal surfaces are easily created and therefore gold is preferred to porcelain. Facings have to be made before the occlusal surfaces are waxed whether with porcelain or acrylic resin. A platform has to be provided for waxing and to be both removable and re-attachable to the facing.

Pontics for removable dentures

Gold occlusal surfaces are still preferred for these surfaces, however unrealistic this may be in terms of cost and the requirements of appearance. Where feasible, the

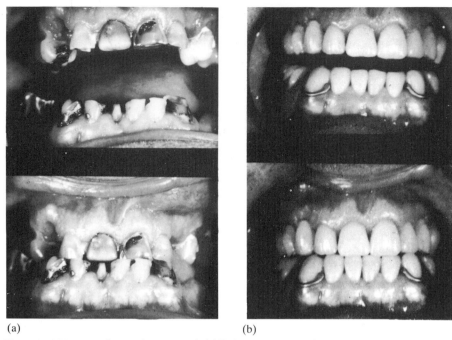

(a)   (b)

Figure 11.8 Two complete arches restored. (a) Before treatment, with increased freeway space. (b) Completed treatment. All upper restorations and lower incisors, canines and one molar were fixed. Partial lower denture with one free-end saddle

waxing is carried out on a removable plaster platform, allowances made for retention to facings and the castings returned to the master cast. When ready for securing to the denture framework, a plaster matrix is made over the cast occlusal surfaces in their correct position and this is used to retain it while processing is carried out.

Class II, division 1 and class III jaw and tooth relations

Canine and incisor articulation is obviously not possible for these mouths and the question of how to protect the opposing buccal segments from parafunctional articulation is not easily answered. It has been suggested that the first premolars should take over this role and that their buccal upper cusps (with normal upper overlap) be waxed and cast to provide the necessary guidance. No experience is available to comment on this solution but the principle is sound.

Positional record articulator

Not every dentist can afford the time for training nor the cost of buying a fully adjustable articulator. Positional record articulators provide an accurate intercuspal position and a reasonably accurate protrusive path angle. Incisal guidance can be introduced with an adjustable incisal table, either by adjusting its angle or adding to it in acrylic resin. Some instruments have adjustable intercondylar distance devices and this improves the accuracy of the facebow transfer. Before using any instrument a knowledge of its features and limitations should be understood so that the dentist and technician alike know what can be achieved and what cannot. Adjustments in the mouth are to be avoided if possible but are almost always inevitable when these instruments are used.

Care of the reconstructed dentition

Two aspects of care are emphasized: hygiene and limited occlusion.

Every cement margin is a potential source of caries recurrence and gingival irritation. In spite of the best operative techniques and the most skilled hands no margin should be left unclean. The most vulnerable regions are between the teeth where the toothbrush cannot reach. The dental woodstick or tape will provide not only clean interdental tooth surfaces but will reduce irritation to the gingival papillae to a minimum.

Instructions to the patient on the use of a new occlusion should centre on the avoidance of abuse. The natural position for the jaw is with the teeth parted. The advice, 'Lips together, teeth apart, never from this rule depart', should be imparted to all people as well as to patients. The avoidance of parafunctional clenching and grinding habits cannot be overstated. As always, prevention is preferable to cure but is often more difficult to prescribe. Irrelevant muscle activity is almost universal and is often directed to the mandibular muscles. Advice to patients should include: 'Keep the tongue between the teeth; move the jaw without touching the teeth'. For clenching while asleep the anterior overlay has proved helpful and its construction will be described in Chapter 13. This can also be worn while driving a car or during other activities which produce stress.

Alternative methods of reconstruction

There will always be attempts to simplify by alternative methods. And there will always be patients whose proprioception and neuromuscular responses will adapt to occlusal positions and articular schemes perhaps less precisely conceived than in the foregoing sections. 'Long centric' which permits sliding contacts between habitual and retruded intercuspal occlusion makes use of this adaptability but promotes parafunction.

Two sources of information in Europe are strongly recommended in the field of complete reconstruction: the experiences and writings of Pameijer (1985) and Wise (1982) should be followed and read. Both writers present expertise, attention to detail and fine illustrations. From the USA, Lundeen (1971) provides wise guidance on the morphological considerations that repay study.

Advantages of anterior guidance

If there are any doubts about the advantages of incisor and canine guidance in contact movements away from intercuspal occlusion, reference is made to Pokorny's (1971) report on the disadvantages of bilateral balanced articulation (i.e. cross-tooth and cross-arch group function) which reveals the following complaints from patients whose dental arches have been restored with bilateral balanced articulation.

1. They bit their cheeks and tongues.
2. The long mandibular cusps hindered chewing.

3. Balancing contacts hindered chewing.
4. Cross-tooth and cross-arch balance prevented chewing freedom.
5. Awareness of friction in those patients who constantly tested their occlusion.
6. They had lost their lower jaw.
7. So many closures were possible that they could not distinguish retruded IP from other positions.

Stuart and Stallard (1960) report from their early procedures which included bilateral balanced articulation that cusp tips wore and ridges became 'faceted' with consequent loss of OVR. They also noted that working side contacts wore faster than non-working contacts.

Many of these complaints would seem to derive from parafunctional grinding habits or from too much occlusal awareness. The latter phenomenon may have been present before treatment but bilateral balance in articulation would seem to accentuate it. The principle of disclusion in all movements from retruded IP will reduce this tendency to a minimum and the tripod contact between cusps and opposing fossae will provide a stable occlusion and ease of movement from it.

Comment

Complete reconstruction and the alloy restoration would seem to be poles apart but the principles involved in rendering patients able to shred and chew their food and to be unaware of their teeth while doing so are the same for all restorative operations. In addition, such a service will provide neuromuscular peace in the masticatory system which is never more desirable than when it is lost. There will always be other concepts and other instruments where difficulties are allied to inventive minds but the gradual attainment of skill in the use of the intruments selected will reward the operator who sustains his interest. The morality of reconstruction is often debated. Is so much care for one patient justified when so much requires to be done for the community at large? Justification lies in its being genuinely necessary, accurately done and for a patient who will maintain it. Thus, one hopes, the need for further treatment is prevented for an indefinite period. Implied in this justification is the need for the work to be carried out by groups of trained specialists working together, in consultation and in performance, for their common benefit and that of the patient.

References

Greenberg, M. J. (1986) Diagnosis of TMJ clicking from pantographic tracing recorded with tooth contact. *MSc. Thesis*, University of Michigan, USA

Lundeen, H. C. (1971) Occlusal morphologic considerations for fixed restorations. *Dental Clinics of North America*, **15**, 649

McLean, J. W. (1980) *The Science and Art of Dental Ceramics*, Quintessence Publishing, New York

Pameijer, J. H. N. (1985) Periodontal and occlusal factors in crown and bridge procedures. Dental Centre for Postgraduate Courses, Amsterdam

Pokorny, D. K. (1971) Current procedures in prosthodontics. *Dental Clinics of North America*, **15**, 685

Shakespeare, W. (*circa* 1602) *Measure for Measure*, I. iv. 77

Stuart, C. E. and Stallard, H. (1960) Principles in restoring occlusion to natural teeth. *Journal of Prosthetic Dentistry*, **10**, 304

Thomas, P. K. (1967) Syllabus on full mouth waxing technique for rehabilitation tooth-to-tooth cusp–fossa concept of organic occlusion. University of California, San Francisco

Wise, M. D. (1982) *Occlusion and Restorative Dentistry for the General Practitioner*, British Dental Association, London, p. 29

Chapter 12

Occlusion in removable prosthodontics

Complete dentures

The importance of occlusion and articulation for maintaining the stability of complete dentures has never been underestimated but is often overlooked. The registration of jaw relations is often cursorily performed, especially when the procedure is combined with setting the incisor teeth. This divides the priorities, usually in favour of appearance. The placing of the posterior teeth is left to the technician who, with more skill than he is credited, often produces the correct positions and occlusions. Here, the dentist and technician should form a team but too often communicate by phone or on hastily written slips of paper. Such a situation is often inevitable for the solo practitioner but is hard on the dentist, technician and patient alike when it comes to setting teeth, making alterations and keeping to time.

There are four properties required by complete dentures which will be briefly defined in order to clarify the objectives of this chapter. *Support* is the property of the residual ridges and mucosa which allows them comfortably to support the dentures. *Retention* is the property of the denture bases which causes them to resist vertical displacement. *Stability* is the property of the dentures which causes them to resist displacement during function and parafunction. *Appearance* is the property which makes the dentures pleasing to the dentist and patient.

Stability is the property chiefly affected by the various occlusions between the teeth. The objectives in this chapter are to discuss the principles involved and describe the methods of registering jaw relations and of setting the teeth for complete and, in the next section, for partial dentures in order to achieve optimal stability in occlusal function.

Jaw relations

In complete dentures the dentist is presented with the ultimate exercise in reconstruction where he can choose innumerable jaw and tooth positions for the dentures. However, if the jaw relation transferred to the articulator is to be reproducible when brought back to the mouth, it should be registered on the retruded axis. If the muscles are healthy and permit this movement the registration presents few difficulties. The difficult patient in this respect is one who has suffered changing intercuspal positions in the decline through diminishing and painful teeth, through insecure partial and complete dentures. The muscles have spent years in adapting to changing tooth positions and are fatigued and sometimes injured. The patient is then blamed for having a 'difficult bite'. When encountered, and before the jaw relations are registered, muscles should receive some rehabilitation and the psyche some tranquillity.

The *mandible on the retruded arc* assures a reproducible horizontal relationship and the remaining problem is to select the correct vertical relation. This should exist at a level 3 mm above that of rest position. This is *not* to say that the relation should be registered with the mandible moving up from rest position, but that rest position is used as the reference level whose distance from the maxilla can be measured.

Permanent bases

One further principle pleaded but seldom heeded is that of registering the required relation using the permanent bases. During the moment of registration the bases must fit the residual ridges with the greatest possible accuracy. If they move, the registration will not represent what was registered. This inaccuracy can seldom be seen to take place and the subsequent diagnosis of what went wrong is made more difficult. The use of wax or processed trial bases (even with fixatives) does not approach the accuracy of using the bases which will be used in the completed dentures. An additional advantage of making the permanent bases before the jaw registration is made is that the bases can be checked for retention before they are subjected to the requirements of stability. Consequently, permanent bases are recommended and mounting casts made before the jaw relation is registered. A thin sprinkling of fixative can be used for the bases if there are doubts about retention but at least the bases will fit the mounting casts as accurately as they fit the residual ridges. The final processing of teeth and gumwork to the bases can be achieved without distortion if time and temperature figures for reprocessing are observed.

Jaw registration

Horizontal and vertical relations. Compound occlusion rims are formed on the bases and a preliminary closure into them allows the rims to be shaped for height.

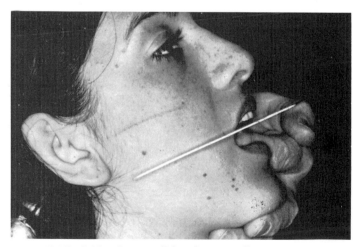

Figure 12.1 Fox's bite plane parallel to alar–tragus line

At this stage the upper rim should be aligned to the alar–tragus plane (see Figure 12.1). The occlusal vertical relation is then decided by measuring the distance between spots marked on the nose and chin with the mandible in rest position (see Figure 9.2). The bases and rims are then replaced in the mouth with the compound on the lower softened and closure stopped at the level of rest position. The lower rim is then reduced by 4–5 mm in height and notches are cut in the upper rim, at the region of the first molars. Movement on the retruded arc of the mandible is then practised by the patient with the assistance of the dentist. The bases are inserted and a compound stop placed on the lower rim in the incisor region to arrest closure at the planned OVR. The posterior segments of the lower rim are then loaded with the registration material (minimal viscosity, rapid setting and dimensional stability after setting) and the registration made. The upper base is held lightly in place by the forefinger and thumb of the left hand while the right is free to guide the mandible on the retruded arc into light closure and held while the registration material sets (see Figure 9.5). Care is required to ensure that the bases do not move during the closure or setting. This aspect of the operation cannot receive too much emphasis.

Facebow transfer

A facebow transfer of the arbitrary retruded axis (condyle studs on marks 12 mm in front of the tragi on lines between them and the external canthi of the eyes) is now made (Figure 12.2). This will permit the maxillary base to rotate on the same retruded axis as the mandibular base rotates, relative to the maxilla, in the mouth.

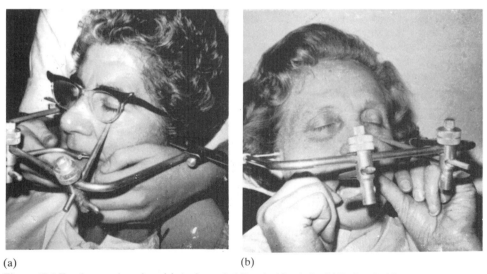

(a)   (b)

Figure 12.2 Facebow registration. (a) Assistant holding the bite-fork. (b) Patient holding

Protruded registration

A preliminary protruded registration can be made at this stage with the mandible protruded 6 mm and using a wax wafer between the compound occlusal rims. The technician can then institute preliminary balance in the articulation of the set-up. However, this registration should be repeated at the try-in stage.

Discussion

The assessment of the OVR in relation to rest position is arbitrary as it is not easy to assess the RVR when the patient is edentulous. The edentulous mouth has no periodontal receptors and this may result in an increased tonus of the mandibular elevators (Attwood, 1956), thus closing the RVR. A further cause of RVR closure may be the lack of lip support by the teeth. It is, therefore, advisable to ask the patient to part the lips (but only slightly) when rest position is being measured. This emphasizes the arbitrary nature of the procedure. Movement of the lips (the 'm' sound) followed by rest is one of many methods. The marking and measuring of this distance are subject to error and the Willis bite gauge can be used if a consistently light touch in method can be achieved. The use of the facebow permits the OVR to be altered on the articulator and this may be done at the next stage when making speech tests.

The screw jack method

An alternative method of registering the jaw relation and, in particular, of determining the vertical height, was devised by Timmer (1968) using a screw jack for self-assessment of the most comfortable position or zone. This utilizes the patient's 'inherent proprioceptive sensation' to determine the optimal interarch relation and was first advocated by Timmer (1964) and Lytle (1964). The method uses a screw and adjustable bolt attached to the mandibular base and a metal plate secured to the maxillary base. By increasing and decreasing the height of the screw by measured amounts (half or full turns) and asking the patient to assess 'better or worse', an optimal vertical level (or comfortable zone) is eventually reached. The device can then be used as a tracing plate to find the apex of the Gothic arch indicating the retruded horizontal position. A pin-hole drilled on the plate at the apex of the arch can then be used to engage the point of the screw. The two bases can then be joined around the screw by fast-setting plaster (see Figure 12.3). This provides the record for mounting the mandibular to the maxillary base, assuming that the maxillary has been previously mounted with a facebow transfer.

McMillan, Christenson and Tryde (1977) devised a new screw jack which proved to be more accurate than the Timmer original. Mean play in the new screw was 0.01 mm, compared with 0.05 mm in the Timmer version. A clinical experiment was carried out on 17 subjects between the ages of 50 and 80 years by comparing pairs of variances for both upper and lower border data from the two screw jacks. The variances of upper border data, collected by the new screw jack, were smaller than those from the Timmer jack. Fujii et al. (1977), using McMillan's screw jack, had 13 edentulous subjects approach the comfortable zone in three different ways: (1) the screw is adjusted from the fully opened and fully closed positions until comfortable positions are reached; (2) the screw is adjusted from the same starting points but crosses the comfortable zone until an uncomfortable position is reached; and (3) adjustments alternate between high and low uncomfortable positions and pass through the comfortable zone. The readings proved to be dependent on the starting positions. Different approaches to the borders of the comfortable zone produced different responses from the perceptual mechanism. The response showing the greatest stability was shown to be from the fully opened to the lower border.

Tryde et al. (1974) had previously established that the method was not dependent on whether the dentist or patient operated the screw jack but that there were

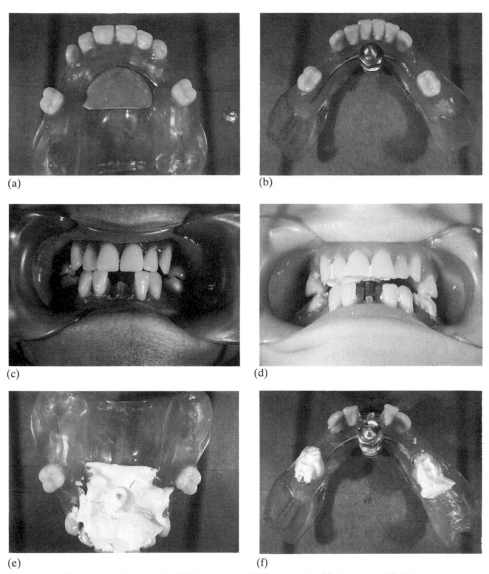

Figure 12.3 The screw jack method. (a) Metal plate. (b) Screw jack. (c) In mouth. (d) Plaster registration. (e) Plaster record: upper. (f) Plaster record: lower

difficulties in achieving reproducibility of the readings. The principle is worth pursuing and has worked favourably in the author's hands. The position of closure for complete dentures is so important for comfort and function that every proposal and idea should be tested and incorporated when found helpful.

Checking the record

Before setting the teeth it is always advisable to check the record transferred to the articulator. The split cast method using three or more records has already been described (p. 189), as has Brewer's pin method applied to reconstruction (p. 190). For complete dentures this latter method is particularly applicable and has proved helpful in the author's hands for 25 years. For this, two sets of four pins are set up on the articulator following the preliminary mounting, with the pins in edge-to-edge contact (Figure 12.4). The bases carrying the opposing pins are transferred (with the cups removed) to the mouth. If the pins do not meet on the retruded arc, the conclusion is that closure on the articulator is different from closure in the mouth. The extent of the difference, in both anteroposterior and buccolingual planes, can be seen as the pins approach each other. To complete the set-up at this relation would lead to unbalanced occlusion on closure in the mouth. Replaceable cups are now screwed on to the lower pins and filled with compound, plaster or acrylic resin and the retruded arc registration made again. The lower base and pins are remounted, the pins reset to touch again and the bases retried in the mouth. This procedure is repeated until the pins meet in the mouth as they do on the articulator (Thomson, 1961). If this method is to succeed, the retruded closing arc must be used each time. Registration on any other arc of closure is certain to produce a difference between the mounting on the articulator and the closure in the mouth since no two habitual arcs of closure will be similar.

The vertical and horizontal jaw relations have now been decided and no re-registration of the retruded relation is made until the dentures are completed.

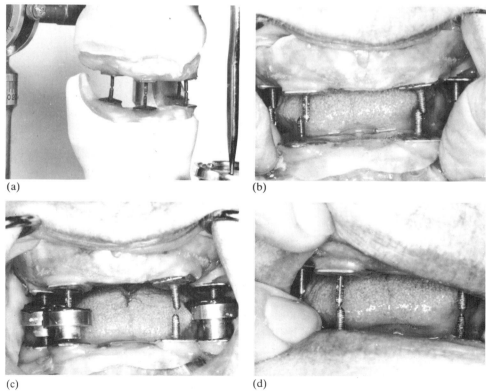

(a)   (b)

(c)   (d)

Figure 12.4 Check jaw record by opposing pins. (a) Pins set on permanent bases as from first jaw record. (b) Try-in: not together. (c) Re-registration. (d) Pins together

Theoretically this should not be necessary but practically it often is due to processing errors and the further seating of the bases after wear.

Setting the teeth

When the bases have been mounted in the correct jaw relation, a preliminary setting of the teeth is carried out by the technician. Sequences vary but the following principles should be observed.

1. The artificial teeth should be set in the positions of their natural predecessors. This can be difficult if it is some years and several dentures since the natural teeth were present. Smiling, pre-extraction photographs can be a help to the skilled technician, and the patient's spouse or relative can provide criticism at the trial stages. Pre-extraction casts, if available, can be invaluable, especially for intercanine and intermolar widths which can be measured.
2. The length, overlap and inclination of the maxillary incisor teeth should be set according to the skeletal classification and a lateral skull radiograph can be helpful by utilizing the SNA–SNB angle (p. 52). The lower lip should partly cover the maxillary incisors in repose, with normal lip competence.
3. The mandibular incisor line should be approved for speech and appearance at the first try-in and the dentist should be prepared to make alterations at this visit.
4. The canines in both arches should be vertical with only the mesial surfaces visible. The maxillary canines should be no longer than the central incisors and often shorter if the requirements of appearance, articulation and lower lip line permit. Lee (1962) set practical standards for the setting of all artificial teeth where the principle of a pleasing appearance is associated with good function.
5. The mandibular canine and premolar teeth should be compatible with the activities of the modiolus effect. If these teeth are in conflict with muscle activity the denture will rise every time the muscles are used. The mandibular second premolars should be at right angles to the occlusal plane.
6. The mandibular molars and premolars should be set in the gap of minimal activity (neutral zone) between the tongue and cheek muscles and below the greatest convexity of the tongue. The technician and dentist should work together on this setting. It can be helpful if only the first molars are set for the first try-in. This makes it easier to see them in occlusion and also to change their positions.
7. The maxillary molars should follow and be set in class I relation to the mandibular molars since they are most efficient in this relation. If the incisor relation has been determined as class II or class III, some attempt at compromise should be made for the premolars, such as a small gap or an additional premolar in order to maintain the class I molar occlusion. The maxillary second molars can often be omitted in the interests of balanced articulation for the protrusive movement if there is difficulty with a flat occlusal plane (Figure 12.5). The tongue should rest comfortably against the lingual cusps of the maxillary posterior teeth and so provide stability for the denture.
8. *Teeth on the ridge.* At no time is it necessary to set any of the teeth over the residual ridge for reasons of stability. Those parts of the ridge which were once occupied by the natural teeth have probably been resorbed and the significant factor is the zone of minimal effort of the cheek and tongue muscles.

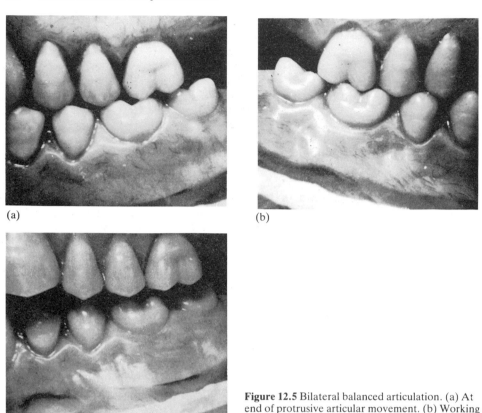

(a)

(b)

(c)

Figure 12.5 Bilateral balanced articulation. (a) At end of protrusive articular movement. (b) Working side. (c) Non-working side

9. *Tripod contact.* The possibilities for developing this most stable of occlusions will depend largely on the choice of posterior teeth. Occlusion will be more secure with 'anatomical' posteriors set in tripod contact.
10. *Porcelain or acrylic resin.* Acrylic posterior teeth are becoming increasingly hard and the need to prescribe porcelain for prolonged wear is less necessary. Patients who habitually grind their teeth will wear porcelain teeth as well as those made with acrylic. Also it is more difficult to adjust the occlusion on porcelain teeth.
11. *Balanced articulation* (see Figure 12.5). As each tooth is set in relation to an opposing tooth the upper arm of the articulator is moved laterally and retrusively, thus allowing the mandibular teeth to move protrusively. The teeth are moved until balance is achieved. This requires a special skill possessed by the well-trained technician. The dentist should know the principles involved and be able to cooperate with the technician in dealing with articulation problems as they arise. These principles are known as the five factors of articulation, namely, condyle guidance, incisal guidance, the plane of orientation, the occlusal curve and cusp height. Some notes on these factors follow.

Factors in articulation

1. The *condyle guidance* has been adjusted but it can be altered. It should be remembered that the protrusive path is usually a few degrees closer to the horizontal plane than the lateral path (Fischer's angle). In adjusting articular contacts for the lateral movements the condyle guidance should be increased by 5° over that used by the protrusive movement.

2. The *incisal guidance* will be determined by the setting of the incisor teeth to conform to tongue and lip activity. This, too, can be altered but care should be taken not to interfere with the latter activity. The vertical incisor overlap and horizontal overlap will also have been determined, where possible, by the natural teeth predecessors but a slight increase in the overlap may be permissible to allow for articular movements. The angle of the incisal guidance table should be set when the inclination of the upper incisors has been decided. This is achieved by moving the table until the incisal guidance pin remains in contact with it while the opposing incisors maintain articular contact in the protrusive movement. The combination of the condyle and incisal guidances thus provides a curved path of motion for all points between the guidances unless the guidance angles are identical.

3. The *plane of orientation* is usually determined by laying a rigid flat plane to touch the lower canines and the retromolar pads on the cast. Alternatively, this may have been decided by the alar–tragus transfer (see Figure 12.1). Such a plane can then be temporarily attached to the upper cast while the height of the posterior teeth are adjusted to it. This level may conflict with the height decided by the tooth positions in relation to the tongue and the latter level must take precedence, if correct. A compromise may be necessary and is justified if the dentist and technician realize the requirements of both neutral zone and plane of orientation.

4. The *occlusal curve* is vital to requirements of free articulation. The steeper the condyle guidance the steeper will the occlusal curve have to be. Monson's curve may be of value if the articulator possesses a centring plate. This method brings a mathematical certainty to the curve but it may not be harmonious with the requirements of the condyle and incisal guidances. However, as these guidances are by no means certain, Monson's curve may yet be revived.

5. The *cusp height* of the posterior teeth is determined by the limited choice of available teeth. Cusp heights can be altered provided the curves of the triangular ridges are not flattened and the teeth allowed to lock into each other like cogs. The occlusion of artificial posterior teeth should be by tripod contact for the supporting cusps and adequate horizontal and vertical overlap by the guiding cusps. This preserves the principle of minimal occlusion and will reduce parafunctional grinding, provided the jaw relationship has been correctly registered. The horizontal overlap will prevent cheek and tongue biting. Stability in IP will be provided and gliding to and from IP during the articular movements will be more easily developed. The occlusal surfaces of artificial posterior teeth have undergone many changes of design but the natural design is still available and, if correctly used, is reliable. Teeth without cusps provide an unstable IP and articulation cannot be balanced. To be successful, the cuspless-tooth denture must have its teeth accurately placed in the neutral zone and its wearer not given to clenching or grinding habits.

Discussion

Many complete dentures are made and comfortably worn without *mechanical balance* in articular movements. The habit of denture doodling (by irrelevant muscle activity) is often blamed on the dentist by the patient and bilateral balance in articulation may encourage it. Unilateral balance is often considered to be the ideal articulation and a compromise solution. Bilateral balance can be created from this articulation by reducing the distal facing buccal cusp ridges of the maxillary teeth and mesial facing lingual cusp ridges of the mandibular teeth (BULL rule, p. 211). Neither unilateral nor bilateral balance is possible with the class II, division 2 jaw relation. Such patients have never been able to achieve it between their natural teeth and it is doubtful if they would benefit from it in artificial reproductions.

Free articulation consists of balanced occlusal contacts during articular movements and the chief difficulty in achieving it is the inaccuracy of the transferred positional records which at best provide an estimate on the articulator of the movements which take place in the mouth between these occlusal positions. Nairn's (1973) three recommendations for occlusion and articulation in complete dentures are worth stating: achieve unobstructed movements into intercuspal occlusion; avoid premature balancing contact in lateral occlusions; do not pay too high a price for protrusive balance.

The much quoted dictum 'enter bolus, exit balance' is often used to discredit the value of mechanical balance. If balance is present the patient will soon discover the reassuring approach of it. However, dentures will be more stable if bilateral chewing can be learned (Figure 12.6).

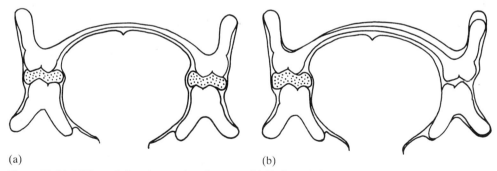

(a)   (b)

Figure 12.6 (a) Bilateral chew in complete dentures. (b) Unilateral chew

The try-in

Many features of complete dentures can be checked at this stage and a helpful reference on this topic and on causes of denture failure is by Lawson (1959). For purposes of checking jaw and tooth relations the following observatons are made.

1. Ask the patient to speak and note the closest speaking space as indication of the occlusal vertical relation. Also, any molar contact during speech will indicate an increased OVR.
2. Ask the patient to close with the chin back and lips 'sneering', and note any deviation between opposing incisor midlines.

3. Ask the patient if the teeth 'feel level' when making retruded closure. The strangeness of the new bases and tooth positions make it difficult for the patient to provide an accurate closure but the horizontal position should have been checked and confirmed by this stage.
4. Compare the contacts, using shimstock or ultrathin articulating paper, between the dentures in the mouth and the dentures on the articulator. If there is a difference a new precontact registration may be necessary but if the original record has been checked, as by the opposing pins method, the discrepancy is likely to be small. The teeth may have moved in the wax. Cooperation with the technician should correct the fault.
5. Ask the patient to close with the front teeth to check the desired protruded occlusion. If the incisors are in contact but not the molars the condyle guidance is not steep enough. In addition, the occlusal curve may be too flat. If the molars only are in contact, the condyle guidance is too steep and the occlusal curve may be too deep. Alternatively, a protruded registration (6 mm in front of intercuspal position and precontact) is remade in quick-setting plaster and the angle of condyle guidance is checked.
6. Ask the patient to open wide and note the mandibular tooth positions in relation to the tongue.
7. Ask the patient to 'close and slide the teeth side to side'. Note any interferences. Compare with the dentures mounted (see Figure 12.7).

Laboratory procedures

Processing of the teeth to the bases must be carried out without any impairment of the dimensional stability of the bases or movement of the teeth. Processing temperatures should be carefully observed. It is always reassuring to return the processed dentures to the mounting casts on the articulator where the occlusion and articulation can be checked. If the incisal guidance pin reaches the incisal table on the articulator the OVR will correspond to the one registered in the mouth. Remount plates joined by a removable pin (Hanau) are a useful aid for returning the mounting cast accurately to the articulator.

The remount

This is carried out if there is any suspicion of unilateral occlusion and is often recommended immediately after the first insertion of the new dentures. It can be more practicable two days later when the bases may have become better seated and occlusal faults (with their associated bruises) have become apparent. The retruded arc of closure is rehearsed and assurance made that the bases are seated, with adhesive if necessary. Faulty occlusion may have led to instability. The registration is made, preferably with plaster, making sure, with correct hand holding, that the bases are seated and remain seated while the plaster sets and that no tooth contact takes place through the plaster. Alternatively, three mounds of fast-setting low fusing wax (Alminax) or Kerr's bite registration paste can be used. The mounting casts will have been preserved (especially if the remount plates are used) and no facebow transfer is necessary. The mounting ring of the mandibular cast is removed and replastered using the new record. Occlusal adjustment can usually be carried out while the patient waits, following the procedure outlined below. Any major

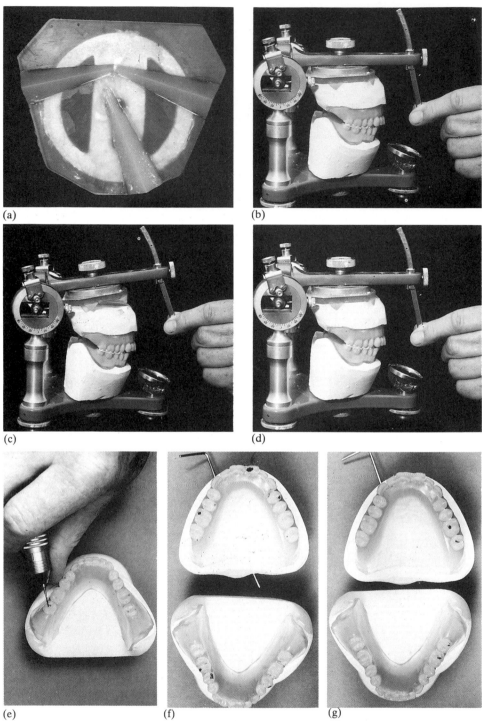

Figure 12.7 Split cast and occlusal adjustment. (a) Notch former. (b) Retruded record used for mounting lower denture. (c) More protruded mounting. (d) Second retruded record: confirms first record. (e) Adjust distal lower of 37 for balance in IP. (f) For balance in protrusion adjust distobuccal of 24; distolingual of 45; lingual of 21 or incisal of 31. (g) For non-working interference adjust mesial inner of buccal lower (MIBL) of 36 and 37

descrepancies may have to be corrected by altering tooth positions and reprocessing but this is rare if care has been taken with the original registrations.

Occlusal adjustment for complete dentures

The objectives are to restore intercuspal occlusion between the opposing teeth of both dentures as the mandible closes to retruded horizontal and correct vertical relation, and to allow free articulation on excursive articular movements.

Registrations required

1. Facebow transfer of the maxillary denture to an adjustable articulator. This ensures that the maxillary denture will rotate on the same axis of opening and closing as the mandible does on its retruded axis.
2. A jaw relation record between the mandibular and maxillary teeth just prior to contact on the retruded axis of the mandible. This will allow the mandibular denture to close on the same retruded axis on the articulator.
3. This record should be checked by three other retruded records by the split-cast method (Figure 12.7).
4. A record, preferably in rapid-setting plaster on each buccal segment, of the protruded relation between mandible and maxilla just prior to contact between the opposing incisors. These records will allow the angle of condyle descent to be adjusted on both sides of the articulator.

Procedure

1. Use ultrathin articulating paper, preferably with the marking stain on one side only so as to prevent confusion of marks on the teeth. Ensure that the upper arm of the articulator is pulled forwards on closing to ensure retruded closure.
2. For interferences on retruded closure into IP, trim *m*esial facing aspect of *u*pper fossae *or d*istal of *l*ower; hence MUDL. This assures a more distal closure of the mandibular teeth (see Figure 12.7e).
3. For protrusive articular interferences, trim the *b*uccal *u*pper cusp ridges (the distal facing aspects) and/or the *l*ingual *l*ower cusp ridges (the mesial facing aspects); hence BULL (Figure 12.7f). Where the interferences occur between the incisors or canines, trim the lingual surfaces of the maxillary teeth unless it is desirable, for appearance reasons, to trim the mandibular labial or incisal surfaces (Figure 12.7f). Note: if the tooth or teeth causing cusp interferences are more than a third of a tooth out of line or in vertical contact it (they) should be replaced.
4. For working side articular interferences, trim *b*uccal *u*pper cusp ridges (the distal facing aspects) and/or *l*ingual *l*ower cusp ridges (the mesial facing aspects); hence BULL again. Again, use ultrathin articulating paper and of a different colour from that used for the IP adjustment.
5. For non-working (balancing) side articular interferences trim *m*esial facing *i*nner aspect of *b*uccal *l*ower cusps *or* the *d*istal facing *i*nner aspect of *l*ingual *u*pper cusps; hence MIBL or DILU (Figure 12.7g).

For working and non-working side adjustments (in the lateral excursions) the condyle guidance should be increased by $5°$. Take care to maintain shape of supporting cusps.

Faults, complaints and denture intolerance

There are few new complete dentures that are free from faults and the complaints vary from the justifiable to the tragicomic. Bruising of mucosa, lack of stability and difficulty in eating can all be attributable to cusp interference and *lack of balance* on closure and during articulation. 'The dentures fit well and look fine, but I can't eat with them' is a not uncommon complaint and can be attributable to a high mandibular occlusal plane. An increased OVR that should have been recognized at the try-in stage can have adverse effects on muscles, joints, mastication and swallowing. There are few stability problems, however, that will not respond to a new precontact, retruded registration and occlusal adjustment following remount of the dentures.

There are, however, patients who have an intolerance to dentures and they may require special if not specialist consideration. Newton (1984) discusses this problem in an article on the psychosomatic component in prosthodontics and refers to 'operantly conditioned symptoms'. These can be defined as behaviour repeated because of desirable results. Patients will use illness to obtain social reinforcement and they may suffer from hysteria. Newton quotes Whitehead *et al.* (1979) who consider the psychological process to be 'operant conditioning' and describes such patients as seeking not only physical relief but official sanction of the illness. They have found, early in life, that social success can be achieved by the manipulation of illness. Newton adds that some denture patients may present a wide spectrum of complaints, show no detectable pathological responses, and often have good residual ridges and healthy mucosa, but are unable to wear their dentures. Many of these patients have been treated by several dentists and have collected many 'unwearable' dentures. Berry and Mahood (1966) showed that these clinically normal patients do not suffer from a sensorimotor impairment. Nairn and Brunello (1971) found that intolerant patients have significantly higher scores on questionnaires designed to reveal neuroticism. This state of sustained arousal may result in muscle tension related to environmental stresses causing sores on mucosa and painful muscles. Dentists, therefore, would do well to consider referring such patients to the care of the appropriate physician before embarking on further prosthodontic treatment.

Intercuspal occlusion on the retruded arc

No doubt this will continue to be arguable as long as dentists make dentures. This occlusal position does involve effort and elderly patients will tend to find a more comfortable habitual position of closure forward of the retruded IP. Consequently, the compromise of providing free articulation between the retruded and habitual positions ('long centric') may be justifiable. On the other hand, if patients can be persuaded to close their teeth only when swallowing and avoid all other parafunctional contacts, the retruded IP is advisable.

Inexpensive complete dentures

The foregoing procedures involve time and therefore expense and will prove unrealistic for dentures which have to be made on a strict budget. As has been implied, more problems derive from failures of occlusion (stability) than of impressions (retention) and emphasis on the following features may prove helpful in low budget dentures.

1. The cost and correct use of a facebow adjustable articulator will soon be offset and rewarded if a large output of dentures is involved. A facebow record, with practice, takes two minutes on the patient in the chair and the same in the laboratory. The upper cast has to be secured to an articulator in any event.
2. The retruded arc interocclusal record can be achieved quickly with practice and a good patient rapport.
3. If wax bases are used for this registration the wax should be hard, when chilled, and trimmed short of the proposed denture borders to reduce displacement. A fixative is advised to reduce displacement of the bases to a minimum when making the registration.
4. If wax occlusion rims are used they should be trimmed short of the OVR. For the registration, plaster or a lower-fusing wax should be used.
5. Before jaw registration the proposed buccolingual position of the posterior teeth may be carved in the wax and the anterior teeth set up. However, the emphasis on the registration should not be diminished.
6. The bite fork of the facebow can then be inserted into the labial and buccal surfaces of the upper wax base.
7. In practices where the laboratory work has to be sent out, there are difficulties of transporting the facebow and articulator. Even if the articulator can be kept with the technician, it is valueless without a facebow. The dental assistant is, however, well able to perform the operation of mounting the casts. There is, of course, the Slidematic facebow for use with the Denar Mark II articulator (p. 132) which prevents the need for transferring the bow. Somehow an understanding between dentist and technician on matters of occlusion must be established in these difficult circumstances.
8. If the plain-hinge articulator is used for complete dentures its limitations must be understood and more emphasis placed on the need to record the correct OVR when making the jaw relation registration. The OVR should *not* be altered on this articulator.

Improvement of existing dentures

It is often more profitable to improve existing complete dentures than to embark on new ones. This is always advised when the tooth positions are correct. Extension of underextended borders can be performed with compound additions which are later processed. This is preferred to the complete rebase because rebased dentures have to be remounted in any event. A retruded axis precontact registration and facebow record will provide the requirements necessary for remounting the dentures. Occlusal adjustment can then be carried out according to the foregoing notes. Any border additions made can be processed at the same time.

Occlusal adjustments carried out in the mouth will be described and discussed at the end of the section on partial dentures.

One complete denture

Jaw registrations for one complete denture opposing an arch of natural teeth (or one including bridgework or partial denture) emphasize the problem of maintaining retention of the denture base while making the registration. They present the problem of obtaining an accurate, hard cast of the opposing teeth and the need to preserve their occlusal surfaces while developing the occlusion. The following procedures are suggested in an attempt to meet the difficulties which are often encountered.

Teeth preparation

The natural teeth should be inspected with a view to emphasizing the fossae and marginal ridges so that intercuspal occlusion can provide the features of tripod contact for the supporting cusps and overlap for the guiding cusps. This may require reshaping of old fillings or flat surfaces on pontic teeth. It need not be pointed out that once the impression has been made the teeth on the cast cannot be altered.

Impression and cast

Plaster is always reliable but seldom preferred. As one teacher at Northwestern University used to say: 'Plaster don't bend'. The difficulties of using plaster for this type of impression can be minimized by recording only the occlusal surfaces and by waxing out undercuts in case the plaster does reach into embrasures or under pontic teeth. Plaster will permit a low-fusing metal cast to be made which is preferable to the hardest stone. Alternative materials are well known and emphasis is placed on accurate retention within the tray of the alginate, reversible hydrocolloid or rubber. If a partial denture is worn it must be accurately seated when the impression is made. This presents the problem of movement not being recognized, especially if the material reaches beyond the denture border. It is therefore doubly desirable that the impression material does not reach beyond the greatest convexity of the teeth.

Base and occlusal rim

The permanent base should be used for the jaw registration for reasons already given and the occlusal rim should be made of hard compound. This can be trimmed and grooved to accept the registration material.

Jaw registration

The OVR is decided and registered into the compound softened on its occlusal surface. This surface is then cut away and grooved to a depth of 3–4 mm with the exception of two stops. The relationship is re-registered using the same hand-holding method (Figure 9.5a) and the material of choice. The lightest contact into the softest material (with the quickest set) at the retruded position are the objectives. If the 'stops' do not show through the record the OVR will be slightly increased and the closure can be completed on the articulator provided a facebow transfer has been made. If more than the 'stops' show it is likely that the base has moved and the registration should be remade.

Setting the teeth

Care in achieving accurate occlusal relations may require cast metal occlusal surfaces for the posterior teeth. If this luxury cannot be afforded, the choice of posterior teeth should be made on a basis of well-shaped cusps and fossae. It can be an advantage to process only two posterior teeth when first completing the denture in order to ensure accurate closure and function. The occlusion between first molars can be seen more accurately from the mesial aspect when the premolars are not present. They can be processed later. The articulation scheme will depend on what is permitted by the opposing teeth.

The remount

One complete denture almost always requires a remount. It is hoped that minimal adjustments are necessary since only the denture teeth can be adjusted. The registration is even more difficult when processed teeth are present since any contact between opposing teeth will result in movement of the base. Plaster is always preferable provided it sets quickly after contact with the teeth. With this material, timing and an accurate knowledge of the setting time will minimize the time required to hold the dentures. A fixative for the base is permitted, even advised.

Comment

Whether the denture in question is upper or lower the difficulties are the same and can be overcome by the closest attention to details of jaw and tooth relations.

Immediate complete dentures

In a mouth where the decision has been made to remove the remaining teeth it is always tempting to utilize the existing intercuspal position, if there is one. This may prove unstable when denture teeth have replaced the natural teeth. The most stable and reproducible jaw position is the retruded and no opportunity should be lost to make use of it if the opportunity arises. Time may have to be spent instructing the older patient in the use of the retruded position and the challenge is often gladly accepted. A reduction in the number of posterior teeth is also advised, especially if the patient has been making do with a molar and premolar on each side for a number of years. Good occlusion can be more easily developed, and seen to be developed with fewer teeth. The tongue will adapt more efficiently to a denture if the teeth correspond in number and position to those just removed. The extra teeth can be added later.

Most denture problems can be anticipated and prevented if every immediate denture can be made as a permanent denture. Additions to acrylic resin dentures can be made with a cooperative and well-planned laboratory service while the patient waits. Then, when the immediate denture is comfortable and acceptable, a duplicate denture can be made (Thomson, 1967). A spare denture is always desirable and provides an assurance for travel and holiday.

Permanent immediate dentures

It is not within the scope of this text to describe the techniques of making these dentures nor the surgery that makes them possible but five principles will be advocated and a brief outline of the techniques used will be given.

1. The maxillary incisor and canine teeth should be retained until the immediate denture is to be made. If possible and practicable all the other teeth should be removed. The object is to provide as much stable residual ridge as possible on which to make the permanent denture. In the case of the mandibular teeth, existing circumstances will determine the plan. Ideally, an edentulous ridge makes for the best denture but temporary loss of teeth is not always acceptable to the patient. If not, mandibular incisor teeth can be retained and removed prior to placing the denture, as for those in the maxilla. A further objective is to free the mandible from the influences of previous occlusions so that a retruded registration can be made.

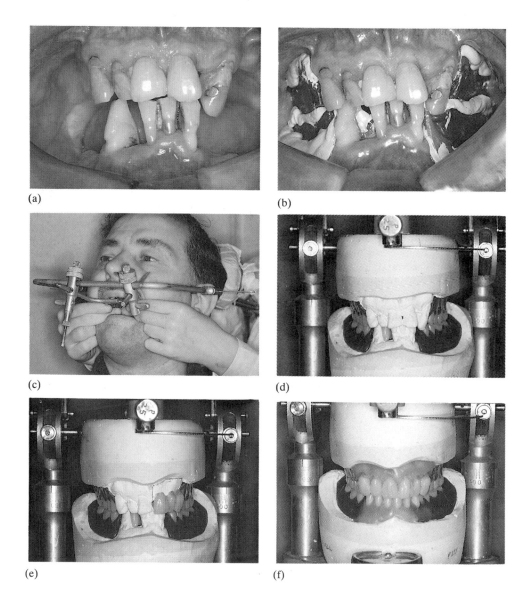

(a)

(b)

(c)

(d)

(e)

(f)

2. Impressions and records are made and the casts transferred to a semi-adjustable articulator. Teeth are selected to copy the characteristics of the existing teeth and should have the approval of the patient. The number of posterior teeth is based on the estimated tolerance of the patient.

3. The artificial teeth should occupy the positions of their natural predecessors. Any improvements are discussed with the patient and related to occlusal and lip tolerance. Migrant and tilted teeth should be restored to their original postions as closely as can be estimated. As a tooth is removed from the master cast, the artificial replacement is seated on a wax base. When all the plaster teeth have been removed and the replacements waxed into position, the base and teeth are removed. Plaster is then removed from the labial surface of the cast which will allow the labial plate of the denture to occupy the same outline as the plaster did previously.

4. Room has now to be made, surgically, for the labial plate of the maxillary denture and the incisor and canine teeth so that they will retain the outlines of the natural teeth and gum and show no appearance of swelling. This is achieved by the operation of intraseptal alveotomy, following the removal of the incisor and canine teeth. Triangular areas of gum are incised and removed from the distal ends of the canine sockets, followed by triangular notches of labial bone using side-cutting rongeur forceps. The interdental septa are then removed

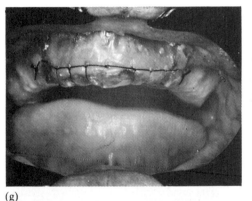

(g)

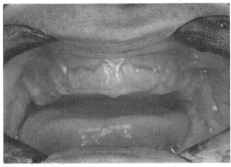

(h)

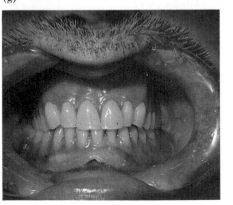

(i)

Figure 12.8 Immediate dentures. (a) Pre-treatment. (b) Impressions. (c) Facebow. (d) Mounted master casts. (e) Part set-up. (f) Completed set-up. (g) Completed surgery 24 h post-op. (h) 6 months post-op. (i) Immediate permanent dentures

using the same forceps and making the first cut from the labial aspect of each septum. The forceps are then directed from the palatal aspect and pointed to the line where it is intended that the labial cortical plate should fracture. On removal of the septa, the fractured labial plate is apposed to the palatal plate and should present a slightly loose fit (in the labial region) for the denture, which is then tried in and the occlusion checked. Postoperative swelling will provide a close fit between denture and tissue and new bone will be deposited from the cortical plate inwards, thus maintaining the fit. This procedure has proved successful in the author's hands for 34 years (Figure 12.8).

5. After three months of healing the extraction areas on the fitting surface can be rebased, although this is not always necessary. The immediate denture thus becomes a permanent denture.

Duplicate complete dentures

It has been said by dentists, sometimes ruefully, that if dentures are successful a duplicate set will be requested. Not always is the success repeated, especially if the policy of starting again is adopted. However, many are the successes claimed for duplicate methods and the one used by this author has stood the test of time. Details were first published (Thomson, 1967) following seven years' use of the method and few changes have been necessary since then. The focus is on tooth positions and occlusion.

The dentures are sent to the laboratory where stone plaster casts are made of the fitting surface and permanent bases are made on them. If there are severe undercuts the casts can be made in three parts, as in the 1967 illustrations, or by using a flexible material (Flexibase). Mounting casts are made and notched and the dentures placed on them. White plaster matrices are formed around the labial and buccal surfaces of the casts and teeth (Figure 12.9). A facebow transfer is all that is required from the patient and the maxillary denture is mounted on an adjustable articulator. The mandibular denture is then mounted at the denture IP using the mandiblar mounting cast. The dentures and new permanent bases are thus interchangeable on the mounting casts and the intercuspal position of the duplicate dentures has been determined by the existing dentures.

The set-up can now proceed using the matrices to seat the maxillary teeth at the duplicated horizontal and vertical positions. The mandibular teeth follow and it may be desirable for the technician to have the existing dentures for an hour while refining the set-up, if this can be arranged before the try-in visit. Much has to be checked at this visit, particularly the patient's approval, but as this is the only appointment before completion when chair time is spent it should not be grudged. OVR bilateral balance, free articulation, appearance, speech, retention and, of course, 'Do they feel the same?' are all checked.

Be prepared. If duplicate dentures are anticipated while making the first set, four points should receive attention.

1. Ensure that the dentures to be duplicated are satisfactory. Enquire if any changes are required.
2. Order a duplicate set of teeth and note any adjustments or alterations made on the original set.
3. Keep the mounting casts used for the original set, with notes on any additions or removals made on the bases.
4. Keep the same technician. He is a key figure.

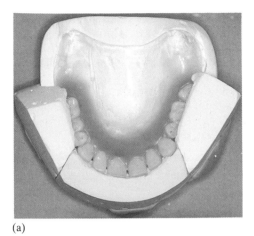

(a)

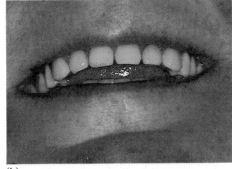

(b)

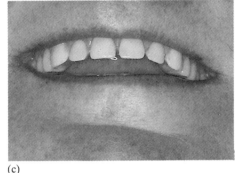

(c)

Figure 12.9 Duplicate dentures. (a) Plaster matrices. (b) Original and (c) duplicate dentures

Unsatisfactory complete dentures

The referred patient complaining of unsatisfactory dentures is so common as to be a blight on the profession. Reference has already been made to denture intolerance which can be associated with psychosomatic problems but, too often, the dentures are to blame. Yet success will not be achieved by immediately deciding on new dentures. A consultation to assess the causes of failure of existing or previous dentures is essential before a decision is made either to improve the unsatisfactory dentures or to start again.

Consultation

This will consist of a series of questions in an attempt to relate the complaints to support, retention, stability and appearance. A sympathetic rapport should be established away from the dental chair. A spouse or friend may want to take part and this should not be discouraged provided he or she does not take over from the patient, in which case the door should be courteously shown.

Questions should begin with: 'What is wrong?' The open in preference to the closed question. If this produces a barrage of complaints the questions can become more specific. 'Sore places?' Often a stability problem caused by cusp interference which may tilt the denture or cause it to slide. 'Can you control your dentures when eating or swallowing?' If not, the cause may be an increased OVR with raised mandibular occlusal plane. 'Appearance?' To which the answer is often: 'They're not me'. The cause is tooth positions, and reference should be made to smiling and pre-extraction photographs. 'Do you clench or grind your teeth?' Perhaps a stress-related problem but maybe an occlusal cause. 'Do they interfere with speech?' Test with words beginning with 's', 'sh', 't', 'f' and 'v', and suspect the incisor or tongue–palate relation.

Examination

There are seven features of problem dentures that should be examined.

1. Rest vertical relation (RVR) with both dentures in place using fixative if necessary. 'Let the lips touch; let the lips part.' Measure. 'Close on your back teeth' (OVR). Measure. RVR to OVR should be ±3 mm.
2. Repeat and measure again. Ask if both sides meet equally. Ask if dentures are in place: if not, more fixative. Repeat and ask again if teeth meet equally.
3. Repeat closure, this time ensure that the maxillary denture is secure and hold the mandibular denture (see Figure 9.5). Close on retruded arc and look for cusp interference. If so, prepare for remount.
4. 'Open wide.' Observe retention and tongue behaviour in relation to mandibular denture. It should stay behind mandibular incisor teeth.
5. Observe speech and any lip problems with 's', 'sh', 't', 'f' and 'v' sounds.
6. Remove the mandibular denture and note RVR. Measure and note any difference. Similarly, with both dentures removed. This usually results in a more closed level of rest position, as has already been suggested, due to an increased tonus of the elevator muscles in the edentulous mouth (Attwood, 1956). This should be taken into account in assessing the OVR.
7. Finally, the residual ridges should be examined for support problems such as sharp mylohyoid ridges, undercut tuberosities and flabby ridges. Although not the province of this text these features should receive attention.

Decisions

A clear clinical picture can be established in half an hour of consultation and examination if the questions are carefully asked and in a kindly manner. The dentist must now ask himself, 'What is genuinely best for this patient: new dentures or improve these ones?' If the occlusion is unbalanced and the bases and tooth positions seem correct, consider remount with facebow transfer and precontact registration followed by occlusal adjustment (see p. 211). If the base or bases are underextended, consider rebasing followed by remount and readjust occlusion (see below). If the tooth positions are incorrect, consider removal and resetting, followed by remount and adjust occlusion. With all complete denture problems improvement will follow readjustment of occlusal relations and it is essential if rebasing is found necessary. It is always preferable to consider improvement before remake because faults are discovered and treated without too heavy a commitment.

Rebasing complete dentures

This procedure can be a saving grace for many dentures provided it is coupled with remounting and adjustment of the IP to the correct level. It will solve nothing if the impression is made by having the patient close to the existing occlusion, the base subsequently processed and returned to the mouth. There will always be alterations to the IP due to the variable closing forces applied by the patient. New problems are inevitable and the old ones are seldom solved.

One denture at a time is recommended and the following steps are suggested.

1. A measurement is made of the existing OVR and a decision made on any correction to this level. This measurement is best done between small marks drilled on the labial gum of each denture, which can be refilled, or between selected points on the incisor teeth.
2. The fitting surface should be cleared of undercuts and allowances made for the free flow of impression material, without allowing the denture surface to penetrate the impression. 'Stops' may be indicated on the impression surface. The patient is allowed to occlude lightly when the denture with impression material has been seated, after which the operator should take over and apply gentle force to retain the impression while setting.
3. After removal and checking the impression it is reseated and the OVR noted. An anterior stop is placed on the maxillary incisors and the mandible guided into the retruded relation on the softened stop, making sure that there is no posterior tooth contact. The occlusal surfaces of the buccal mandibular teeth are then loaded with the registration material (fast-setting plaster or bite registration paste) and the retruded jaw registration completed.
4. A facebow registration, avoiding contact on the bite fork with the anterior stop, completes the chairside procedures.
5. In the laboratory the dentures are mounted and the OVR distance is measured.
6. The denture to be rebased is removed from its cast and the impression material removed. The impression surface is scoured and the denture seated on the mounted master cast. The OVR is decided (by dentist and technician together) and the incisal guidance pin figure noted. The denture for rebase is then placed in intercuspal occlusion against the opposing denture (or cast of the natural teeth) and the articulator closed to the OVR previously decided. If the upper denture is being rebased the palate should be cut out. Waxing of the denture to its cast is carried out while making sure that intercuspal occlusion is maintained. The denture is then processed.

A refinement in this procedure is to provide a device for removing and replacing the master to the mounting cast so that the processed denture and cast can be returned to the articulator for checking the occlusion.

Procedural problems

These are concerned chiefly with ensuring the correct jaw position for remount, in both vertical and horizontal relations, and with secure seating of both dentures on the residual ridges. Neither problem may be seen to be correctable and the fingers of the operator are the only guide. The mandible must be felt to be retruded and the bases not to have moved. These are key and critical aspects of occlusion in complete denture prosthodontics. The rest is technique and is chiefly in the hands of the technician who must, however, work under the instructions of the dentist. Plaster for mounting casts, facebow and jaw record transfers must show minimal expansion. Articulator parts must have tight screw fittings. Attention to details of occlusal adjustment must be strict; in particular, there must be no reduction of supporting cusps in IP or articular movements.

Implants

The advent of these aids to complete and partial dentures, and chiefly to complete lower dentures, has brought a new expertise to restorative dentistry, and with it a heavy responsibility on the prosthodontist for estimating, recording and maintaining the correct occlusal vertical and horizontal relations. The vertical relation must be correct to a millimetre and tension by muscles on osseointegrated implants through the medium of the teeth must be eliminated. Considerable skill and judgement are therefore required of the prosthodontist.

Comment

Many elderly patients want only carpet slippers for dentures; comfortable, loose-fitting, easily removable covers for their gums to be worn occasionally when eating and when their grandchildren come to tea. But even these never-to-be-despised dentures require teeth which are not displaced by lips, cheeks and tongue and whose appearance does not shock. If, in addition, they can be provided with an intercuspal position which does not cause nibbling habits and sore places they can often be worn outdoors. Immediate dentures provide the opportunity to make permanent dentures with teeth where they are best tolerated, and at a time when changes are expected and new movements can be learned. If replacement dentures are being made where others have failed, attention to the vertical level of occlusion relative to the rest position and a retruded horizontal intercuspal position of the mandible will solve many problems. Before new dentures are planned, however, an attempt should be made to improve the existing dentures by border additions, to improve retention and, by occlusal adjustment, to provide stability.

Partial dentures

The decision to make partial dentures is often bedevilled by 'for' and 'against' factors. Appearance, occlusal function and the containment of food being masticated are those in favour, against which there are the factors of design, skill, understanding of the problems, the health or otherwise of the supporting tissues, doubtful tolerance and possible rejection by the patient. Then there is the possibility of failure to wear the appliance by the patient, and whose is the fault?

Several studies have been carried out in the past twenty years, on an epidemiological basis, to discover the existence of tooth loss problems and the need for restoring these losses. Battistuzzi and colleagues (Battistuzzi, Käyser and Kanters, 1987; Battistuzzi, Käyser and Peer, 1987) examined and questioned 750 people between the ages of 25 and 54 and classified them according to socioeconomic class and age. In all strata the percentage of antagonistic contacts was higher in the premolar than in the molar areas. More teeth were missing in the lower than in the higher socioeconomic group. Only 40% of 'open tooth spaces' were restored and 33% of 'free-end spaces' were filled with removable partial dentures. The distribution of opposing contacts was more important to the patients than the relation between missing teeth and function.

Bjorn and Owall (1979) examined 543 industrial employees for the location of toothless areas and the extent of replacement. The frequency of untreated spaces was almost the same for mandibular as for maxillary teeth. Premolar and molar spaces did not constitute a primary indication for replacement and there was more prosthetic treament in the higher age groups, probably due to a greater loss of anterior teeth.

Mohlin *et al.* (1979) examined 389 military males with a mean age of 32. By means of an index for dental status 39 (10%) were judged to be in great need of dental replacements for aesthetic as well as for occlusal reasons. The authors established three indices which could be helpful for further studies: ER (aesthetic), PT (prosthetic) and OR (oral rehabilitation), all on a scale of 1 to 5, with 5 representing the greatest need.

Smith and Sheiham (1980) conducted structured interviews with 254 elderly people living at home and compared dental (normative) needs with expressed needs. Two age groups were examined: between 65 and 74, and 75 and over. There was a wide discrepancy between the two and only 42% of those clinically assessed as needing treatment felt that they required it. Only 19% had tried to obtain it. The causes of not wanting nor seeking treatment were given as cost, fear, immobility, age and 'not want to bother the dentist'.

These studies are four out of many and details of others are given in the references of the four. The findings may not affect decisions or designs but should give indications for treatment needs.

The application of the principles of occlusion to partial dentures may be complicated by two factors, namely, a displaced IP of the existing natural teeth, and the differing movements of natural and denture teeth during occlusal function. The IP of the mandible may be incorrect in terms of retruded arc closure and an occlusal analysis is always worthwhile in order to assess if it should be corrected. If allowed to persist, the additional adaptive demands made by the denture on muscles, joints or teeth may lead to a disorder. On the other hand, the policy of letting well alone is always tempting and the decision on pretreatment occlusal adjustment is never easy but is worth consideration. The forces of occlusion acting jointly on the periodontia of the teeth and the mucosa of the residual ridges usually result in a greater displacement of the denture bases than of the natural teeth. This results in two potentially damaging forces. Firstly, the residual ridges may resorb in response to masticatory and parafunctional movements and will cause a change of supporting tissue outline, particularly in the buccal segments. This may result in a more prominent mylohyoid ridge and be a cause of denture sore in the lower arch. It will also predispose to a support problem if and when a complete lower denture has to be made. Secondly, there will be an added pull by the retainers (attached to the denture bases or metal framework) on the abutment teeth. This differin᷈ response of teeth and mucosa also makes for difficulties in the registration of ja᷈ relations.

Difficulties

In order to provide good occlusal function by partial dentures, the following difficulties may be encountered and attempts should be made to overcome them before the final impressions are made.

1. The existing intercuspal position may be causing a disturbance and potential disorder. These include cusp interferences on closure to IP and during articular

movements. If necessary, corrections should be made before making the denture.
2. Altered occlusal curve by exfoliation of unopposed teeth. A decision may have to be made to reduce the height of such teeth by occlusal adjustment or by crowning at a reduced level.
3. High caries incidence and periodontally disturbed abutment teeth. These may have to be crowned and splinted to sound adjacent teeth. This treatment may also apply to teeth whose occlusal surfaces have been worn and are required for improved function.
4. Differing responses of mucosa and teeth in the registration of jaw relation.
5. Method of making the jaw registration and the materials used in order to obviate (4).
6. Laboratory errors. Most of these can be resolved by correct design of the denture and its return to casts mounted on an adjustable articulator.

In order to assess and deal with these difficulties before the dentures are made, an analysis and treatment plan should be carried out.

Analysis and treatment plan

Analysis prior to partial dentures should be comprehensive (Chapter 9) and a planning session with the technician essential. Radiographs and hand-held casts should be available for decisions on corrections to the occlusal curve, the acceptance (or not) of the habitual IP and articulation, the removal or treatment of any doubtful teeth (especially those selected as abutments), the type of teeth to be used which will provide the best function with the opposing natural teeth, and the method to be used in transferring the jaw relations. In addition, the technician will want to discuss the design of any cast framework which may be required, and the preparation of any teeth for occlusal rests and retention areas. The plan may therefore call for extractions, root canal and periodontal therapy, inlays and crowns, splinting of teeth, occlusal adjustment and a further consultation with the patient if any of these radical measures are advised. Premolars are not satisfactory abutment teeth and consideration should be given to extracting those with inadequate bone support or to splinting two premolars by soldered crowns. With the exception of the canine, an abutment tooth for a partial denture should have two roots and this can be achieved by two premolars joined together. If occlusal adjustment is advised in order to correct a potentially harmful intercuspal position of the mandible, a retruded arc mounting of casts on a semi-adjustable articulator will be necessary.

Procedures

Before the final impressions are made, the jaw relations registered, and the teeth set (the last two of which are the subject of this text), the following procedures are carried out if required by the treament plan: extractions, root canal and periodontal therapy, preparation of the abutment teeth including crowns splinted to adjacent teeth (as for lower premolars) and occlusal adjustment if required (see Chapter 10).

IP jaw registration

The IP having been determined by the existing teeth, it is recommended that the registration be made with the existing teeth lightly touching in this position. A facebow transfer of the upper cast to a semi-adjustable articulator is followed by a choice of five methods for mounting the lower to the upper cast.

1. *Hand placement* of the lower cast against the upper provided that there is a triangle of contact between teeth of opposing arches. The requirement is that the angles inside the triangular tripod be as close as possible to 60°. This will provide a stable equilateral triangle of contacts with little chance of the casts tipping. Opposing molar–central–molar would be stable while canine–canine–premolar would not. All plaster bubbles must be removed and a reminder about the problems arising from the two phases of contact (p. 177) is given.
2. *Trial bases.* Fast-cure acrylic bases (joined preferably by a lingual bar connector) with compound occlusal rims are advised especially where there are free-ending saddles. The rim is reduced by 3–4 mm from contact in IP and the registration made using the material best suited to the dentist, while the existing opposing natural teeth maintain light contact. The material should have the properties, previously mentioned, of minimal viscosity, rapid set and minimal dimensional change after setting. The bases must not move during the registration and must fit the mouth as accurately as the cast. The use of the casting seated on the teeth for this registration is not advised since the casting is seldom fully seated at this stage nor is it comfortable (exception: see (5)).

    In making the registration, care should be taken to ensure that the lightest contact is made between the registration material and the opposing natural teeth and simultaneously with the natural tooth contact (Figure 12.10b). If this contact is made before that of the opposing natural teeth, especially if softened wax is being used, setting of the wax may take place before the teeth meet. This will result in the mounted casts being further apart on the articulator than the opposing arches are in the mouth. An increased OVR ('high bite') will be the result. Alternatively, and if wax is used, the force of closure may induce strains in the wax which will cause it to expand on removal from the mouth with the

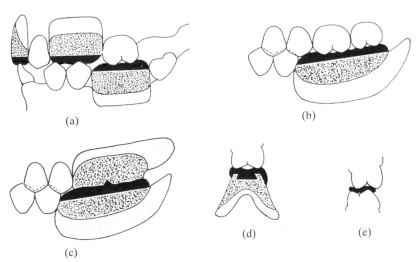

(a)

(b)

(c)

(d)

(e)

Figure 12.10 Jaw registration for partial dentures. (a) No opposing teeth. Pre-register position on anterior stop if possible. (b) Natural teeth opposing base. (c) Two free-end saddles. (d) Undercut occlusal rim to carry plaster. (e) Warning: if register pre-contact use facebow transfer

same result. It may not be enough for the technician to ensure that the plaster teeth engage the wax at the same time as the opposing plaster teeth as the base will not move on the plaster residual ridge as it does in the mouth. It is a complex problem. The use of plaster or zinc-oxide–eugenol paste will help to solve this aspect of the problem but both these materials take time to set when movements of the jaw or base can take place and inaccuracy on the articulator result. Bite registration paste (Kerr) has a fixed setting time and can be seated in the mouth just prior to set.

The converse of this problem is the registration made with the material barely in contact or where the base has been raised from the residual ridge, either by the dentist's fingers or the patient's tongue. The effect of this error on the mounted casts will be to bring them closer together than in the mouth. The completed denture teeth will then be *short of occlusion* in the mouth. Neither of these inaccuracies can be seen on the finished denture even if mounted on the articulator and the technicians should not be blamed.

3. *The wax wafer.* This established method of registering a precontact mandibular position has two sources of error: the release of strains from the wax following registration can cause deformity, and the tendency to penetration of the wax during registration resulting in tooth or mandibular displacement. The following procedure should prove helpful.

(a) Two sheets of hard wax are softened in a water bath and laid against the maxillary master cast. The wax is cut to the outline of the buccal surfaces of the teeth with minimal overlap.

(b) The wax is resoftened and pressed gently against the maxillary teeth, holding it there with the left forefinger and thumb.

(c) The mandible is coaxed into closure on a rehearsed retruded path and made to tap lightly on to the wax, making sure that the teeth do not penetrate the wax. The nurse chills the wax with cold water while teeth remain in contact with the wax.

(d) The record is transferred to the maxillary cast and the mandibular cast is placed gently into the tooth marks.

(e) If there is any doubt about the instantaneous contact of the teeth into the wax, the tooth marks (maxillary and mandibular) should be filled with a zinc-oxide–eugenol paste (Temp-Bond) and the desired position re-registered.

As has been said, this method has its limitations and should be confined to situations where there are opposing teeth. The wax sheet can be strengthened by a metal plate (Figure 9.7b). A facebow is essential in order that the closure be completed on the retruded axis.

4. Another situation which can cause inaccuracy in registration is that of *opposing free-end saddles* (Figure 12.10c). The chief difficulty is that of ensuring contact between the trial bases and the residual ridges while the registration is being made. A fixative is advised and careful holding of opposing bases, as illustrated for complete dentures (see Figure 9.5), is advised. These problems are made more difficult where there are only natural teeth opposing artificial teeth in dentures being made for both arches (Figure 12.10a, c). Jaw registrations have then to be made as for complete dentures, with the added difficulty of natural teeth dislodging the occlusal rims. Several attempts should be made to ensure even contact between the teeth and opposing compound rims at the correct OVR. The rims are reduced in height to allow for the registration material but

keeping one tooth in contact with the rim on each buccal segment to act as a stop. After registration, the contact areas should be inspected to ensure even penetration and contact by the 'stop' teeth.

5. *Casting and base only*. An alternative method where a casting is being used is for the patient to wear the casting with the final processed base added (but not the posterior teeth) for a few days. This will premit the casting fully to seat itself on the teeth, after which the registration can be made as in the previous section but using the casting and processed base. Alternatively, immediate fast-cure plastic has been successfully used for securing teeth to the base in the mouth while the patient maintains light contact in IP.

Protrusive registration

The registration of protrusive and lateral positions now follows if an articulation scheme is planned. This will be determined by the incisal guidance and articulation scheme of the existing natural incisor and canine teeth. If these teeth are being replaced, articulator adjustment to the positional records is made as for complete dentures.

Setting the teeth

The factors involved are tooth positions, the number of teeth to be used, the shape and material of the occlusal surfaces, the development of the occlusion and articulation, and the return to the articulator after processing in order to assess and correct any previous errors.

1. *Tooth positions* will usually be determined by adjacent and opposing teeth but it may be helpful, in case of doubt, to place soft, easily displaced, wax on the base at the try-in stage. A few swallows will displace the wax until the position determined by equal and opposite muscle force is achieved.
2. The *number of teeth* should be minimal compatible with adequate function and the prevention of any drift of opposing teeth. The patient may complain at this thrift but he or she can be assured of additional teeth if necessary and if requested.
3. *Plastic will wear more quickly than porcelain* but a decision on this choice can be reversed if one type proves unsatisfactory. If there is a difficult occlusal relation to resolve, the waxing and casting of a thin gold occlusal surface can be made and processed to the denture. The principle of tripod contact between well-shaped supporting cusps with adequate overlap by the guiding cusps applies. The *articulation* of the teeth will be determined by the requirements of the existing natural teeth.
4. *Processing errors*. The return of the processed denture to the master casts mounted on the articulator is always advisable. Processing errors in occlusion can be seen and adjusted and the dentist cannot blame the technician for 'high' or 'low' bite. It should be possible to estimate the cause of occlusal errors more easily when processing errors can be excluded.

Stress breakers

The use of these applicances is arguable since the displacement of the saddle on closure is determined by a hinge which does not necessarily conform to the direction of force caused by the opposing teeth. Nevertheless, they may provide a useful method of distributing the forces of occlusion between the base and the connector or framework, depending on the design used. Tooth positions on the affected base may have to be altered from time to time as the base moves or the supporting residual ridge resorbs.

Rebase or new teeth

If the teeth on a saddle are seen to be separating from their opponents on closure and the patient complains of a 'lack of support' the decision to increase either the height of the teeth or the thickness of the base has to be made. If resorption of the ridge has obviously taken place, the indication is for rebase but this should be accompanied by remounting the denture and readjusting the occlusion. If wear of the teeth is the cause, remounting is recommended and new teeth added. A change of teeth will make adjustments easier and will be more acceptable to the patient than a new base.

The inexpensive partial denture

As with complete dentures, not every patient can afford these time-consuming procedures and castings, and many dentures without retainers have proved comfortable and functional. Many partial dentures succeed by restoring appearance or by providing a space filler and support for the tongue, but good occlusal relations and tooth positions will help to maintain the low budget denture.

An extension of this theme is the question of the need for a partial denture in the first place. In view of the number of dentures which are worn in the top drawer, this is a question which should receive an answer. The replacement of maxillary molar teeth when only the mandibular first molars are present is one of many such debatable questons. Lack of suport by posterior teeth and the possible effects on the muscles and joints will indicate the need for replacements. On the other hand, many dentitions provide adequate function without this support. The variable factors that may help this decision are the presence of free-end saddles and the admission of parafunctional habits, both of which will prejudice the success of partial dentures. Front teeth must be replaced and certain functionless teeth restored to function sooner rather than later (Figure 12.11).

Treated mouth. The casts illustrated in Figure 12.11 were shown, before treatment, in the first edition of this book. Brian Parkins joined the author in the treatment procedures and these are illustrated in Figure 12.12a–g. There had not been any joint dysfunction or pain.

A temporary partial maxillary denture was made with an acrylic resin plane behind the incisor teeth. This allowed the OVR to be adjusted, by addition or reduction, until acceptable to the patient, after which a mandibular permanent denture was made, supported by a gold crown on 46. The mandibular incisors were then crowned to occlude with the bite plane. In the maxillary arch, 16,15 and 27,26 were crowned and each pair was soldered together. Dalbo attachments to support the maxillary denture were soldered to the mesial aspects of 15 and 16 and the denture was made at the OVR determined by the mandibular incisors and maxillary bite plane. The maxillary incisors (11 and 21) were extracted prior to immediate insertion.

This case illustrates the method of gradual build-up to complete reconstruction

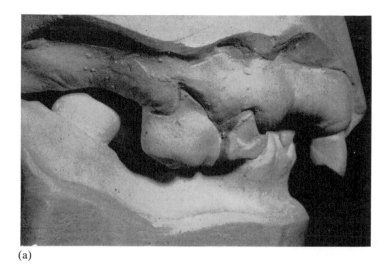

(a)

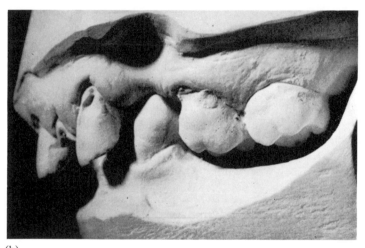

(b)

Figure 12.11 Overclosure overlooked. Treatment necessary. (a) Right side. (b) Left side

and of using a trial denture to establish the OVR. This was also used for registering the jaw relation. The work has been in function for fifteen years, with routine visits for hygiene and occasional repairs to the Dalbo attachments on the acrylic maxillary denture.

If existing isolated teeth are stable and functional, if potential abutment teeth are unstable, and if the patient has neither functional nor appearance complaints, then Punch's celebrated advice to those contemplating marriage may not be out of place: 'If in doubt, don't' (Figure 12.13). The genuine need of the patient remains the justification.

Empirical occlusal adjustment

Many, if not most, postinsertion occlusal adjustments for both partial and complete dentures are performed on a trial and error basis in the mouth. This can prove

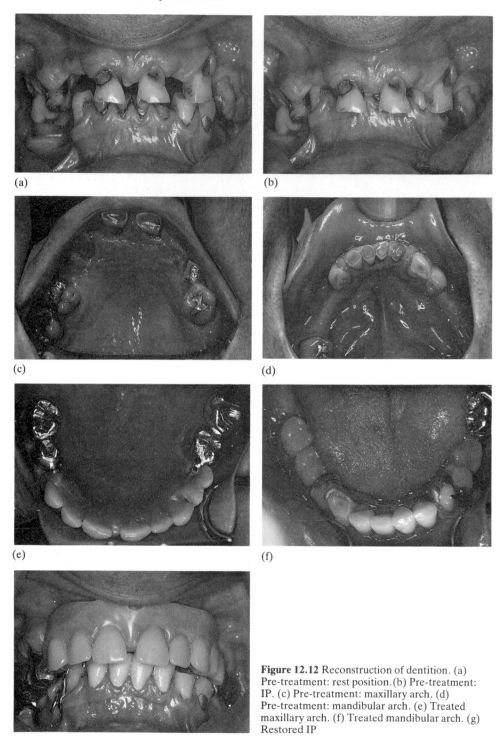

(a)

(b)

(c)

(d)

(e)

(f)

Figure 12.12 Reconstruction of dentition. (a) Pre-treatment: rest position.(b) Pre-treatment: IP. (c) Pre-treatment: maxillary arch. (d) Pre-treatment: mandibular arch. (e) Treated maxillary arch. (f) Treated mandibular arch. (g) Restored IP

(g)

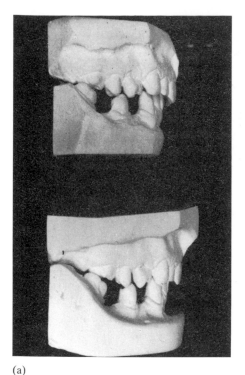
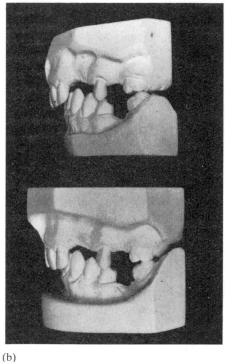

(a)   (b)

Figure 12.13 Missing teeth not missed. Study casts of mouth made at an interval of 11 years. (a) Right side. Above, 1962; below, 1973. (b) Left side. Above, 1962; below 1973. 1989: no change; patient male, now aged 80

successful if done with the objective of maintaining cusp–fossa contact at IP. The flattening of cusps and fossae leads to loss of certainty in finding a comfortable occlusion and to adverse forces being directed on the residual ridges and abutment teeth. These forces cause bruising of the mucosa, which is often wrongly diagnosed as being caused by overextension of the denture base or by processing errors in the denture bases. The chief difficulty in making occlusal adjustments in the mouth is that of being able to hold the dentures in position while placing the articulating paper between the teeth. The method recommended is to hold both upper and lower dentures with the left forefinger and thumb between the posterior segments and so allow the right hand to place the articulating paper. However, this does not leave a hand free to guide the patient on the required arc of closure. If this is necessary, either the assistant can be trained to place the articulating paper or remounting is advised. Disclosing paste may reveal an area of heavy contact on the supporting surface which is confirmed by a bruise on the mucosa and a premature contact on the denture (Figure 12.14).

Occlusal adjustments in the mouth require the certainty of stable bases and the assurance that the correct jaw closure is being used. Articulating paper should be thin and cut into strips the length and breadth of the posterior segment being tested. Spring-loaded forceps for holding the paper are advised. Three colours are advised: one for IP, one for working side contacts, and the third for balancing contacts. Premature contacts in IP will penetrate the paper and leave a clear

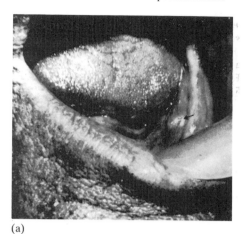

(a)

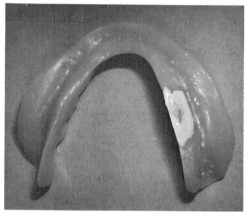

(b)

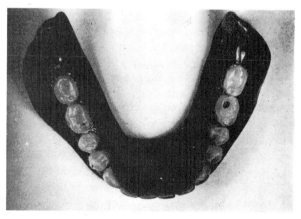

(c)

Figure 12.14 (a) Bruise on mucosa as result of premature contact. (b) Confirmed by displacement of disclosing paste. (c) Associated penetrating contact of articulating paper

punched-out mark on the teeth. Sliding contacts leave a blurred mark. The fossa mark should be removed, leaving the supporting cusp untouched. The triangular ridge in the fossa should retain its ridged surface if possible and tripod contact is thus maintained. Lateral and protrusive articular movements may then be adjusted using the incoming movements, if possible, since these correspond more closely to the functional pathways used. These will be blurred marks.

Comment

Good occlusal function in partial and complete dentures is a service that will cure many complaints. It will reduce to a minimum the persistent nibbling activities which are often caused by cusp interferences and which, in turn, cause pain and loss of stability. It will reduce parafunction and allow occlusion to be minimal and therefore optimal.

References

Attwood, D. A. (1956) Cephalometric study of the clinical rest position of the mandible. Part 1. Variability following removal of occlusal contacts. *Journal of Prosthetic Dentistry*, **6**, 504

Battistuzzi, P., Käyser, A. and Kanters, N. (1987) Partial edentulism: prosthetic treatment and oral function in a Dutch population. *Journal of Oral Rehabilitation*, **14**, 549

Battistuzzi, P., Käyser, A. and Peer P. (1987) Tooth loss and remaining occlusion in a Dutch population. *Journal of Oral Rehabilitation*, **14**, 541

Berry D. C. and Mahood, M. (1966) Oral stereognosis and oral ability in relation to prosthetic treatment. *British Dental Journal*, **120**, 179

Bjorn, A. L. and Owall, B. (1979) Partial edentulism and its prosthetic treatment. A frequency study within a Swedish population. *Swedish Dental Journal*, **3**, 15

Fujii, H., Stoltz, K., Tryde, G. *et al.* (1977) Short term changes in the perception of comfortable mandibular occlusal positions. *Journal of Oral Rehabilitation*, **4**, 17

Lawson, A. W. (1959) Analysis of the commonest causes of full denture failure. *Dental Practitioner and Dental Record*, **10**, 61

Lee, J. H. (1962) *Dental Aesthetics*, Wright, Bristol

Lytle, B. B. (1964) Vertical relation of occlusion by patients' neuromuscular perception. *Journal of Prosthetic Dentistry*, **14**, 12

McMillan, D. R., Christenson, J. and Tryde, G. (1977) The fallacy of facial measurements of occlusal height in edentulous subjects. *Journal of Oral Rehabilitation*, **3**, 353

Mohlin, B., Ingerval, B., Hedegard, B. *et al.* (1979) Tooth loss and dental treatment habits in a group of Swedish men. *Community Dentistry and Oral Epidemiology*, **7**, 101

Nairn, R. I. (1973) Lateral and protrusive occlusions. *Journal of Dentistry*, **1**, 4

Nairn R. I. and Brunello D. L. (1971) The relationship of denture complaints and level of neuroticism. *Dental Practitioner and Dental Record*, **21**, 156

Newton, A. V. (1984) The psychosomatic component in prosthodontics. *Journal of Prosthetic Dentistry*, **52**, 871

Smith, J. M. and Sheiham, A. (1980) How dental conditions handicap the elderly. *Community Dentistry and Oral Epidemiology*, **7**, 305

Thomson, H. (1961) A method of checking jaw relationships in full dentures. *Dental Practitioner and Dental Record*, **11**, 196

Thomson, H. (1967) Duplication of complete dentures. *Dental Practitioner and Dental Record*, **17**, 173

Timmer, L. H. (1964) De dynamische beetbepaling. *Nederlands Tandheelk*, **71**, 174

Timmer, L. H. (1968) A reproducible method for the determination of the vertical dimension of occlusion. *Journal of Prosthetic Dentistry*, **22**, 621

Tryde, G., McMillan, D. R., Stoltze, K., Morimoto, T., Spanner, O. and Brill, N. (1974) Factors influencing the determination of the occlusal vertical dimension by means of a screw jack. *Journal of Oral Rehabilitation,* **1**, 233

Whitehead, W. E., Fedoravicus, A. S., Blackwell, B. and Wooley, S. (1979) A behavioural conceptualisation of psychomatic illness. Psychosomatic symptoms as learned responses. In *Behavioural Approaches in Medicine* (ed. J. R. McNamara), Plenum Press, New York

Chapter 13

The mandibular dysfunction syndrome

In Chapter 7, disturbances and disorders of mandibular function were separated according to pathological response. In this chapter the dysfunction syndrome will be described as a disorder, followed by an outline of the literature. This will be an attempt to trace the history of this still unresolved pathological problem. Clinical features will be discussed and current treatment measures described. The title of 'mandibular dysfunction syndrome' (MDS) was chosen in 1971 to conform with Scandinavian and many American investigators. Since then many other titles have been suggested, most of them presuming a diagnosis or tissues involved. As the pathology and cause of the condition is not yet clear, the less suggestive the title the easier it may become to understand it.

The syndrome

Patients complain of one or more of the following symptoms: limitation of jaw movement. impaired joint function (click, crepitus, deviation on opening), pain in the muscles, pain in the joint and side of the face, pain on movement of the mandible. This list follows Helkimo's (1974a) index of mandibular dysfunction, albeit criticized for providing insufficient evidence (by van der Weele and Dibbets, 1987), with which to establish a syndrome. However, these are the symptoms which appear on most investigators' questionnaires. The pain and tenderness are usually unilateral but can change from one side to another. Patients may complain of difficulty in opening the mouth or in eating and this may result in 'locking' of the mandibular joint. More generalized headaches and pains in the neck and shoulders may be mentioned. The patient can usually point to painful areas on the face and neck and on the condyle itself. The symptoms are usually intermittent and often subside, for example, during holiday periods. Thus, a psychological factor is introduced and this will be developed in the review of literature which follows.

Review of literature: 1835 to date

Historically, Hunter (1835) referred to 'nervous pains in the jaws sometimes brought on by affections of the mind'. This aspect of the disorder attracts support today, as has been mentioned. However, it was Costen (1935) who brought the condition to the dentist by noting that ear and sinus symptoms (as facial pain) were often dependent on 'disturbed function of the mandibular joints'. He claimed that they were 'frequently observed in patients with edentulous mouths and marked overbite'. This led to alterations of occlusal levels by dentists but not always with benefit to the patient. Nevertheless, Costen's syndrome held its appeal for dentists who believed that pressure by the condyles on the nerves and vessels within and behind the joint capsule was the cause of this puzzling pain. Eventually, Sicher (1948) protested that there was no anatomical support for this reasoning and suggested that a more likely cause of the pain was a disturbed interaction of muscles around the joints. This pain in the muscles was then thought to be caused by cusp interferences which resulted in altered jaw positions and movements during function. Thompson (1954) referred to premature and initial contacts in mouths where excessive attrition patterns had resulted from malocclusion. Premature contacts occurred within the interocclusal space and with some force. Initial contacts took place at the normal level of occlusion, following which the mandible was directed to an abnormal path and intercuspal position with consequent disturbed interaction of the muscles. Ballard and Grewcock (1956) explained the condition as a 'reflex disturbance of endogenous patterns of muscle behaviour' such as could be caused by a displaced occlusion of the teeth, with a sudden trauma acting as the precipitating factor. Thus the need for occlusal adjustment arose; the principles and practice of these procedures were described in Chapter 10.

Schwartz (1959) reported on 20 patients treated for painful jaw movements by the application of an ethyl chloride spray over the area of the masseter muscle, in the belief that the pain was due to spasm of this muscle. He based his reasoning on the work of Travell (1960), who described the condition of myalgia and associated it with 'trigger areas in skeletal muscle' that provided small hypersensitive regions from which impulses were sent to the central nervous system, causing pain. Svein (1954) also discussed myalgia and mentioned psychic contributory factors. Anxiety and nervous tension were emphasized by Vaughan (1954) and Campbell (1957) as causative factors. In the following year Campbell (1958), in a study of 1109 patients, concluded that pain could be induced in muscles by vasoconstriction, cold, anoxia, acidosis or fatigue. Blood supply was therefore considered to be a factor and this could be disturbed by tension.

Psychological considerations

This suggests a tension component and it is now widely believed that a stress response produces the muscle tension that causes the pain. Newton (1984) says that the most common sites for tension syndromes are the posterior muscles of the neck and the occipital region, those of the lower back, and some of the shoulder muscles. He adds that the term 'temporomandibular joint syndrome' is inaccurate as the joint itself is seldom pathologically involved.

Moulton (1957), a psychiatrist, studied 35 patients with mandibular joint pain. 'At least half', she stated, 'were aware of long-standing bruxism and had reached a climax of some life dilemma.' The remainder of this group associated this pain with 'excessive trauma in the dental region'. Thus, anxiety and stress were being associated with the syndrome, and psychogenic pain with facial effects became a clinical entity. Appliance therapy was used to restore occlusal defects and to control parafunctional habits (bruxism). Thomson (1959) examined and treated 100 patients, many with appliances, and with 70% success. At the same time he examined 100 people with similar age distribution and found a similar incidence of occlusal dysfunction but without pain symptoms, except in 18 cases where pain in one or other joint had occurred but had subsided without treatment. This was repeated in 1971 with similar results, but adding an awareness of emotional stress in the histories, as given by the patients.

Rugh and Solberg (1976) discussed the psychological implications in mandibular joint disorders at length but could not relate them to any single 'frame of reference'. They could find little evidence to indicate that they were 'correlated with one specific personality trait', and that they had a 'multifactorial etiology acting on a target organ'.

Molin (1973a, b) made comprehensive studies on psychological and psychiatric aspects of the syndrome. Further, he estimated pain tolerance and measured the muscular forces used by electromyography. Pain and control groups were also examined. Molin found that higher scores were recorded in the pain group for 'anxiety-proneness' and 'muscular tension'. Related to this problem of how to relieve parafunctional jaw movements, the biofeedback system was introduced. This allowed patients to see (or hear) what was happening in their muscles and how the harmful movements could be controlled. When applied by Berry and Wilmot (1977), using the Myotron 220, 24 out of 35 patients were relieved in less than 2 months, 7 in 3–5 months, 2 relapsed after an initial good response (they were possible depressives) and 2 failed appointments. More recent success has been reported by Carlsson and Gale (1977), Stenn, Mothersill and Brooke (1979), Wepman (1980), and Hijzen, Slangen and van Houweligen (1986). A study of a combination of biofeedback and antidepressants by Gessel and Alderman (1975) also made a helpful contribution. Further proof of a pathological response in the facial muscles was provided by Berry and Yemm (1974) and by Yemm (1976) who reported that experiments to measure the temperature of the skin overlying the masseter muscle (by measuring infrared emission) showed that the skin overlying a tender region of muscle was hotter than the corresponding area on the opposite side. Yemm (1976), however, pointed out that whereas pain and discomfort of mandibular joint dysfunction could arise solely from jaw muscles, this does not exclude the possibility of joint damage, as by injury or disease.

Juniper (1987) contributes to this aspect of the discussion by quoting Yemm (1969a,b) and Rugh and Solberg (1976), who showed conclusively that patients who suffer the signs and symptoms of temporomandibular joint dysfunction react to stress by excessive contraction of the masseter muscles. He goes on to say that the medial pterygoids are also contracting and loading the menisci at their tendons of insertion. As hyperactivity continues, progressive damage occurs, often in episodes related to increased psychological stress. This is an article on the pathogenesis of temporomandibular joint dysfunction and repays further study.

Finally, Lundeen, Sturdevant and George (1987) indicate a link between muscle hyperactivity and muscle pain that has a significant correlation with depression and activity impairment. Examination of these patients should include assessment of stress, depression and activity levels.

Theoretical assumptions

Berry (1963) asserted that all treatment methods produced an alteration of masticatory movement and that any of them could be helpful. Franks (1965) described a compromise pattern of movements due to altered occlusion that would result in a change in the excitability thresholds of the neurones governing jaw movements. He suggested that this threshold could be changed by influences from the central nervous system (such as emotional stress) resulting in hypertonic activity. On the other hand, Yemm (1969a,b) suggested that premature contacts between opposing teeth may be secondary to muscle or joint disorders. Newton (1969) said that the reflex protective action of the masticatory muscles can be disturbed by stimuli from the higher centres acting through the reticular formation and initiating strong contractions in the elevator muscles. Berry (1969) suggested a possible connection between chronic minor illness and joint pain and that a common origin exists for these conditions, indicating a central perception of a state of stress mediated by hypothalamic function. Thus, pain occurs in some people from a joint or muscle disturbance but not in others.

Laskin (1969) suggested a psychophysiological cause comprising muscle fatigue produced by chronic oral habits, often involuntary and tension relieving. Because the initiating factors are usually emotional rather than physical, treatment should be directed towards this aspect of the condition. Correction of underlying conflicts causing the oral habits may be difficult, even with psychotherapy. A team approach to treatment is indicated.

Muscular fibrositis

A pathological reponse to overactivity was demonstrated by Christensen and Moesmann (1967) from human and animal experiments. They concluded that a condition of 'muscular fibrositis' could be caused by muscular hyperfunction producing a mechanical lesion of interfibrillar connective tissue and resulting in an aseptic serious inflammation. Thus, a pathological reaction in the muscles was demonstrated and has provided the only histopathological evidence to date.

Appliances, counselling and medication

It could be said that there are as many designs of appliance for controlling parafunctional habits as there are dentists designing them; and this author is no exception. There are those that cover all the maxillary or the mandibular teeth and those that cover certain teeth. There are those that are adjusted by removal or addition until even contact can be achieved and sustained and those that keep certain teeth apart. There are warnings against their use; there are controlled experiments to prove them successful and to prove them less than successful.

With the increasing awareness of psychological involvement in the aetiology, counselling has become a favoured approach to treatment. However, dentists are trained to cure by doing or making and are lacking in the skills of knowledge leading to enlightenment. But it can be said that they are learning. In cooperation with the prescription of antidepressant or muscle-relaxant drugs, counselling has proved a valuable aid to treatment and post-treatment care.

Feinmann and Harris (1984) made a study, with treatment, of 93 patients with 'psychogenic facial pain' and made the diagnosis of facial arthomyalgia or atypical facial pain. The treatment was based on a 9-week two-centre double-blind controlled clinical trial to test the efficacy of dothiepin (Prothiaden) against placebo and a soft bite guard. The results confirmed the superiority of dothiepin, although no examination for dysfunction was reported. Previously, Jagger (1974) had conducted similar double-blind cross-over trails using diazepam and a placebo on 61 patients. The results proved diazepam 'significantly better' than the placebo.

Kopp (1979) examined 30 patients with clinical and subjective dysfunction according to Helkimo's (1974b) five grade scale. At the first visit all patients received counselling. At the second they were divided into two groups, one receiving occlusal adjustment and the other receiving no treatment. Sixty per cent of the patients improved after counselling. No effect on the clinical dysfunction score was found. The score of clinical dysfunction was significantly reduced following occlusal adjustment and 67% of the patients improved.

Atypical facial pain and migraine

In terms of differential diagnosis these two conditions merit study and understanding by dentists concerned with joint and facial pain, if only to know when and where to refer the patients. Moore and Nally (1975) contributed an analysis of 100 patients with atypical facial pain and stated that in every case the pain was diffuse and not localized to a definite site. Most of the patients were 'poor historians' and frequently changed the descriptions of their symptoms and site of pain. Two patients developed paroxysmal trigeminal neuralgia with facial trigger zones, but only two. Hypnotics and analgesics did not provide relief but chlordiazepoxide and amitriptyline were 'highly effective in the majority of cases'.

A comprehensive study of classic and common migraine is presented by Ruff, Moss and Lombardo (1986) and describes the classic version as a true vascular headache and leaves unanswered the cause and pathological process in common migraine, except to suggest that 'oral behavioural patterns, facial pain and temporomandibular joint dysfunction relate to head pain'. The basic proposal is that common migraine might be better viewed as a muscular rather than a vascular disorder. The authors were able to eliminate migraine symptoms effectively in 28 patients by infiltrating tender areas with either a local anaesthetic or saline, thus suggesting a possible aetiological role of localized muscular tenderness in common migraine.

Failures

Ash (1986) examined a substantial number of patients at an orofacial pain clinic where treatment had failed. He described the failure of repositioning appliances, the high percentage of patients who should have had orthodontic therapy and/or restorative reconstruction, the need for surgery as a result of repositioning and the failure of mandibular joint surgery. Terminology, aetiology, diagnosis and treatment are illustrated and discussed. Confusion about the syndrome is related to lack of information about the natural history of the various categories of dysfunction, to the difficulty of making a precise diagnosis, to the complexity of the causes, and to the problem of rendering definitive treatment. A valuable list of references is appended.

Rheumatoid arthritis

Ettala-Ylitalo, Syrjänen and Halonen (1987) have tackled the question of whether the high frequency of temporomandibular joint disorders in patients suffering with rheumatoid arthritis is predisposed by malocclusion. A longitudinal study is under way but they are unable to answer the question of 'why some individuals with signs and symptoms of mandibular dysfunction become disabled while others do not'. Another long list of references is given.

One final reference is given here and this provides a return to psychological considerations. It concerns a report by Hughes *et al.* (1989) on 138 consecutive attenders at a psychiatric clinic in a dental hospital. The importance of using a standardized psychiatric interview was stressed and this took the form of a multiaxial classification known as DSM-111. This gives specific codes to certain pain syndromes and is designed to categorize the pain complaint as to site, nature, severity, system and presumptive aetiology. All patients were seen jointly by the psychiatrist and oral surgeon. The rate of psychiatric disorder in these patients was over 90%. This high rate of treatable psychiatric disorder indicates the need for close liaison between dentists in pain clinics and the psychiatric services.

It may be that this review is too long, yet many questions remain unanswered and investigations unquoted. Apologies to those authors may be more in order than regret at inordinate length. Too much may be made of this syndrome and this is indicated in a recent letter from California (Pogrol, 1987) entitled *The Wonders of the Temporomandibular Joint*. If nothing else, it is a chastening exposé; on the other hand, these patients must not be neglected.

Epidemiological surveys

Several surveys of dysfunction of the masticatory system have been made in Sweden. Helkimo (1976) refers to them and introduces a dysfunction index which classifies the symptoms numerically according to their severity. This survey has already been mentioned in the review of the literature and the criticism of it by van der Veele and colleagues. Different types of occlusal interferences did not differ significantly between different classes of dysfunction. The state of the dentitions examined, however, was poor and there were, on average, fewer residual teeth and a higher frequency of complete dentures among those with symptoms than in those without. There were no significant differences in degree of dysfunction between males and females or between age groups.

Symptoms

One or more of the following symptoms are diagnostic: a dull ache in the preauricular area; pain during mastication; pain on opening wide; tenderness over and in front of the condyle; limitation of opening; fixation of the mandible; stiffness of the mandible on waking; clicking of the joint on opening or closing; and crepitus or cracking in the joint cavity. To this list should be added the factors of emotional stress, mentioned in the Review, and fear of pain in the face, which adds greater concern. The acknowledgement of stress can often be elicited by discreet questions, such as: Do you feel tense when driving? When late? Does this make you clench your teeth? In addition, cold or damp weather may be associated with recurrences of the pain, as with other conditions involving muscles and joints.

Clinical signs

On examination of the patient, one or more of the following features may be observed by the dentist or acknowledged by the patient: displacement of the mandible from the rest position to habitual IP; lateral displacement of the mandible from retruded occlusion to habitual IP; the preference for one side in mastication; a clenching or grinding habit and associated ridging of the cheek mucosa; facets of wear on the teeth; lack of posterior tooth support; deviation of the mandible on opening wide to the affected side; and difficulty in placing the lips together at rest position.

These features can often be elicited from the dentitions of many people examined (Thomson, 1959, 1971) and cannot be considered causative. However, on correction of these features in affected patients the condition often subsides. This aspect will be discussed in the section on 'Explanations'.

Onset

This may be sudden or gradual. If sudden, there may be an association with a yawn or laugh, or with a visit to the dentist. If gradual, the association may be eating tough foods or posturing the mandible forwards in order to make a lip seal, as in, say, class II, division 2 jaw relations.

Age and sex

Many surveys of MDS reveal a predominance of young females. There are many exceptions to this incidence and Helkimo (1976) reports 'no great differences of frequency of dysfunction between men and women in the general population. Why women dominate in patient material has not been convincingly explained'.

Pathology

The assumption that the causes of MDS are to be found in the muscles has had scant support from pathological studies. Fatigue, spasm, intramuscular injury and disorders of muscles were discussed (Chapter 3) as possible causes of pain and dysfunction. Histopathological studies were carried out by Christensen and Moesmann (1967), already mentioned in the literature review, where a diagnosis of aseptic serous inflammation of the muscular connective tissues was made. This was given the more general title of 'muscular fibrositis' and was attributable to muscular hyperfunction. Osteoarthritis (Blackwood, 1963) was diagnosed from post-mortem studies on patients with joint symptoms but the age group was considerably older than usually found in the muscular dysfunction syndrome.

Alteration in the viscosity of the synovial fluid may represent a pathological response to a circulating toxin and provide a cause of crepitus. It is unlikely that this could be associated with mandibular dysfunction, although protrusive condylar movements may aggravate such a condition. On the other hand, effusion of tissue fluid into the joint space, causing swelling and tenderness, may represent a response to injury or to prolonged dysfunction. Occlusal relations may be temporarily altered and rest from occlusal function may be required to prevent deterioration.

Radiographic examination

Many radiographs of the temporomandibular joint have been taken for this syndrome, and considerable radiation absorbed, with little diagnostic evidence to show for them. This author is as guilty of sending patients for radiographs as any other clinician in this respect and consequently makes this reflection.

Most joints with infective or degenerative conditions and having likely radiographic signs have received diagnosis and treatment before reaching dental departments. Further, the only reliable radiographic projection for viewing the condyle is the tomograph as there is no space in the joint capsule to act as a comparison with the usual projections.

Differential diagnosis

As the condition is neither infective not degenerative, it is necessary to make a differential diagnosis from the following conditions: rheumatoid arthritis, oesteoarthritis, trigeminal neuralgia, specific infective arthritis, headache of systemic origin, sinus and ear infections, pain of dental origin, facial migrainous neuralgia, lesions in the central nervous system, and atypical facial pain. Migraine and atypical facial pain have been discussed in Review of the Literature and, whereas it has been suggested that common migraine should be viewed as a muscular rather than a vascular disorder, these two conditions should be assessed separately from the MDS.

Explanations

Some explanations of click, locking, pain and tenderness experienced in MDS will be offered, on the assumption that they are speculative.

Click and other mandibular joint sounds

This phenomenon can be described as an interference to the established translatory movements of the condyle and meniscus during the opening and closing movements of the mandible. The superior ridge on the condyle makes it possible for interferences to occur between condyle and meniscus as each moves. Normally the muscle activity is such that the flexible meniscus moves smoothly between condyle and eminence. If the starting position of the condyle is altered (as by altered intercuspal position) its path of movement can be altered and the thicker posterior zone becomes momentarily trapped between condyle and eminence. The neuromuscular response will usually provide the necessary adaptive movement to complete the opening. A deviation of the opening movement to avoid the click may follow and a further sequence of click and adaptive movement may be the result. Due to the absence of pain fibres in the meniscus, click is seldom painful, but if the resistance is increased (as by an increased viscosity of the synovial fluid) the movement required to continue the opening may result in torn muscle fibres (lateral pterygoid). A further adaptation follows with pain and stiffness as accompanying symptoms.

Click generally takes place during the opening movement but can occur just before closure as the meniscus moves backwards on an altered pathway.

The fact that click can be made to disappear by having the mandible open and close on its retruded axis or by placing a bite plane to engage the lower incisor teeth just before closure supports this explanation. Thus, an alteration of the intercuspal position is a possible cause of click. Other causes are an excessive and sudden opening of the mandible displacing the meniscus or prolonged clenching of the teeth with consequent altered opening by fatigued muscles.

Click may also occur intermittently in the adolescent due to adaptive movement while growth is taking place. But here, too, it can be avoided by retruded opening and closing.

Watt (1980) has made a study of 191 patients with mandibular joint dysfunction using synchronous records of joint and occlusal sounds from gnathosonic recordings. He points out that temporomandibular joint sounds vary between opening and closing cycles as well as between different visits of the patient. Joint sounds can be identified from occlusal sounds by their position on the occlusal record: sounds occurring 30 ms before the main occlusal sound can be interpreted as joint sounds. Watt classifies them into clicks and crepitus and both groups as soft or hard, depending on their quality. He further classifies them as 'near', 'middle' and 'wide' which indicate the jaw positions when the noises occur. He explains soft clicks as sudden movements of ligaments; *soft* crepitus (which comes and goes) as a surface effect and not necessarily associated with an anatomical feature; *hard* clicks may indicate a joint disorder and is often accompanied by hard crepitus suggesting specific defects on the joint surfaces; hard crepitus (likened to a footstep on gravel) is almost always diagnostic of arthritic changes.

Van Willigen (1979) made an analysis of sagittal condylar movements of the clicking mandibular joint using a pantograph attached to the maxillary and mandibular anterior teeth (labial surfaces) without disturbing the existing occlusion and lip closure. Both bows were provided with photoreceptors, with the mandibular bow being placed over the retruded axis point and the stationary maxillary bow providing the reference point. By means of movement scanners, the positions of the photoreceptors in the sagittal planes were determinable by optical electronics. Five dysfunction patients with clicking joints were compared with five subjects with symptom-free mandibular joints. The results indicated that in the 'clicking' group there were deviations from the patterns of movement seen in the healthy group. It was suggested that a dislocation of the disc might be the cause.

The fact that click seldom produces a pathological response, either in the joint tissues or the musculature, speaks well for the adaptability of these tissues. Thus, while click justifies its inclusion in the syndrome it may be wrong to label it a disorder.

Locking (or fixation of the mandible)

This disturbing symptom, which usually takes place at an open position, may be an extension of click. A muscle spasm following persistent click can fix the mandible at the position where the click usually takes place, and therefore can be associated with an altered intercuspal position. Two other causes of locking are, first, muscle spasm following injury to the mandible by either a blow or excessive stretch; and secondly, by spasm at a subluxated position associated with an articular eminence developmentally shaped to permit the condyles to slide forward in front of the eminence. Dislocation is an extension of this latter condition. An infective condition in the masticatory system may also produce spasm (trismus) which may seem to be protective, but this has been questioned. Alarm rather than pain is a feature of jaw fixation and reassurance as well as therapy to reduce the muscle spasm is required.

Pain

There are three factors which may be associated with pain in the MDS: cusp interference resulting in alterations in the established activity of the masticatory muscles, parafunctional activities and emotional disturbances. The last two are usually interrelated. A combination of all three may even provide the explanation.

Such alterations are more likely to cause pain in the mandibular muscles if there has been previous injury to them. Within the joints, pain fibres ramify with the blood vessels in the synovial membranes and adjacent periosteum, but the menisci are not supplied with pain fibres. Thus, only when the menisci are displaced against the joint membranes can they cause pain. Non-infective intracapsular joint pain is, therefore, the result of relatively violent injury, such as dislocation or distraction of the meniscus (by muscle spasm) against the joint membranes. It is likely that the less spectacular joint pain in this syndrome is the result of muscle injury followed by scar tissue which is subsequently stretched during jaw movements. The unilateral feature of this pain indicates that excessive chewing or parafunction on one side has caused the injury and that similar unilateral movements have sustained the injury.

The part played by *cusp interference* can vary between minor displacements during occlusal function and mandibular overclosure at intercuspal position. Cusp interference can be the result of parafunctional habits or of missing or incorrectly restored teeth, but *irrelevant muscle activity* would seem to be the exciting cause. The effect of altered muscle activity on the teeth is an upset of the proprioceptive stimuli to the reflex centres involved. This could result in either tolerated adaptive movements (as in a limp) or in incoordination and spasm (as in any painful or stiff joint). When a muscle lesion has been established, it constitutes a weakened region of activity to which impulses from the higher centres tend to be directed. The factor that determines a response of adaptation or incoordination may be the degree of activity in the limbic system. This group of structures in the brain provides intensity to stimuli from the cortex by emotions such as anger, fear, panic and aggression. Stimuli from the limbic system combine with those from the cortex and determine the direction and intensity of the action to be taken. The parts of the body affected by these stimuli must be prepared for the appropriate level of physical activity and this is the function of the hypothalamus. The tissues of the limbic system and the hypothalamus are thought to have connections in such activities as physical effort resulting from anxiety.

Thus *cusp interferences*, *parafunctional habits* and *emotional upsets* are interrelated in the pathological responses involving the muscles of the masticatory system. The part played by emotional disturbances was first emphasized in two original studies by Moulton (1955a, b) on the oral and dental manifestation of anxiety. Further studies by Molin (1973b) reported on two series of patients with the MDS and a control group who were investigated for personality traits and tolerance to experimentally-induced pain. He concluded that personality traits and emotional disturbance play an important part in the aetiology.

Orofacial pain as a manifestation of psychiatric disorders is reported by Harris and Davies (1980). They assert that 'it is a gross clinical error to assume that such pains are imaginary' and that in many cases they arise from biochemical disturbances in blood vessels, muscles and nerves, having no connection with irrelevant muscle activity. Equally, there are many people grinding their teeth who are neither victims of joint pain nor subject to psychiatric disorders. It remains for dentists to cooperate with psychiatrists in order to evolve methods for investigating this syndrome without necessarily referring the patients for psychiatric care.

In spite of these opposing views on the cause of facial pain there would seem to be a link between emotional stress and irrelevant muscle activity, with occlusal disturbances acting as a peripheral stimulus to initiate or perpetuate the syndrome.

Tenderness

Pain on palpation is most common over or in front of the condyle and this points to the insertions of the lateral pterygoid muscles or the masseters. The condyle itself may be tender, suggesting synovitis. Tenderness may also be felt inside the mouth, behind and lateral to the maxillary tuberosities where the lateral and medial pterygoid muscles have their origins.

Association with chronic minor illness

As already mentioned, Berry (1969) noted the existence of certain minor illnesses in 100 cases of mandibular dsyfunction pain. These included migraine, back, neck and shoulder pain, pruritic skin diseases, hay fever and asthma. Sixty-four percent of the samples had two or more of these diseases. Berry suggests that the common origin for these conditions may be a central perception of stress mediated by hypothalamic function.

Treatment

Treatment begins with the consultation and continues with the examination, occlusal analysis and preliminary counselling on the control of harmful jaw movements. Further treatment will depend on further needs, which may include appliances to control parafunction, replacement of missing teeth, occlusal and, at every visit, counselling on corrective movements and the prevention of harmful habits.

First visit

Consultation and examination

Carefully phrased questions will establish good rapport with the patient, who will then have the confidence not only to describe the condition accurately but also to feel that he or she is already being treated. The often quoted dictum of Sir William

Osler applies: 'Listen to the patient, he is giving you the diagnosis'. Questions should be open (What is wrong?) rather than closed (Does your joint hurt?). The description by the patient of what is wrong then gives the responsibility for treatment to the practitioner and this tends to remove the worry of it. Questions on site, time of occurrence and onset of pain, associated functions and any periods of remission should help to establish a preliminary diagnosis. The patient can then be reassured that the cause of pain (or click) is probably 'muscle strain' or 'muscle stiffness' or fatigue due to the way the jaw is being used. Thus the emotional content of the pain is removed and the examination can be carried out without apprehension.

Specific questions and examination should follow those outlined in the Appendix, from which it should be possible to make a diagnosis of one or more of the following.

1. Lip incompetence and uncertainty of rest position due to conflict between lip seal and tooth positions. Result: fatigue of muscles as they insert into joints.
2. Altered intercuspal position.
3. Recurrent parafunction.
4. Unilateral mastication.
5. Working and non-working cusp interferences during mastication and during parafunctional grinding.
6. Site of pain.

Reference is made to the eight questions and five features to be examined on pages 277 and 278.

Mounted study casts

Impressions of both arches are also made at the first visit, together with facebow transfer of the arbitrary condyle axis. An interocclusal precontact record should also be made if cusp interference is suspected, otherwise the lower can be placed against the upper cast for mounting. Thus, a preliminary inspection of the occlusal relations can now be made and a decision taken on whether to make a pantographic tracing of the mandibular border movements. This can be helpful in deciding the reproducibility of the movements by comparison with tracings made after treatment. Injured muscles will not provide reproducible or border tracings (see Figure 11.1). The mounted casts can also be used for making an overlay appliance.

Diagnosis and treatment plan

A diagnosis of MDS can be made on the basis of the symptoms described and of altered or excessive function. This can result in fatigue or low-grade injury. Tenderness over the condyle or ramus may indicate areas of spasm in the muscles. Infective and degenerative conditions are excluded by the differential diagnosis, with laboratory tests if necessary. In addition some form of emotional tension is usually present. Based on this diagnosis the treatment plan will consist of:

1. Explanation of the condition and reassurance to relieve anxiety.
2. Advice on rehabilitation to provide a physiotherapeutic basis for further treatment.
3. Appliances to prevent parafunctional habits.
4. Occlusal adjustment.
5. Appliances to restore teeth and/or lost OVR.

Treatment prescribed at first visit

Counselling

Explain to the patient that the pain, difficulty in eating and noises in the jaw are probably caused by an alteration in the established (usual) way of using the muscles. 'You have been chewing with a limp and the joint is suffering.' 'Small wonder that your muscles are hurting.' 'It is the same problem with a sprained ankle, a frozen shoulder or tennis elbow.' Explain that the cause was probably too wide a yawn, eating tough foods or prolonged opening of the mouth at the dentist, and that the muscles are 'torn' or 'tired'. Such explanations will reassure the patient, relieve anxiety and can be curative.

Question the patient discreetly about tense situations (being late, driving in traffic, frustration with work, studies or relationships) and explain that emotional conflicts and tensions can have outlets through hyperactivity of muscles. Pacing the floor is one example, fighting is another, but one of the most common is clenching and grinding the teeth. These impulses arise in the reticular system of the brain-stem and facilitate contraction of the masseters while inhibiting that of the digastrics (see also p. 42). The patient should be counselled on this aspect of everyday life, emphasizing self-help.

Advice on rehabilitation

Advise the following movements for rehabilitation of the muscles.

1. 'When eating chew with the chin back and on both sides at once.' This will restore bilateral function of the muscles, especially the lateral pterygoids which are seldom allowed the luxury of stretching. 'Try to avoid letting the teeth touch when shredding food and to close them only when swallowing.'
2. 'When not eating keep the teeth apart. In particular, avoid clenching and grinding movements which tire the muscles and wear the teeth.' The golden rule for all functional problems of the mandibular muscles is: 'Lips together teeth apart, never from this rule depart.' In other words, adopt the rest position at all times when not using jaw muscles for relevant activity. An aid to prevention of irrelevant muscle activity and tooth clenching is a small cotton pellet placed between the posterior teeth on one side and 'Don't flatten it.'
3. 'On waking and before eating, open and close with the chin back a few times so that your teeth touch behind their usual contact position.' A helpful suggestion for this movement is made by Juniper (1986) who advises sitting comfortably and with the tongue resting behind the incisor teeth. The tip of the tongue is then curled backwards while touching the hard palate. This is the retruded arc of opening and closing and prepares the muscles for bilateral back teeth mastication. In addition, it provides passive gentle stretching for the lateral pterygoid muscles. These can be called conditioning movements and can be likened to an athlete limbering up before a race. The suprahyoid muscles (behind the chin and under the tongue) should be felt to contract. Opening and closing on this arc will also arrest any click and will reassure the patient that this disturbing symptom can be cured.
4. For the incompetent lip seal, 'Relax the jaw and let the lips part.' In other words, adopt the true rest position and forget the lip seal. This will reduce the

fatigue and pain caused by persistent efforts to maintain a seal. To provide a lip seal orthodontics may be indicated and, failing that, instruction on maintaining a mouth seal between lower lip and tongue or upper teeth may prove an effective alternative.

The overlay appliance

A decision should be made at the first visit on the need for an appliance to control clenching of the teeth while asleep. This will be indicated by the patient's acknowledgement of waking with the jaw fixed or that the habit is uncontrollable by day. The appliance which has proved most effective (in the author's hands) is that which covers the maxillary incisors and canines and makes level contact on a flat polished plane with the mandibular incisors and canines (Figure 13.1). The posterior teeth are thus kept apart (discluded). The removal of all posterior tooth occlusion seems to be helpful in breaking the cycle of periodontal stimulus (feedback) and impulses which cause fatigue, injury or spasm in the mandibular muscles.

Complete coverage of either maxillary or mandibular arch by acrylic or other material has proved helpful in other hands, as has been suggested in the review of literature, and even a cover for the palate (with no overlay) has reduced symptoms. But the procedure recommended above has proved effective in the author's hands in forty years of clinical practice.

Treatment at the second visit

The response of the patient to the question 'How are you?' should be noted and should be seen by the patient to be noted. This adds importance to their reply and will encourage accuracy of statement. It is seldom that the symptoms will have completely subsided but an improvement is often acknowledged. Questions on clenching and grinding, the preference for one side in chewing and the awareness of tooth contact when eating will confirm the need (or otherwise) for use of the overlay, tooth replacement and occlusal adjustment respectively. Questions on emotional tension will often be acknowledged and further counselling may call for medication (see p. 250), preferably prescribed by the patient's doctor. The following treatment can then be carried out.

Fitting the overlay appliance (Figure 13.1)

This should ensure even contact by the mandibular incisors on the overlay and should disclude the posterior teeth while making sure that the retention cribs are not in contact. The patient should be made to place and remove the appliance and be advised on hygiene and storage (in water) in a covered container through the day. Care should be taken to prevent too much coverage of the incisor teeth which might cause damage to restorations, or to thin enamel margins and crowns. Advice should be given to wear the appliance on going to bed and through the day at such times as driving, when alone, and in anticipated tense situations where it can be worn without embarrassment.

As the intention with this appliance is to disclude all teeth, including the incisors, there is little chance of depressing the lower incisors.

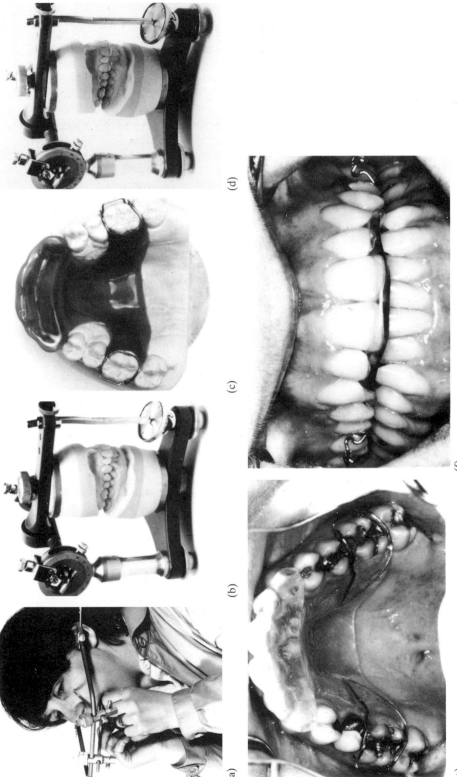

Figure 13.1 Overlay appliance. (a) Facebow record. (b) Casts mounted and maxillary arm raised 2 mm. (c) Overlay waxed. (d) Overlay returned to articulator. (e) In mouth. (f) Overlay permitting free movement with disclusion of posterior teeth

Encourage physiotherapy

No further treatment measures, save physiotherapy, should be prescribed until the effects of the overlay appliance are known. This should be a period of one month after fitting. During this time the patient should be advised to chew on both sides with the chin back and without the teeth touching, to maintain the 'lips together, teeth apart' posture when the mandible is not in function and to perform the retruded opening and closing movements on waking and before meals.

Treatment at the third visit

If the overlay treatment has proved successful in reducing the symptoms and dysfunction, a further analysis of occlusal function is necessary. The successful wearing of the appliance will have relieved the muscle fatigue and stiffness and will have allowed any injury in the muscles at least partially to heal. If cusp interference is still present, it is pointed out to the patient who is advised to assess any discomfort or annoyance it may cause. The patient is advised to remove the appliance for one night and report any recurrence of the symptoms. If none, continue for a second night without it, and so on. He is also advised to assess the need for more chewing surfaces with a view to replacing lost teeth or altered intercuspal positions. The following factors should now be considered.

1. The effect of missing teeth, which is often described by patients as 'a loss of support for my jaw'. Even the reduction of acrylic occlusal surfaces on the teeth of partial dentures can be described as a loss of teeth. Replacement should be considered.
2. An increase in the OVR should be viewed with critical concern. Where there has been an obvious loss of OVR, by loss of teeth with consequent repositioning of remaining teeth or by dentures made at overclosed vertical relation, this should be restored but the practice of empirical 'bite raising' is contraindicated. Three patients treated with appliances to restore lost OVR are described and illustrated in Chapter 14, p. 261.
3. The recognition of cusp interferences on the retruded arc of closure in a deviation to one side or the other should be corrected by occlusal adjustment (see Chapter 10).
4. A plan should be made to reduce any emotional tension which has seemed to be a cause of muscle hyperactivity. This may be provided by carefully selected medication or by referral to the patient's physician for further, and perhaps specialist, care.

Henceforth, treatment will depend on the decisions made from the foregoing factors and the symptomatic requirements of the patient.

Medication

With little or no experience in the prescription of drugs for the MDS, it would be unwise to write on the subject save to pass on the experience of others. Undoubtedly, drugs have proved helpful in pain alleviation and the relief of muscle spasm. In the use of analgesics and muscle relaxants, recurrence of the symtoms following the withdrawal of the drug has been reported in almost all cases treated.

On the other hand, some drugs have proved to be a useful adjunct to treatment. Of the analgesics, mefenamic acid (Ponstan) and pentazocine hydrochloride (Fortral) have been helpful. Muscle relaxants used have included mephenesin (Myanesin), orphenadrine citrate (Norflex), chlormezanone with paracetamol (Lobak), methocarbamol (Robaxin) and diazepam (Valium) with intermittent success. With the emphasis on emotional stress, tranquillizers and antidepressants would seem to be indicated. The use of fluphenazine hydrochloride and nortriptyline (as Motival) is providing encouragement (Harris and Davies, 1980) for facial arthromyalgia, to the exclusion of all other therapy. This drug elevates the mood and improves the vascular tone. Side-effects are minimal but do include an increased tendency to fall asleep which is not helpful for students, in whom the syndrome is common. More recently, Feinmann and Harris (1984) have shown that dothiepin (Prothiaden) is successful in reducing symptoms in a double-blind clinical trial against a placebo and a soft bite guard. The experienced practitioner, skilled in combining reassurance and muscle rehabilitation with minimal occlusal therapy, may yet be grateful for the use of these drugs and their improved successors. A review of dental sedation by Ryder and Wright (1988) might also prove helpful. Perhaps if these agents were referred to as medicines they would be viewed with less suspicion by both dentists and patients.

Surgery of the joint

Rowe (1972) has made a list of conditions which may require surgical intervention. In addition to the more severe pathological problems, such as ankylosis, intolerable arthritis and neoplasms, he includes arthrosis (intractable to conservative methods of treatment). He describes the bases for the majority of problems involving the mandibular joint dysfunction as 'a disturbance in the coordinated activity of the musculature, arising generally from malocclusion and often accentuated by psychological factors including neuromuscular tension'. The applied anatomy and operative techniques are precisely described. Surgical procedures on the joint may often be a last resort for patients with genuine despair because of a disordered joint but resort to them should not be made without dispassionate and careful consultations between dentist, surgeon and patient.

After care

After the establishment of good function by physiotherapy, occlusal adjustment or restorative dentistry and the elimination of signs and symptoms of dysfunction, the patient should be recalled within four months to ensure that the correct movements of the mandible are being maintained and that the teeth are parted when not in function. Avoidance of tooth contact during mastication is emphasized and the patient counselled on prevention by the use of conditioning movements for the mandible (passive gentle stretching) on waking and before eating. The best preventive therapy is to chew on both sides at once and with the chin back. Unilateral chewing tends to cause unexpected cusp contact on the non-working side and possible injury to the lateral ptyergoid muscle on that side. Finally, a positive attitude to good function is encouraged.

Comment

It has been acknowledged that the literature on the mandibular dysfunction syndrome is expanding, which means that the demand for treatment of it is increasing. Yet fifty years ago there was no such syndrome, at least for dentists to treat. Were all these cases treated with ear drops, aspirin or Sloan's Linament? There surely was as much occlusal dysfunction. As to emotional stress and parafunctional habits, there are few revealing records. So there would seem to be a case for counselling to establish and maintain bilateral back teeth function with the restorative dentistry necessary to make this possible, yet comfortable. Parafunctional clenching and grinding habits have to be controlled, if not abolished. As to psychogenic, atypical facial and migraine pains, dentists in practice have to learn to recognize these clinical conditions and to hope that there are clinics with enlightened consultants to whom the patients can be referred.

References

Ash, M. M. (1986) Current concepts in the aetiology, diagnosis and treatment of TMJ and muscle dysfunction. *Journal of Oral Rehabilitation* **13**, 1

Ballard, C. F. and Grewcock, R. J. G. (1956) Clinical aspects and physiological mechanism of abnormal paths of closure. *Dental Practitioner and Dental Record*, **6**, 259

Berry, D. C. (1963) Temporomandibular syndrome. *Journal of Prosthetic Dentistry*, **13**, 1122

Berry, D. C. (1969) Mandibular dysfunction pain and chronic minor illness. *British Dental Journal*, **127**, 170

Berry, D. C. and Wilmot, G. (1977) The use of a biofeedback technique in the treatment of mandibular dysfunction pain. A preliminary report on the Myotron 22. *Journal of Oral Rehabilitation*, **4**, 255

Berry, D. C. and Yemm, R. (1974) A further study of facial skin temperature in patients with mandibular dysfunction. *Journal of Oral Rehabilitation*, **1**, 255

Blackwood, H. J. J. (1963) Arthritis of the mandibular joint. *British Dental Journal*, **115**, 317

Campbell, J. (1957) Extension of the temporomandibular joint space by methods derived from general orthopedic procedures. *Journal of Prosthetic Dentistry*, **7**, 386

Campbell, J. (1958) Distribution and treatment of pain in temporomandibular joint arthroses. *British Dental Journal*, **105**, 393

Carlsson, S. G. and Gale, E. N. (1977) Biofeedback in the treatment of long-term temporomandibular joint pain. *Biofeedback and Self-regulation*, **2**, 161

Christensen, V. and Moesmann, G. (1967) On the aetiology, pathology, pathophysiology and physiology of muscular fibrositis due to hyperfunction. (In Danish with English summary.) *Tandlaegebladet*, **71**, 230

Costen, J. B. (1935) A syndrome of ear and sinus symptoms dependent upon disturbed function of the temporomandibular joint. *Aurology and Otology*, **43**, 1

Ettala-Ylitalo, U-M., Syrjänen, S. and Halonen, P. (1987) Functional disturbances of the masticatory system related to TMJ involvement by rheumatoid arthritis. *Journal of Oral Rehabilitation*, **14**, 415

Feinmann, C. and Harris, M. (1984) Psychogenic facial pain. *British Dental Journal*, **156**, 165, 205

Franks, A. S. T. (1965) Conservative treatment of temporomandibular joint dysfunction: a comparative study. *Dental Practitioner and Dental Record*, **15**, 205

Gessel, A. H. and Aldermann, M. M. (1975) Management of myofacial pain dysfunction syndrome of the TMJ by tension control training. *Psychosomatics*, **12**, S302

Harris, M. and Davies, G. (1980) Orofacial manifestations of psychiatric disorders. In *Oral Medicine* (eds D. C. Mason and H. Jones), Saunders, Eastbourne

Helkimo, M. (1974a) Studies on function and dysfunction of the masticatory system. *Svensk Tandlakare-Tidskrift*, **67**, 101

Helkimo, M. (1974b) Studies on function and dysfunction of the masticatory system. Analyses of anamnestic and clinical recordings of dysfunction with the aid of indices. *Svensk Tandlakare-Tidskrift*, **67**, 165

Helkimo, M. (1976) Epidemiological surveys of dysfunction of the masticatory system. *Oral Sciences Review*, **1**, 54

Hijzen, J. L., Slangen, J. L. and van Houweligen, H. C. (1986) Subjective, clinical and EMG effects of bio-feedback and splint treatment. *Journal of Oral Rehabilitation*, **13**, 529

Hughes, A. M., Hunter, S., Still, D. and Lamey, P-J. (1989) Psychiatric disorders in a dental clinic. *British Dental Journal*, **166**, 16

Hunter, J. (1835) *The Works of John Hunter*, Vol. II, Longman, Rees, Orme, Brown and Longman, London

Jagger. R. G. (1974) Diazepam in the treatment of temporomandibular joint dysfunction syndrome. A double blind study. *Journal of Dentistry*, **2**, 37

Juniper, R. P. (1986) Temporomandibular joint dysfunction: facts and fallacies. *Dental Update*, **Nov.-Dec.**, 479

Juniper, R. P. (1987) The pathogenesis and investigation of TMJ dysfunction. *British Journal of Oral and Maxillofacial Surgery*, **25**, 105

Kopp, S. (1979) Short term evaluation of counselling and occlusal adjustment in patients with mandibular dysfunction involving the TMJ. *Journal of Oral Rehabilitation*, **6**, 101

Laskin, D. M. (1969) Etiology of the pain-dysfunction sydrome. *Journal of the American Dental Association*, **79**, 147

Lundeen, T. F., Sturdevant, J. R. and George, J. M. (1987) Stress as a factor in muscle and temporomandibular joint pain. *Journal of Oral Rehabilitation*, **14**, 447

Molin, C. (1973a) Vertical isometric muscle forces of the mandible. A comparative study of subjects with and without mandibular pain dysfunction. *Acta Odontologica Scandinavica*, **30**, 485

Molin, C. (1973b) Psychological studies of patients with mandibular dysfunction syndrome. *Acta Odontologica Scandinavica*, **66**, 1

Moore, D. S. and Nally, F. F. (1975) Psychogenic, diagnostic and therapeutic aspects of temporomandibular joint pain. An analysis of 232 patients. *Journal of the Canadian Dental Association*, **41**, 402

Moulton, R. E. (1955a) Oral and dental manifestations of anxiety. *Psychiatry*, **18**, 26

Moulton, R. E. (1955b) Psychiatric considerations in maxillo-facial pain. *Journal of the American Dental Association Dental Cosmos*, **51**, 408

Moulton, R. (1957) Psychologic considerations in the treatment of occlusion. *Journal of Prosthetic Dentistry*, **7**, 148

Newton, A. V. (1969) Predisposing causes for temporomandibular joint dysfunction. *Journal of Prosthetic Dentistry*, **22**, 647

Newton, A. V. (1984) The psychosomatic component in prosthodontics. *Journal of Prosthetic Dentistry*, **52**, 871

Pogrol, M. A. (1987) Letter from California: the wonders of the temporomandibular joint. *British Dental Journal*, **163**, 207

Rowe, N. L. (1972) Surgery of the temporomandibular joint. *Proceedings of the Royal Society of Medicine*, **65**, 383

Ruff, G. A., Moss, R. A. and Lombardo, T. W. (1986) Common migraine: a review and proposal for a non-vascular etiology. *Journal of Oral Rehabilitation*, **13**, 499

Rugh, J. D. and Solberg, W. K. (1976) Psychological implications of temporomandibular pain and dysfunction. *Oral Sciences Review*, **7**, 3

Ryder, W. and Wright, P. A. (1988) Dental sedation. A review. *British Dental Journal*, **165**, 207

Schwartz, L. L. (1959) Management of disorders of the temporomandibular joint. *Journal of the Canadian Dental Association*, **20**, 219

Sicher, H. (1948) Temporomandibular articulation in mandibular overclosure. *Journal of the American Dental Association*, **36**, 131

Stenn, P. G., Mothersill, K. L. and Brooke, R. I. (1979) Biofeedback and cognitive behavioural approach to treatment of myofascial pain dysfunction syndrome. *Behavior Therapy*, **10**, 29

Svein, E. (1954) Temporomandibular joint disorders. *Dental Digest*, **60**, 361 (abstract)

Thompson, J. R. (1954) Concepts regarding function of the stomatognathic system. *Journal of the American Dental Association*, **48**, 626

Thomson, H. (1959) Mandibular joint pain. *British Dental Journal*, **107**, 243

Thomson, H. (1971) Mandibular dysfunction syndrome. *British Dental Journal*, **130**, 187

Travell, J. (1960) Temporomandibular joint pain referred from muscles of the head and neck. *Journal of Prosthetic Dentistry*, **10**, 745

van der Weele, L. Th. and Dibbets, J. M. H. (1987) Helkimo's index: a scale or just a set of symptoms? *Journal of Oral Rehabilitation*, **14**, 229

van Willigen, J. (1979) The sagittal condylar movements of the clicking temporomandibular joints. *Journal of Oral Rehabilitation*, **6**, 167

Vaughan, H. C. (1954) External pterygoid mechanism. *Journal of Prosthetic Dentistry*, **5**, 80

Watt, D. M. (1980) Temporomandibular joint sounds. *Journal of Dentistry*, **8**, 119

Wepman, B. J. (1980) Biofeedback in the treatment of chronic myofascial pain dysfunction. *Psychosomatics*, **21**, 157

Yemm, R. (1969a) Variations in the electrical activity of the human masseter muscle occurring in association with emotional stress. *Archives of Oral Biology*, **14**, 873

Yemm, R. (1969b) Temporomandibular dysfunction and masseter muscle response to experimental stress. *British Dental Journal*, **127**, 508

Yemm, R. (1976) Neurophysiological studies of temporomandibular joint dysfunction. *Oral Sciences Review*, **7**, 31

Chapter 14

The treatment of disturbances and disorders

The decision to treat disturbances before they become disorders is not an easy one to make. Many mouths, particularly in middle age, show signs of secondary malocclusion and the effects vary widely between healthy adaptation and breakdown of the dentition. Mobility and migration of the teeth are often arrested by stable repositioning. Parafunction and attrition of the occlusal surfaces can sometimes be controlled by stern warnings to, and cooperation by, the patient. Cusp interferences and displacing activities can result in adaptation by healthy muscles unaffected by parafunction. Mandibular overclosure is often normal in many class II patients, especially if there is no loss of teeth. Knowledge of the tissues and their behaviour, experience, and an awareness of the need for treatment may provide a better basis for treatment than ability, enthusiasm and optimism, to say nothing of the power of persuasion by patient or dentist. On the other hand, disorders represent a pathological response to disturbances and when the patient complains of pain in the teeth or face, when teeth are drifting and the periodontia is diseased, when gums are being ulcerated by opposing teeth or food stagnation, the time has come to treat.

Treatment for the following disorders will be discussed and described.

- Mandibular overclosure
- The mandibular dysfunction syndrome
- Progressive wear of the occlusal surfaces
- Mobility and migration
- Pulp necrosis
- Gingival ulceration from food stagnation
- Developmental anomalies

Mandibular overclosure

Treatment of mandibular overclosure has to be based on an accurate assessment of the occlusal vertical dimension in relation to rest position and the disorders which may be caused by it (p. 112). The cautionary conclusion made by Bergström (1950) to his study on the reproduction of the dental articulation is worth quoting: 'We do not know if and to what degree we can prevail upon joints and muscles to adapt themselves to new central positions, heights of bites and movements, but everyone probably agrees that our possibilities in this respect are very limited.' Nevertheless, there are occasions when it is necessary to restore rather than to raise, to correct rather than to open the occlusal vertical relation. Thus the terms 'raising the bite' and 'bite raising appliance' are discounted since they suggest an indiscriminate alteration rather then a planned restoration.

Plan

The plan will be based on an analysis and diagnosis of the signs, symptoms, rest position and interocclusal distance of the masticatory system. Preliminary treatment should include minimal removal of injurious incisor contacts on opposing mucosa, rehabilitation of painful muscles (see next section), the institution of good hygiene, and decisions to deal with problems of mobile teeth and altered occlusal curves. A decision will have to be made on the use of fixed restorations or removable appliances for the permanent restoration of the OVR. An overlay temporarily to restore the OVR is always recommended. The patient should be advised that the muscles will have to adapt to changes of chewing level and that this may not be easy. However, if the planned OVR is correct, the change will prove comfortable and more efficient, particularly if this involves pain in the mandibular joints. (see Figures 14.2–14.4).

Fixed restorations or removable appliances?

This decision is usually easy to make since the decision to restore lost OVR cannot be so assured as to risk the costly and irreversible crown and bridge work required. Even if the patient resists the idea of wearing a removable appliance, he or she should be prevailed upon to wear one as an interim measure in case the alteration is not, in the event, tolerated. A removable appliance for this purpose will cover the supporting cusps of the teeth and can be called an onlay denture; metal is preferred to acrylic resin. However, a temporary acrylic appliance is advised as a primary measure and this takes the form of an overlay. Fixed restorations can follow if the need and the demand are justified.

The overlay appliance or bite guard

Reference to this appliance and its illustration has been made (see p. 248). As a temporary measure, it serves four purposes: first, to test the tolerance to increase in OVR by the joint tissues and muscles; secondly, parafunctional jaw movements can be controlled often with relief of pain in the muscles and joint tissues; thirdly patients can be encouraged to find and use the retruded closure and position, thus providing some rehabilitation of the lateral pterygoid muscles which are seldom permitted the luxury of stretching; finally, it can be used as an anterior stop in making a jaw registration.

The level of closure can be adjusted by removal of the resin or addition to it until an acceptable position is determined but the plane should be kept flat and polished so that retrusion can be reached as a gliding movement. Requirements for making the appliance are impressions and a facebow record. After the maxillary cast has been secured to the upper arm of the articulator, using the facebow, the mandibular cast can be placed against the maxillary one at intercuspal occlusion and plastered to the lower arm. However, the facebow transfer is essential in order to keep the degree and direction of the opening on the retruded arc the same on the articulator as in the mouth. One also requires a careful and caring technician.

This appliance can provide a further service in the reduction of *clicking joint*. If the patient complaining of this disturbing symptom can be persuaded to pull the chin back at each opening and closing of the mandible, the click will almost always disappear. The overlay appliance will help to promote this movement.

Comments

It will be noted that the mounting of the lower cast was made at the existing IP and that no wax record was used, thus possibly transferring a displaced mandibular position. The flat bite plane, however, permits the mandible to adopt its own horizontal position. Encouragement should be given to 'pull the chin back' and so get the feel of the retruded position. This will also give the lateral pterygoid muscles the luxury of stretching.

The overlay will remove all occlusal stimuli which may have been causing displacing activities and any consequent hyperactivity of the muscles. It will therefore provide a cure for any muscle pain caused by this activity and confirm the diagnosis of the dysfunction syndrome. It can thus be called a *diagnostic appliance*.

The overlay will also provide an inhibition to any clenching or grinding habits, particularly during sleep. The symptom of jaw stiffness on waking usually subsides if the appliance is worn conscientiously while asleep.

The disclusion of the posterior teeth by the overlay, allowing the muscle force of mandibular closure to be directed on the lower incisors and canines, will tend to depress these teeth rather than cause the posteriors to erupt. This is difficult to measure or prove and the statement is made on a basis of experience and on the assumption that it is more likely for teeth to depress under force than to erupt through lack of it.

Why not a posterior overlay? Many acrylic resin overlays are made to cover the posterior teeth. Since the posterior teeth are going to be covered in the eventual treatment, why not use the principle as a temporary measure? The answer lies in the importance of allowing the mandible to find its correct horizontal relationship to the maxilla. This can be found more easily using the incisal overlay. It is used as a diagnostic appliance. Posterior overlays are clumsy and tend to fix the teeth in one occlusal position. Even if they have flat surfaces and permit lateral gliding the posterior teeth are not freed from contact and mandibular activity is often increased.

The permanent appliance (the onlay denture)

This should be delayed for more than a month for reasons made in the comment regarding depression or raising of the teeth. It now becomes necessary to cover one or other of the arches in order to restore intercuspal occlusion at a level determined by the overlay. Two principles of design are advised.

1. The coverage of the posterior teeth should be limited to the supporting cusps, thus reducing the possibilities for food stagnation and subsequent decalcification (Figure 14.1).
2. All teeth should be restored to function to prevent unequal depression and eruption between posterior and anterior teeth. Thus, if the mandibular arch is chosen, the incisiors and canines should either be covered or the appliance should have support arms (mesial and distal rests) on these teeth. An exception

to this principle is the assurance that the anterior teeth will make gliding contacts with each other or with the food bolus in function. Tongue posture may be helpful in this respect. Another exception is an edge-to-edge incisor occlusion with lack of development of the posterior dentoalveolar tissues. In such a patient there is usually a forwards and upwards displacing activity to IP (pseudo-class III) and the onlay denture serves to restore the posterior occlusion at the level determined by the anterior occlusion (Figure 14.2).

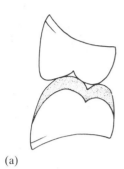 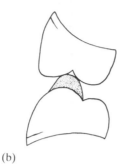

Figure 14.1 Onlay denture coverage. (a) Incorrect. (b) Correct

(a)   (b)

Choice of arch

This is usually determined by the site and number of missing teeth. Overclosure is usually associated with missing mandibular teeth and narrowing of the lower arch with consequent overclosure. In such a case the mandibular arch is chosen. Patients usually adapt more easily to lower onlay dentures and the factor may be gravity. However, the problem of the free standing mandibular anterior teeth mentioned above remains and has to be solved without disturbing the appearance of the mandibular teeth. If the maxillary arch is chosen, this problem is solved by incorporating a bite plane behind the incisor teeth (see p. 262). Two appliances should be avoided and individual circumstances will determine the choice.

Registration and transfer

Accurate casts of the arches should be available before these records are made so that they can be fitted on the casts and mounted at once. An arbitrary facebow transfer is made for mounting the upper cast. The actual retruded axis is not required since the vertical level of closure will be determined by the overlay, as will the horizontal position of the mandible. A semi-adjustable articulator is necessary, however, in order to introduce freedom from interference in protrusive and lateral movements. The interocclusal registration is made with the overlay in place and with the anterior mandibular teeth lightly in contact with the bite plane. The mandible should be withdrawn backwards as far as is comfortably possible. The registration material should have the requirements of low viscosity, rapid set and dimensional stability on removal. Quick setting plaster-stone is always the material of choice, especially if the precise setting time is known, when it can be placed on the teeth with a known time for working and correct closure. Kerr's bite registration paste serves well except that it is brittle when thin. Practice of the retruded closure should precede the registration and the nurse should be on hand to retract the cheeks for visibility, if necessary.

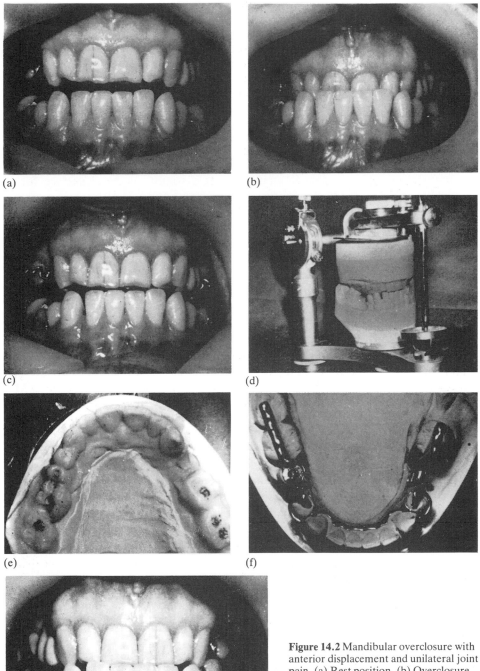

(a)

(b)

(c)

(d)

(e)

(f)

Figure 14.2 Mandibular overclosure with anterior displacement and unilateral joint pain. (a) Rest position. (b) Overclosure at IP. (c) Overlay. (d) Mounted casts (upper made in acrylic resin). (e) Marks for contact of opposing supporting cusps. (f) Metal onlay denture. (g) Denture in place at restored OVR

(g)

Waxing

This is directed at making contact between the supporting cusps of the segments being restored (buccal lower or lingual upper where normal vertical and horizontal overlaps exist) and the opposing central fossae. These areas on the opposing teeth should be marked by the dentist (Figure 14.2e) and the technician advised to build the wax up in cones to contact these areas with a tripod of contact on the triangular ridges forming the central fossae, if this is feasible. The practice of closing the opposing teeth on to a mound of soft wax and carving away the excess should be avoided. This procedure will make the supporting cusps of the onlay denture an exact fit of the opposing fossae or ridges. This fixes the intercuspal occlusion too rigidly and prevents free articular movements. The tripod contact with cusp tip free of contact provides a stable IP and presents a smooth occlusal surface for the avoidance of interfering articular movements (see Figure 14.1b).

Other requirements in the design of the onlay denture are emphasized:

1. Limitation of coverage to the supporting cusps already mentioned.
2. Adequate retention arms extending from the onlays.
3. A rigid connector bar to join the two onlay segments.
4. Coverage of mesiodistal rests on the anterior teeth.
5. Sandblasting of the onlay segments so that any premature contacts in function can be readily seen. This procedure will also reduce the shine of the appliance and make it less conspicuous.

Choice of metal

The gold and chrome–cobalt alloys are the current alternatives. The gold alloys have qualities which make them more suitable for onlay dentures. Their surface hardness is less than in chrome cobalt and less likely to cause wear on the opposing teeth, although the control of clenching and grinding will reduce this as a factor.

Why not plastics? Acrylic resin has provided many onlay dentures but, whereas they are easily made and adjusted, they wear and break and cannot be considered permanent. Also, for purposes of strength, they have to be made to cover the whole occlusal surface of each tooth. This not only promotes greater food stagnation but is more bulky than desirable. One use of plastics, however, is as a pattern prior to casting in metal. The onlay surfaces can be made in resin, according to the principles laid down for waxing, and joined temporarily by the connector eventually to be incorporated in the denture. The denture can then be worn in the mouth for a short period and the occlusal surfaces adjusted. The appliance is subsequently cast and soldered to the connector. Care should be taken to ensure that the resin used will not leave a residue when burnt out prior to casting.

Instructions to patients

There are three instructions which apply to all wearers of dental appliances.

1. Simultaneous bilateral mastication on the posterior quadrants. 'Chew with the chin back and on both sides at once.'

2. Avoidance of parafunctional contacts and movements. 'Keep the teeth parted except when eating. The teeth should touch only when swallowing.' 'Try not to fiddle with the appliance.'
3. Strict hygiene before and after meals. 'It is good prevention to eat with clean teeth.' Explain plaque. 'Clean the teeth and appliance after meals.' This may be too strict a discipline for many patients but the opportunities to encourage preventive hygiene should never be missed. Nowhere does it apply more stringently than when wearing removable onlay appliances.

Appliance therapy for the mandibular dysfunction syndrome

It is worth repeating that the decision to provide permanent fixed or removable appliances for the treatment of mandibular dysfunction and associated joint or facial pain should be made with caution and not until provisional overlays or replacements have proved such provision to be justified. The patient must be made aware that the appliances will have to be retained indefinitely and that routine inspections will be necessary. There will be no going back.

Reference has already been made in the previous section to one patient treated with a permanent mandibular overlay. The symptoms in and treatment for this patient and two others will now be described.

Patient 1 (Figure 14.2): a 38 year-old female physiotherapist. Her symptoms (in 1971) were unilateral pain associated with mastication and while treating patients. The symptoms subsided within the week after wearing the overlay. There was no waking jaw stiffness or joint noises. The permanent overlay appliance covering all mandibular posterior teeth (as illustrated) restored the overclosure to a freeway space of 4 mm and reduce the quasi class III malocclusion completely. After five years of symptom-free wear, the patient dropped the appliance and accidentally trod on it. It was unwearable and the pain returned in 48 hours. The appliance was remade and the pain subsided within a week and has not recurred to date. The patient exchanges the overlay denture for the acrylic maxillary overlay appliance for overnight wear.

Patient 2 (Figure 14.3): a 42-year-old male in the export business. He had unilateral pain (1979) following hard mastication which lasted 1–2 hours. He became afraid to eat any but soft foods and often awoke with jaw stiffness and pain. In addition, the overclosure caused bruising of labial mandibular mucosa. Pain on mastication subsided in three days after wearing a provisional bite plane to restore overclosure to 3 mm above rest position. A metal partial denture was made at this level to restore the missing maxillary teeth and to engage the mandibular posteriors. Also incorporated was a bite plane to occlude with the mandibular incisors (Figure 14.3d). The patient was checked six-monthly for five years without recurrence, after which he went abroad.

Patient 3 (Figure 14.4): a 44-year-old female teacher of physical education to teenage children. She had unilateral facial pain (1970) and acknowledged clenching and grinding her teeth and often found herself waking with the teeth clenched and having tension dreams. Responded to palatal appliance restoring lost OVR due to incisal wear. A mandibular overlay denture maintained freedom from pain but the patient missed the use of her incisor teeth. These were subsequently crowned. No recurrence in 15 years.

262

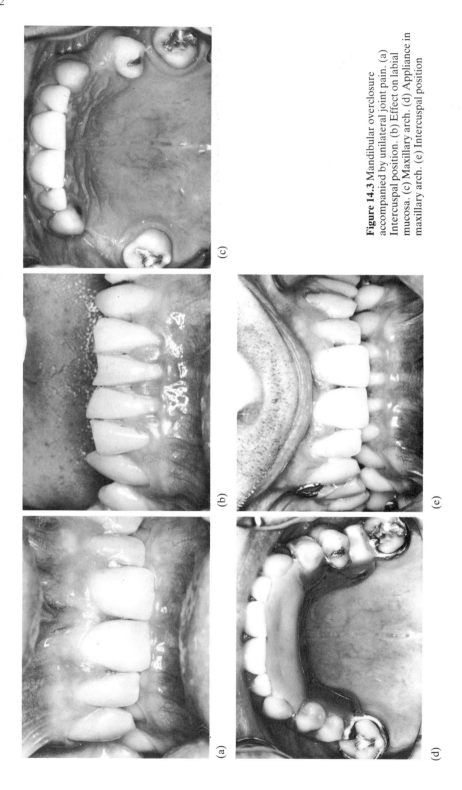

Figure 14.3 Mandibular overclosure accompanied by unilateral joint pain. (a) Intercuspal position. (b) Effect on labial mucosa. (c) Maxillary arch. (d) Appliance in maxillary arch. (e) Intercuspal position

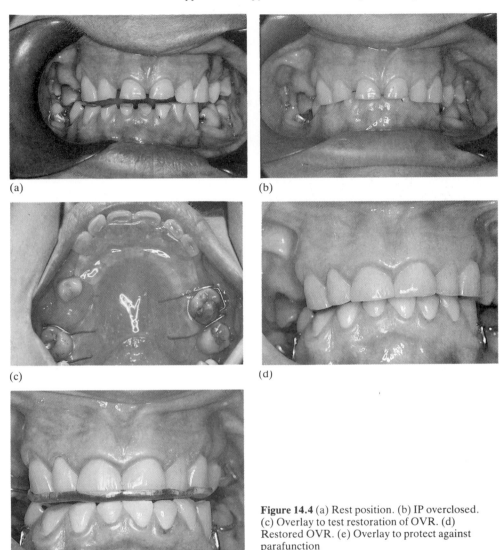

(a)

(b)

(c)

(d)

Figure 14.4 (a) Rest position. (b) IP overclosed. (c) Overlay to test restoration of OVR. (d) Restored OVR. (e) Overlay to protect against parafunction

(e)

Comment

These three patients represent success in treatment by restoring overclosure to an OVR 3–4 mm above rest position. However, not all patients demonstrating overclosure suffer the symptoms of these patients (Figure 14.5, and see also Figure 12.12). Conversely, many sufferers from this syndrome have complete or near complete dentitions (Figure 14.6). This patient was a restaurant owner and suffered severe facial pain while working. He acknowledged grinding his teeth but could not control it, and showed no improvement with overlays, muscle relaxants or tranquillizers.

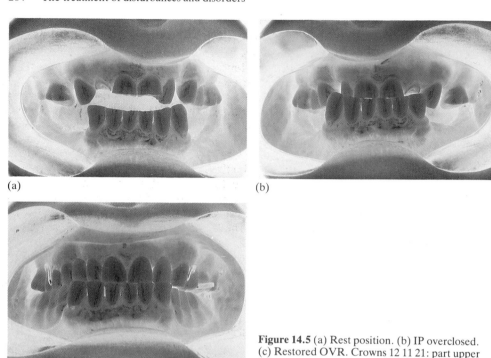

(a)

(b)

(c)

Figure 14.5 (a) Rest position. (b) IP overclosed. (c) Restored OVR. Crowns 12 11 21: part upper and lower dentures. No joint symptoms

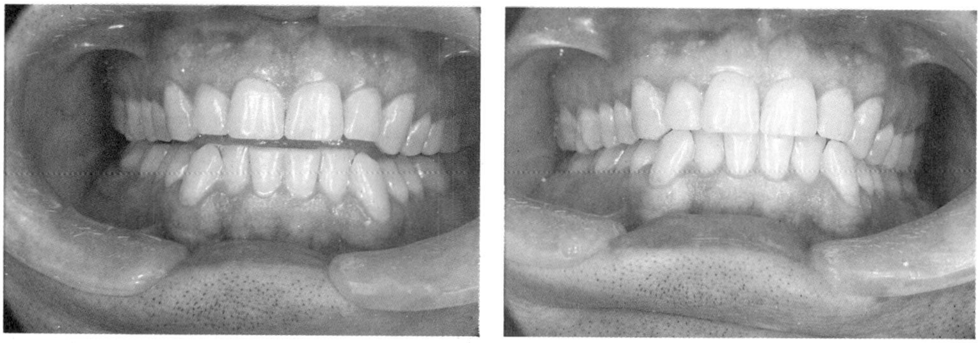

(a)

(b)

Figure 14.6 (a) Rest position. (b) IP with parafunction and severe joint pain

Progressive wear of the occlusal surfaces

Whether this disorder is abrasion or attrition, parafunctional grinding habits usually play a part. Attrition may be initiated by the chewing of tough foods and, when the dentine is exposed and hollowed, lodgements of food will cause further loss of tooth tissue and can be blamed for turning this disturbance into a disorder. As the occlusal surfaces change, the parafunctional habits will cause further wear and sharpen the enamel margins. In many patients the condition suffers from watchful therapy or from no therapy since many of these patients are caries-free and do not attend the dentist. Advice on treatment has to be aimed at prevention and, where possible, any penetration of dentine should be restored by restorations. Amalgam has proved its worth over the years but the composite resins and glass ionomer cements can be used to halt the progress of wear. However, when this condition advances beyond the stage of small dentine replacements into flattened tooth surfaces, with reverse Monson curves, there is often no choice between palliative and reconstruction therapy.

Reconstruction therapy can prove a massive task (Chapter 11) and should not be undertaken without a full realization of the time and cost involved. It can, however, be performed in units. For example, the four first molars can be restored and subsequently other groups of four teeth. If lost OVR has to be restored, an interim appliance for the remaining teeth may be necessary in order to share the load of occlusion and prevent depression of the restored teeth. Onlay dentures by themselves have not proved satisfactory.

This disturbance can affect young adults and the emphasis on prevention cannot be too strongly made. The avoidance of grinding habits, supported by the use of overlays if necessary, is advised. Strict hygiene of the occlusal surfaces (with a soft toothbrush) and care in the eating of carbohydrates and citrus fruits are measures which should be enforced. No patient is too young to embark on a programme of preventing this long-term destructive disturbance and likely disorder.

Mobility and migration

The part played by occlusal disturbances in the disorders of mobility and migration is probably one of aggravation and represents a deterioration of what is essentially a periodontal or orthodontic problem. Nevertheless, an assessment of occlusal function is essential in the treatment planning and in the after care following treatment.

Mobility of a tooth or teeth can be caused by occlusal forces but if the cause is removed the affected teeth will recover their stability, provided that there is no gingival or periodontal lesion. Mobility is usually caused by a loss of periodontal support and is aggravated by occlusal forces either in IP, if there is any extrusion of the affected tooth, or during lateral movements when the affected tooth causes an interference. This presupposes a gingival lesion with subsequent loss of periodontal tissue and alveolar bone. Mobility without migration also implies the condition of jiggling, whereby the tooth is moved by an occlusal or muscle force and is restored to its original position when these forces are removed (p. 115). It is therefore necessary to make a habit analysis of the circumoral and tongue muscles, in addition to the factors of occlusion and periodontal loss, before planning treatment.

Treatment consists, firstly, of assessing the periodontal condition and arresting it if this is possible and, secondly, of removing the aggravating causes. When the periodontal treatment has been completed the occlusion and articulation are reassessed. Occlusal adjustment is performed to remove interferences in closure to habitual IP and during articular movements. If habitual IP has become displaced forwards or laterally from retruded occlusion in excess of what is considered normal for the patient (possibly as a result of the periodontal condition), then

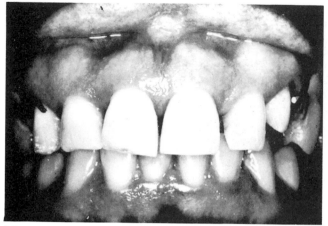

(a)

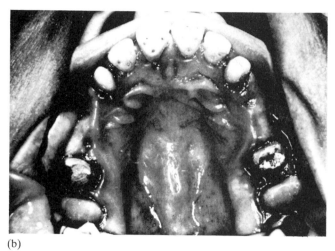

(b)

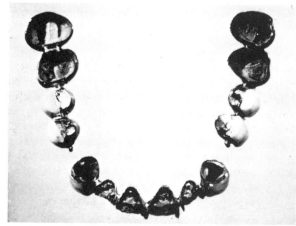

(c)

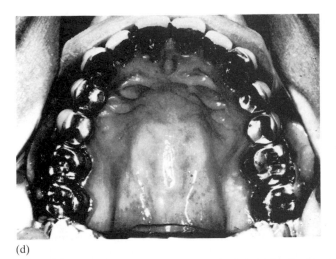

(d)

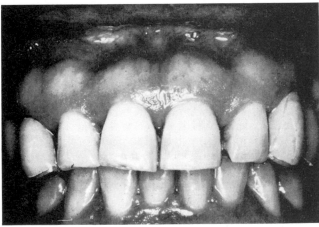

(e)

Figure 14.7 Splinting for migration after orthodontic and periodontal treatment. (a) Preparations begun and temporary partial denture in place. (b) Teeth prepared. (c) Splint and bridgework. Segments soldered (d) Work in place. (e) IP

consideration should be given to restoring IP on the retruded arc. The removal of premature contacts caused by tooth extrusion will accompany the periodontal treatments. Tongue and lip habits have to be pointed out to the patient and efforts made to control them. This alone has proved successful in treating mobility, there being no treatment like self-treatment. Often, however, it is too much to expect and if an irritant mobile tooth is present it can seldom be left alone. Thus, incisor teeth may have to be shortened and irritant edges smoothed. In general, the objectives are periodontal health, teeth in good alignment and an IP in good relation to the rest position.

Migration of a tooth or teeth exists when they have become repositioned and may still be on the move. The commonest example is the drift of the mandibular second molar following the loss of the first. Of more concern to the patient, and by no means uncommon, is the forward drift of maxillary incisors. This is difficult to treat because in many cases the mandibular incisors have followed them. Lip and tongue adaptations to these altered tooth positions can result in aggravation of the condition, as when the lower lip gets behind these maxillary incisors in order to restore the lip seal but tends to promote the drift. The phenomenon of adaptation was seldom better illustrated but less welcome. As with mobility, migration of incisor teeth generally begins with a periodontal lesion which reduces the stability of the tooth and renders it liable to movement by unopposed forces. An exception is that of lip seal in the young adult maintained by voluntary effort which is relaxed in later years. This permits the tongue in function to push the incisors forward until they reach a position of stability with the weaker lip muscles. In the case of tilted mandibular second molars following the loss of first molars, there is seldom a periodontal lesion since the mesial gingival margin is more accessible to hygiene and therefore tends to remain intact. Here again, the tooth will drift until it reaches a stable position, although not in orthodox occlusal function.

Treatment of migration is difficult and debatable. It is difficult because of the adaptive drift of adjacent and opposing teeth and debatable because the teeth may have moved into stable positions. If the condition is progressive, treatment is directed at arresting the migration or restoring the original tooth positions, if this is possible. Treatment consists firstly of measures to restore periodontal health and its maintenance. Then follows orthodontic treatment, if this has been prescribed, which includes retention. Retention will generally require more than a removable appliance worn at night and may call for permanent fixed or removable splinting of the affected teeth. Whether or not orthodontic treatment has been performed, adjustment of the occlusion is necessary in order to promote bilateral occlusion and freedom from interferences into IP. Such interferences will tend to promote recurrence of the migration. Unilateral function will tend to cause drift diagonally across the arch (Thielemann's phenomenon; Thielemann, 1956). Finally, a reassessment of the circumoral and tongue muscle behaviour is made with a view to keeping the teeth stable within the pattern of activity and to preventing habits, both muscular and occlusal.

Splinting as a treatment measure to retain orthodontically moved teeth can be used to support periodontally involved mobile teeth. Without periodontal treatment, splinting will only delay the inevitable loss of severely affected teeth but it can be a successful supporting measure. In cases of postorthodontic retention in adults, and where there is a tendency for recurrence, the incisor teeth should not only be splinted together, preferably by cemented restorations, but this splint should be joined to the posterior segments (Figure 14.7).

Pulp necrosis

This can be the result of prolonged, intermittent occlusal forces between opposing teeth and is an effect of occlusal trauma. Such a case is illustrated in Figure 7.6 where the patient acknowledged such a habit and had no memory of other accident to the tooth. Treatment is by root canal therapy and prevention of recurrence which may require the sevices of an overlay, especially if the habit occurs during sleep. Occlusal adjustment may be necessary if, in protruded occlusion, this is the only contact.

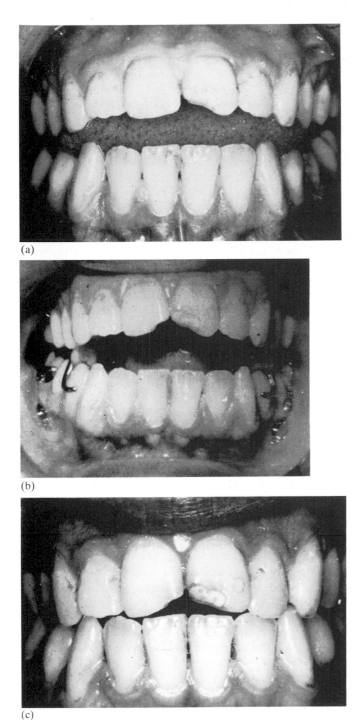

(a)

(b)

(c)

Figure 14.8 Anterior open bite associated with mandibular dysfunction syndrome. (a) IP pre-treatment. (b) Lower onlay denture. Symptoms relieved but appliance clumsy. (c) IP following surgical correction of mandible at Eastman Dental Hospital

Gingival ulceration from food stagnation

Gum bleeding in association with food stagnation suggests ulceration of the interdental epithelium and faulty contact points. The causes and effects of this disorder have been described on page 113. This may have been the result of incorrectly restored class II restorations or crowns. In the case of replacing a faulty restoration, the emphasis is not only on ensuring a 'tight' contact area, but on embrasure shape, on the placement and shape of the marginal ridge above the contact point, on food spillways from the marginal ridge, and on the approximal contour below the contact point. These requirements are best appreciated by looking in a young, caries-free mouth, both clinically and radiographically. The embrasure shape should conform to the norm for that tooth and its neighbour. The marginal ridge should be above and central to the contact area, thus allowing the ridge to be a masticating tool and allowing the food to slide into the embrasure area. A food channel across the ridge into the embrasure area exists on the lingual aspects of the maxillary posterior teeth and buccal of mandibular ones. The shape of the approximal surfaces below the contact areas is more concave than convex, thus permitting access for woodstick, tape or floss hygiene. The approach to interdental health is one of prevention. This disorder can be cured and its recurrence prevented provided that the teeth are close enough to restore the features mentioned.

The plunger cusp is a common cause and aggravating factor of food stagnation and even of tooth separation. It is, however, often seen as the effect of an incorrectly restored contact area, where the marginal ridge has been lowered and the embrasure widened with the result that the opposing supporting cusp loses effective contact and tilts into the space, thus causing the plunger action. It then becomes difficult to treat as, in order to restore the correct relationship, the cusp has to be tilted back and it would be an understatement to say that this presents difficulties. Reducing the cusp size is the regrettable conclusion unless the affected marginal ridge can be reshaped with especial skill.

When the posterior teeth are so separated that 'top heavy' restorations would be necessary to restore the contact point, it may be justifiable to make the space even wider so that food is easily removed. Alternatively, a bridge with sanitary pontic is indicated.

Developmental anomalies

As was said in Chapter 7, developmental anomalies are disturbances which seldom cause disorders. When, however, the anomalies are of occlusion associated with a parafunctional habit in cases of anterior 'open bite' and where there are displacing activities in posterior 'open bite', pain from fatigue or muscle injury in the masticatory muscles may develop and require treatment. The treatment objectives are to prevent the habits and to restore IP. In the case of the former, overlays are large and adaptation to them is difficult (Figure 14.8b). Surgery by mandibular resection has proved beneficial in these cases where the MDS has proved untreatable by conservative or restorative measures (Figure 14.8c). For the latter, appliances to correct posterior open bite are often welcome for purposes of mastication but not always well tolerated (Figure 7.1a,b). Design of these appliances is determined by requirements and the principles outlined for appliances to correct overclosure apply in these cases. Adaptation and tolerance to these appliances may have to be of a high order, since cusp heights are increased and the appliances are bulky, but the needs of the masticatory system may demand this form of treatment.

References

Bergström, G. (1950) On the reproduction of the dental articulation by means of articulators. *Acta Odontologica Scandinavica*, **9** (Supplement 4)

Thielemann, K. (1956) *Biomechanik der Paradentose, insbesondere Artikulationsausgleich durch Einschleifen*, 2nd edn, Barth, Munich

Chapter 15

Comments and an exhortation

There is some truth for the teeth in the proverb: 'Constant dripping wears away the stone'. In more scientific terms this is understood as the cumulative effect, and can be applied to the life and hard times of the teeth in relation to each other. The mastication of food by contemporary humans may decay their teeth if the oral bacteria are pathogenic for caries but it will seldom wear them away. The occlusion and articulation of opposing teeth in the empty mouth will, over the years, do this for him and the effects are cumulative. The occlusal surfaces of the teeth do not repair themselves and their relations to each other are, therefore, continually changing. The effects may cause few complaints in the youthful years and give the dental profession little apparent concern. Adaptation to change and ageing is a feature of all tissues but this is not unlimited. In the case of the tissues of the masticatory system the borders between change, disturbance and disorders are guarded by dentists and their skills often lie in protecting the teeth against disorder by advice and sometimes by treatment.

In their studies of occlusion and practices to achieve good occlusal function dentists have come a long way from Angle's assertion that the key to occlusion is the relative positions of the first molars. This static solution to the problems of malocclusion still has its place as a sign to be noted on the way to a comfortable and efficient relationship between the teeth in the empty mouth. But the movements and positions of the mandible in relation to the maxilla during the varied functions of the masticatory system require a wider range of explanations than are supplied by two molar teeth on either side of the mouth. These movements and positions depend on the muscles which move the mandible, the joints which permit the movements and the shapes of the teeth which control the occlusal function in both the empty mouth and the one filled with food, in both good function and bad. These tissues are interdependent and the stimuli from their functions elicit responses and impulses in the central nervous system which, in turn, governs their functions and health but can lead to disturbances of the tissues.

Teeth wear, tip, become carious, lose their support and are removed. To these declining features can be added restorations that do not always contribute to good function. At each and every stage of change the muscles adapt and maintain the best possible occlusal function but they may tire, become injured or respond with degrees of painful spasm. Meanwhile, the flexible joints provide the movements required but they, too, are subject to unfavourable paths of movement resulting in dysfunction.

To diagnose and treat these disturbances of function and their consequent disorders, dentists are required to watch, advise and treat when necessary. No advice to limit occlusal activities in the mouth is premature. All proposed treatment to prevent or cure is subject to the possibilities of harm and every dentist is his own specialist in watchful therapy while taking care to avoid supervised neglect. But some specialists are more specialized than others, and patients are sometimes warned that when they choose a specialist they may be choosing a diagnosis and treatment plan. It has been said of astrophysicists that they are often in error but never in doubt and this gentle gibe might apply to specialists in occlusion. Treatment of occlusal disorders is best carried out by more minds than one, by groups of dentists with specialized skills and each with knowledge, integrity and a clear appraisal of what is genuinely required for each patient. Practitioners of occlusal problems are often imbued with enthusiasm but this admirable quality is best tempered with a sense of clinical justice.

The studies and practices of occlusion are often criticized for the emphasis placed on the use of articulators, some too complex and some too simple. The articulator will only transfer to the laboratory bench what the dentist wants to transfer and each instrument provides no more than a mechanical copy, not always accurately, of a series of mandibular movements and positions governed by neuromuscular function. And the more this complex function is understood the greater is the need to employ accuracy. The more limited the possibilities of accurate transfer to and from the articulator the more adjustment will be required in the mouth. The training and discipline required to use a fully adjustable articulator will bring the reward of a better understanding of jaw and tooth movements than can be provided by any amount of peering between lips, jostling with hand-held casts, or clamping them together on inaccurate hinges. Students entering this field of study and practice should consider attaching themselves to a teacher or study group where such an instrument is being used. The rewards may even include a reduced need for it in routine practice.

The practitioners of occlusal problems are often unjustly criticized for confining their procedures to reconstruction and grinding the teeth. Such procedures are often the last resort for neglected dentitions and further neglect may involve untreatable disorders and dismay. To rehabilitate a disturbance is preferable to the reconstruction of a disordered dentition. Rehabilitation has been defined in the text as the restoration of muscle and joint function, but in orthopaedic circles it has been referred to as the progressive withdrawal of facilities. The application of this sane but severe definition for the dentist is to treat his crippled patient with the minimum of appliances compatible with adequate function. Reconstruction procedures are for the extreme case and most dentitions will survive a life of adequate function with regular preventive care and advice.

The treatment of most disturbances of occlusion are often for the most part carried out without alterations to the existing intercuspal position of the mandible. Such treatments include alloy and composite restorations, the crown, bridge and various combinations of multiple restorations where the occlusal or proximal surfaces of the teeth require improved shapes but where the existing IP does not require alteration. The objectives are to achieve intercuspal occlusion without deflexions of teeth or mandible and to abolish articular interference during mastication or in the empty mouth. When a change of IP is required, however, there can only be one position for intercuspal occlusion and this is on the retruded arc at a level 3 mm above that of rest position. Here there will be stability and repoducibility of the intercuspal position. For those who like a quickly spoken objective, IP at RC is easily said. But it requires qualification since RC (retruded contact or retruded occlusion) exists at a level slightly below the optimal vertical level for IP. To reach the retruded IP requires effort and the intention is to limit intercuspal occlusion to the act of swallowing. The effort also provides the beneficial stretching of the lateral pterygoid muscles. At all other times and during all other functions let not the teeth touch.

These principles apply to the occlusal adjustment of the natural teeth with the restated warning that the teeth, once adjusted (ground), will not repair themselves. While giving great benefit, occlusal adjustment can lead to iatrogenic disorders of a most distressing nature. Careful planning with a clear objective is encouraged. The suggestion that a generalized reduction of cusp height be carried out as a prophylactic measure (Berry and Poole, 1974) is challenged. This proposal is based on observations that occlusal wear was a constant feature of mammalian and primitive human dentitions and its association with low caries incidence. It is true that the refined diet of contemporary humans has reduced the wear on teeth and that this diet and the absence of occlusal wear have contributed to the disease of caries. With care, however, teeth can now be retained as they evolved and so benefit from more efficient mastication, a reduced need to occlude the teeth and a secure intercuspal position for the mandible when required. It would seem that to make the best use of these unworn tissues is preferable to a haphazard attempt to copy past abuses in spite of environmental hazards. Survival depends on the optimal adaptation of function to form.

The puzzle concerning the association between mandibular dysfunction and facial pain has not been solved. Why it is that some sufferers have this pain relieved by occlusal adjustment while much mandibular dysfunction is unaccompanied by facial pain is not yet clear, despite the claims of those who believe the pain is a psychopathic condition. Adaptation to a musculoskeletal disturbance being more effective in some people than in others may be an avenue worth investigating.

The emphasis in the text on achieving protection for the posterior teeth by providing anterior guidance in all articular movements arose from the deductions of D'Amico (1961). He asserted that the canines and incisors were there to disclude the posteriors and protect them from wear. He also claimed that the shock contact between opposing canines lessened the tension in the mandibular muscles. This scheme of articulation was taken up by Stuart and the gnathologists in California and has proved to be a successful treatment measure where and when such reconstruction is indicated.

There will continue to be debate over the best IP for complete dentures. To make elderly patients thrust backwards every time they want to occlude may seem a harsh and unrealistic discipline and it will be argued that they will slide forwards to a more comfortable and habitual position in any event. So why not allow the more comfortable IP within the parcel of movement? Or at least give them a 'long centric' to slide there? Or flat cusps? The answer lies in the difficulty of transferring to an articulator any other mandibular position than one on the retruded arc. The registrations of all other positions are liable to adaptation by neuromuscular response to bases, occlusal rims, fingers and thumbs. No two will be the same. Somehow the denture patient must be given one secure position at which to occlude the teeth, being allowed freedom to articulate them without interferences. Only then can the patient be realistically advised to 'Leave your teeth alone'.

Let us return briefly to the robin and see it pick up the seed without touching the path. Let our patients chew their food without touching their teeth. Let us dentists make this possible by providing the best possible occlusion, with cusps and fossae making secure contact in one reliable position and freed from interferences in getting there. Let our patients be freed from the aimless, endless and exhausting search for a stable occlusion by giving them one. Let them have an occlusion which they can forget.

References

Berry, D. C. and Poole, D. F. G. (1974) Masticatory function and oral rehabilitation. *Journal of Oral Rehabilitation*, **1**, 191

D'Amico, A. (1961) Functional occlusion of the natural teeth in man. *Journal of Prosthetic Dentistry*, **11**, 899

Appendix

Criteria for good occlusion

1. Two complete arches of teeth with secure contact points and occlusal surface contours adequate for function required.
2. Root shape and alignment adequate to resist occlusal forces.
3. Rest position stable with adequate lip seal.
4. An interocclusal distance of 2–4 mm between rest position and intercuspal position.
5. Simultaneous and bilateral intercuspal occlusion between all teeth of maxillary and mandibular arches at intercuspal position. No deflective contacts.
6. Simultaneous and bilateral occlusion on the retruded arc between one or more opposing posterior teeth.
7. Cusp–fossa and cusp–ridge occlusion having tripod contacts where possible.
8. Each tooth returns to its original position on removal of the occlusal force.
9. Articulation between retruded and intercuspal position free from any interferences causing lateral deflexion.
10. Stable vertical and horizontal overlap.
11. Empty-mouth articular movements free from deflective contacts.

Criteria for good occlusal function

1. Simultaneous bilateral mastication.
2. Light contact in intercuspal position while swallowing.
3. Incoming and outgoing chewing movements free from working or non-working side deflective contacts.
4. No adaptive lip or chin movements on swallowing.
5. No clenching or grinding (parafunctional) movements.
6. No joint noises in mastication or wide opening.
7. No deviation of mandible on wide opening.
8. No tooth contacts in speech or facial expression.
9. Pleasing appearance.

Ten-point test for occlusal function

1. Patient's assessment of function and parafunction.
2. Stability of rest position and lip competence.
3. The interocclusal distance and any cusp interference from rest position.
4. The incisor midlines and any altered tooth inclinations.
5. Palpation and sounds of intercuspal occlusion on firm closure.
6. Length and direction of slide from retruded to intercuspal occlusion.
7. Wear facets as indicators of parafunction.
8. Articulation movements to and from intercuspal position.
9. Maximum active opening of mandible: deviation and noises.
10. Palpation of joints and muscles.

Mandibular dysfunction sydrome

A. Information required from patients and suggested form of questionnaire

1. *Social*
   Name, age, sex, occupation, marital status (and children), source of referral.

2. *Current symptoms or nature of complaint*
   Patient's own description and site of pain is desirable and the open question is preferred to the closed one.
   Such questions are helpful:
   (*a*) Tell me about the problem, discomfort.
   (*b*) Can you point to the place where it starts?
   (*c*) How would you describe the pain (if pain is mentioned)? Note adjectives used, e.g. 'dull', 'neuralgia', or 'burning', etc.
   (*d*) What area is covered by the pain?
   (*e*) Any complaints while eating? Hard chewing? Laughing? Yawning?
   (*f*) How widely can you open your mouth? Make a measurement with, say, Willis gauge.
   (*g*) Do you notice anything about your jaw when you wake up? If so, describe. (Information required regarding any stiffness.)
   (*h*) Do you notice any noises in your jaw? If so, describe.

3. *History of pain or disturbance and nature of onset*
   (*a*) How long have you had it?
   (*b*) Tell me how it first began.
   (*c*) Do you remember if it began suddenly or gradually?
   Information required as to any accident or unusual activity of the jaw such as prolonged opening, or side opening at onset, without suggesting this to the patient.

4. *Progress of pain and/or joint noises*
   (*a*) Has it subsided and recurred without apparent cause?
   (*b*) Has it kept you awake?
   (*c*) Do you take pills? What are they? Are they effective?
   (*d*) Does the weather affect it? Cold day? Damp day?
   (*e*) Have you been treated for it before? What was the treatment? Was it successful?
   (*f*) Is it getting better or worse?

5. *Emotion as factor*
   Assess by tactful straightforward questions:
   (*a*) Are you easily upset at present? Pressed for time? Too much to do?
   (*b*) Have you noticed that you get the pain when you are upset?
   (*c*) Do you clench or grind your teeth when you are pressed for time or concentrating or when you are preoccupied?
   (*d*) Does the pain make you grind your teeth?
   (*e*) Does the pain go away while you are free from worry? On holiday?

6. *Weather*
   Does the weather seem to affect your pain?
   Cold, Damp, Heat?

7. *Past medical history*
   Questions directed towards assessing systemic causes:
   (*a*) Do you have pain or stiffness in any other joints?
   (*b*) Treatment for other joint conditions?
   (*c*) Headaches? Colds? Sinus affections?
   (*d*) Are you under treatment for anything at present, or recently?

8. *Dental history and current function*
   Questions directed towards discovering any recent injury to joint, cause of alteration to tooth relationship or wear on teeth:
   (*a*) Recent extraction dates? Any jaw injury at the time or subsequently?
   (*b*) Injuries: fall, blow, wide yawn or laugh?
   (*c*) Denture history, if any.
   (*d*) Orthodontics.
   (*e*) Clenching and grinding habit? Do you keep your teeth together?
   (*f*) Side preferred in function? Tough foods? Food traps?

9. *Clinical examination*
   (*a*) Missing teeth.
   (*b*) Wear on the teeth.
   (*c*) Closure analysis from rest position:
       Assess displacing activity due to cusp interference and which tooth causative?
       Light tapping – fremitus?
   (*d*) Retruded closure analysis: forward or lateral displacement.
   (*e*) Wide-open analysis:
       Deviation.
       Limit of opening: measure by Willis gauge.
       Palpation ⎫
       Auscultation ⎭ assess noises and pain incidence.

10. *Differential diagnosis*
    Exclude:
    (*a*) Rheumatoid arthritis.
    (*b*) Osteoarthritis.
    (*c*) Trigeminal neuralgia.
    (*d*) Facial pain of dental origin.
    (*e*) Migraine or headache of systemic origin.
    (*f*) Central nervous system disturbance.

(*g*) Sinus disturbance.

(*h*) Specific infective arthritis.

11. *Radiographic examination of both mandibular condyles*
Take at intercuspal position and maximal opening.
Based on radiologist's report, examine:
(*a*) Joint space. Compare sides for increased or decreased space (see Figure 4.10).
(*b*) Extent of opening. Compare spaces.
(*c*) Irregularities of condyle outline. Referral.

B. Some suggestions for treatment

1. Explain and reassure.
    Physical therapy:
    (*a*) Advise bilateral chew.
    (*b*) Avoid chewing and grinding; keep your teeth parted when not in use.
    (*c*) Open movements.
    (*d*) Head, neck and back posture.
    Impressions and records for casts.

2. Note progress: better, same, worse?
    Comments of patient.
    Check on and repeat physical therapy measures.
    Decide if occlusal adjustment necessary:
    Plan and carry out procedures.
    Grinding procedures to correct displacing activities.
    Activity of mandible: (*a*) from rest position; (*b*) on retruded closure.
    Decide if appliance therapy necessary:
    Overlay for night wear.
    Prosthesis to restore lost teeth.
    Prosthesis to restore lost OVR.
    Impressions and records.

3. Note progress.
    Check on and repeat physical therapy measures.
    Place appliance and advise on use and hygiene.

4. Continue as previously.
    Consider referral if no success.
    Awareness of a condition more serious.

Glossary

Anterior guidance – That which takes place when the incisors or canines alone take part in lateral and protrusive articular (excursive) movements.

Arbitrary retruded axis – see Retruded condyle axis.

Articulation – The contact that exists between the teeth of opposing arches while the mandible is moving.

Articular movements – The mandibular movements while two or more opposing teeth are in contact. Alternative term: excursive contact movements.

Balanced articulation – The simultaneous contact between teeth of two or three opposing segments during an articular movement.

Free articulation – The absence of cusp interferences to lateral and protrusive articular movements.

Balancing side – The side from which the mandible moves in lateral articular movement or unilateral mastication. It is the side opposite to the working side. Alternative term: non-working side.

Bennett angle – The angle between the medially translating (orbiting) condyle and the median sagittal plane.

Bennett movement – The bodily lateral component in the rotation of the working side condyle as the mandible makes a lateral movement. Alternative term: lateral shift.

Border movements – see Envelope of motion.

Canine guidance – see Guidances.

Centric occlusion – see Intercuspal occlusion.

Centric relation see Retruded relation.

Condyle guidance – see Guidances.

Cross-arch balance – Simultaneous contact between opposing teeth of working and non-working sides as the mandible makes a lateral articular movement.

Cross-tooth balance – Simultaneous contact between opposing buccal and lingual cusp ridges on the working side of an articular lateral movement.

Cusp – The apex of cusp and triangular ridges of a tooth.

Cusp angle – The angle made by the slope of a cusp ridge or triangular ridge with the plane of occlusion.

Cusp interference – The premature or initial contact which takes place between two opposing teeth in a functional or parafunctional movement (see p. 109).

Cusp ridge – see Ridges.

Determinants – Anatomical features that influence jaw movements.

Anterior – The lingual surfaces of the maxillary incisors and cannines.

Posterior – The paths of condyle movements.

Disclusion – The separation of all posterior tooth contacts when the mandible moves away from intercuspal position and articulation is maintained between the opposing anterior segments (anterior guidance).

Displacing activity – The reflex movement made by the mandible when a mandibular tooth encounters an initial cusp contact on a maxillary tooth.

Envelope of motion

Horizontal – The outline traced by a point between the mandibular central incisors as the mandible moves laterally to the left, forwards, laterally to the right and backwards as far as it can go in these directions. This envelope is usually traced with a central bearing device that keeps the teeth parted but it can also be traced during articular movements in these directions. Alternative term: horizontal border movements. See Chapter 4.

Vertical – The outline traced by a point between the mandibular central incisors as the mandible moves in the median sagittal plane through all possible tooth contacts from retruded to fully protruded position and then downwards, upwards and backwards as far as the mandible can go in these directions. Alternative term: vertical border movements.

See also Space parcel.

Fischer angle – The angle made between the paths of the medially and protrusively translating (orbiting) condyle.

Gothic arch – The outline made by a stylus attached to the maxilla on a tracing plate attached to the mandible with the teeth parted, as the mandible makes retruded lateral movements from one side to the other. The apex of the arch represents the retruded relation of mandible to maxilla and this outline corresponds to the posterior half of the horizontal envelope of motion.

Guidances – The influence on mandibular movement created by the occlusal surfaces of the teeth or condyle paths.

Canine – The guidance provided by the lingual surfaces of the maxillary canines in lateral articular movements.

Condyle – The guidance provided by the paths of the translating (medially or laterally) condyles.

Cuspal – The guidances provided by the cusp ridges of opposing posterior teeth.

Incisal – The guidance provided by the lingual surfaces of the maxillary incisor teeth as the lower incisal edges make contact with them in protrusive articular movements.

Guiding cusps – The buccal upper and lingual lower cusps of the posterior teeth. The surfaces which provide the guidance are the inner facing triangular ridges and their slopes. The lingual surfaces of the maxillary incisors and canines are guiding surfaces.

Horizontal overlap – The horizontal distance between the labioincisal edge of a maxillary incisor and the labial surface of the opposing mandibular incisor when the teeth are in intercuspal occlusion. This overlap also applies to posterior teeth.

Intercuspal occlusion (IO) – The contact between the greatest number of opposing teeth (usually cusps and opposing fossae or marginal ridges) while the mandible is stationary. Alternative term: centric occlusion.

Intercuspal position (IP) – The position of the mandible when the teeth are in intercuspal occlusion. Alternative terms: centric position or muscular position if the mandible has closed in a reflex pattern from rest position.

Habitual intercuspal position – IP following a displacing activity from rest position. Alternative term: tooth position. In this text, however, all intercuspal positions are considered habitual when they are not on the retruded arc of closure.

Retruded intercuspal position – The position of the mandible when it is in retruded relation to the maxilla and the teeth are in intercuspal occlusion.

Interocclusal distance (IOD) – The distance between the maxillary and mandibular teeth when the mandible is in rest position. Alternative term: freeway space.

Marginal ridge – see Ridges.

Oblique ridge – see Ridges.

Occlusal table – The area on a tooth bounded by the mesial and distal marginal ridges and the buccal and lingual cusps.

Occlusal vertical relation (OVR) – The vertical relation (or distance) between points marked on the nose and chin when the teeth are in intercuspal occlusion. Alternative term: occlusal vertical dimension.

Occlusion – Any contact between the teeth of opposing arches. The term is usually qualified as by intercuspal, retruded, lateral, protruded (see Chapter 1).

Plane of occlusion – The imaginary surface that touches the incisal edges and cusps of the lower teeth. It is a curved surface and, when in the sagittal plane, is called the compensating curve (or curve of Spee). When continued distally it is said to run through the condyle (curve of Monson). When viewed in the coronal plane it is called Monson's curve and these two aspects together combine to make Monson's sphere (see Chapter 5).

Parafunction – Disordered function (*Oxford English Dictionary*, 1971). In the masticatory system it implies clenching or grinding habits between the teeth in the empty mouth or between the teeth and various outside agencies such as pens, hair-grips, finger-nails. Alternative term: bruxism.

Plane of orientation – The flat surface which touches the cusps of the mandibular canines and the distobuccal cusps of the mandibular second molars.

Rest position – The position adopted by the mandible when the muscles between mandible and maxilla are in minimal contraction. Alternative terms: resting posture, endogenous posture.

Habitual posture – The position adopted by the mandible when the requirements of lip seal cause the mandible to move away from rest position.

Rest vertical relation (RVR) – The vertical relation (or distance) between mandible and maxilla when the mandible is in rest position. This is usually measured between marks on the nose and chin. Alternative term: rest vertical dimension.

Retruded arc – The arc of opening and closing made by the mandible while it is rotating on the retruded condyle axis.

Retruded condyle axis (RCA) – The imaginary axis which runs through both condyle regions when the condyles are in retruded (most superior and posterior) relation to the maxilla. Alternative term: terminal hinge axis or hinge axis.

Arbitrary retruded axis – The imaginary axis running between points marked on the skin over the condyles, each one 12 mm in front of the tragus of the ear and on a line between it and the external canthus of the eye. Alternative term: arbitrary hinge axis.

Retruded intercuspal position – see Intercuspal position.

Retruded relation – The relationship between mandible and maxilla when the condyles are most superiorly and posteriorly placed in their respective glenoid fossae. Alternative term: centric relation.

Ridges – The crests of tooth slopes that run from cusps on a posterior tooth and are contiguous with other ridges or end in central fossae (see Figure 2.8).

Cusp – ridges that run mesially or distally from a cusp to marginal ridge or contiguous cusp ridge.

Marginal – ridges that are contiguous with the cusp ridges and form the mesial and distal margins of the posterior teeth. The slopes from ridges run towards the central foassae and contact areas respectively.

Oblique – ridges that run from the mesiolingual cusps of all maxillary first molars (and some second molars) and join the distobuccal triangular ridges. They may be continuous or be separated by a fissure.

Transverse – ridges that run across the tooth between the buccal and lingual cusps as in the mandibular first premolar or they may join two other ridges.

Triangular – ridges that run from the cusps to the central fossae of all posterior teeth except the mandibular first premolar.

Rotation centres – The imaginary vertical, coronal–horizontal and sagittal–horizontal axes of rotation which run through both condyle regions and about which the mandible rotates in order to provide three-dimensional movement (Chapters 5 and 8).

Space parcel – The volume occupied by the median vertical and horizontal envelopes of motion at all levels of jaw separation. This is depicted by a point between the two mandibular central incisors and represents the circumductory (or border) movements of the mandible in three dimensions of that point. See Chapters 5 and 8.

Supporting cusps – The lingual upper and buccal lower cusps of the posterior teeth. These cusps and their ridges occlude in opposing central fossae (where they are wholly enclosed within the opposing occlusal table) or marginal ridge areas. The incisal edges of the mandibular incisors and canines act as supporting cusps. Alternative terms: centric holding cusps or stamp cusps.

Tripod contact – The contact between three surfaces of a supporting cusp and an opposing central fossa or marginal ridge area. The cusp tip itself does not make contact with the fossa or ridge surface.

Vertical overlap – The vertical distance between the incisal edges of opposing incisor teeth when the teeth are in intercuspal occlusion.

Working side – The side to which the mandible moves in lateral articular movement or in unilateral mastication. It is the side opposite the non-working (balancing) side.

Index